POWER AND THE PSYCHIATRIC

T0249990

Power and the Psychiatric Apparatus

Repression, Transformation and Assistance

Edited by

DAVE HOLMES

JEAN DANIEL JACOB

AMÉLIE PERRON

University of Ottawa, Canada

Routledge
Taylor & Francis Group

LONDON AND NEW YORK

First published 2014 by Ashgate Publishing

2 Park Square, Milton Park, Abingdon, Oxfordshire OX14 4RN
711 Third Avenue, New York, NY 10017

Routledge is an imprint of the Taylor & Francis Group, an informa business

First issued in paperback 2018

Copyright © 2014 Dave Holmes, Jean Daniel Jacob and Amélie Perron

Dave Holmes, Jean Daniel Jacob and Amélie Perron have asserted their right under the Copyright, Designs and Patents Act, 1988, to be identified as the editors of this work.

All rights reserved. No part of this book may be reprinted or reproduced or utilised in any form or by any electronic, mechanical, or other means, now known or hereafter invented, including photocopying and recording, or in any information storage or retrieval system, without permission in writing from the publishers.

Notice:
Product or corporate names may be trademarks or registered trademarks, and are used only for identification and explanation without intent to infringe.

British Library Cataloguing in Publication Data
A catalogue record for this book is available from the British Library

The Library of Congress has cataloged the printed edition as follows:
Power and the psychiatric apparatus : repression, transformation, and assistance / edited by Dave Holmes, Jean Daniel Jacob, and Amélie Perron.
p. ; cm.
Includes bibliographical references and index.
ISBN 978-1-4724-1731-2 (hardback : alk. paper)
I. Holmes, Dave, 1967– editor of compilation. II. Jacob, Jean Daniel, editor of compilation. III. Perron, Amélie, editor of compilation.
[DNLM: 1. Psychiatry--methods. 2. Coercion. 3. Mentally Ill Persons. 4. Power (Psychology) 5. Repression, Psychology. WM 100]
RC454.4
616.89--dc23

2013039236

ISBN 978-1-4724-1731-2 (hbk)
ISBN 978-1-138-36705-0 (pbk)

Contents

PART II TRANSFORMATION

PART III ASSISTANCE

List of Tables

Notes on Contributors

Emmanuelle Bernheim, PhD is Assistant Professor in the Department Law and Legal Sciences at the Université du Québec à Montreal. During her graduate studies, in addition to her thesis, she looked at various aspects of psychiatric practices: expert testimony, use of seclusion and restraint, commitment, care without consent and rights of psychiatric patients. Dr Bernheim's research examines the role of law and the justice system in the establishment and maintenance of social inequalities. She recently began a project funded by the Social Sciences and Humanities Research Council of Canada on the intervention of child protection services and the courts with mothers who have been committed. She also works on the impact of the privatization of Quebec's healthcare system on access to care for groups such as children and people with mental illness, consent to and refusal of treatment in physical and psychiatric care, psychiatrists' understanding and use of legal mechanisms, the adequacy and use of procedural mechanisms in psychiatrists' and judges' decisions, and the evolution of case law on commitment and psychiatric care.

Sarah Burgess, PhD received her PhD from the University of California, Berkeley in Rhetoric. She is currently Assistant Professor of Communication Studies and the Director of Gender and Sexualities Studies at the University of San Francisco, USA. Working at the intersections of rhetorical, legal, political, and queer theory, her research focuses on the operations and effects of legal recognition for populations who traditionally do not have a voice in law. Her current book project, tentatively titled *Making a Scene: Scandals of Legal Recognition,* examines the possibilities and limits of recognition for transgender people in international law. Her recent work can be found in *The International Journal of Law in Context* and *Critical Interventions in the Ethics of Healthcare* (Ashgate, 2009).

Paula J. Caplan, PhD is a clinical and research psychologist and associate at Harvard University's DuBois Institute. She is the author of twelve books, including *They Say You're Crazy: How the World's Most Powerful Psychiatrists Decide Who's Normal* (her disturbing insider's story of how the Diagnostic and Statistical Manual of Mental Disorders is put together), *Bias in Psychiatric Diagnosis* (which she edited), *The Myth of Women's Masochism*, *Don't Blame Mother: Mending the Mother-Daughter Relationship*, *You're Smarter Than They Make You Feel: How the Experts Intimidate Us and What We Can Do About It*, *When Johnny and Jane Come Marching Home: How All of Us Can Help Veterans* (which was chosen best psychology book of 2011 by the Association of American Publishers in their PROSE Awards competition and was given the Independent Publishers' Silver

Medal in the psychology/mental health category) and *Thinking Critically About Research on Sex and Gender* (co-authored with her son, Jeremy B. Caplan). She is a longtime activist for the rights of people who have been harmed because of being given psychiatric labels and for war veterans whose understandable human suffering is too often being mislabelled as mental illness, with disastrous results. She is an advocate of nonmedical, alternative, humane approaches to helping reduce human suffering.

Jennifer Chandler, PhD is Associate Professor of Law in the Faculty of Law at the University of Ottawa, Canada, where she teaches a course in mental health law and neuro-ethics. She also teaches courses in general medical law and tort law and has taught legal theory at the graduate level. Her research interests focus on the socio-legal and ethical implications of advances in biomedical science and technology with a particular interest in neuroscience and the law.

Pascale Corneau, BSc is a research assistant in the University Research Chair in Forensic Nursing at the School of Nursing, University of Ottawa. She has worked on projects related to psychiatric nursing and also on research projects exploring violence in nursing practice.

John R. Cutcliffe, RN, PhD was appointed to the Acadia Professor of Psychiatric and Mental Health Nursing Chair at the University of Maine in 2010; he also holds adjunct professor positions at universities in the United Kingdom, Portugal, Malta, Turkey and Canada. John's research interests focus on hope, suicide and clinical supervision; in 2003 he was recognized by the Federal Government of Canada and cited as one of the top 20 "Research Leaders of Tomorrow" for his research focusing on hope and suicidology. He has published extensively—over 190 papers/chapters, eleven books and over 70 abstracts/conference proceedings. His work has been translated into German, Japanese, Dutch, Spanish, Mandarin Chinese, Portuguese and Turkish. He is currently working with colleagues from the University of Ulster, Dublin City University, the University of Coimbra and Vestfold University College, Norway on an international program of research focusing on suicide. He has recently served as the national Canadian Representative for the International Association of Suicide Prevention and the Director of the International Society of Psychiatric Nurses: Education and Research Division: he is the Associate Editor for Psychiatric/Mental Health Nursing Journal as well as serving on the boards of eight other health or education focused journals. And in 2012 was invited by the Director of Medicine at Yale University to join the first international advisory board on Clinical Supervision. He retains his interest in clinical work, particularly around care of the suicidal person, inspiring hope, clinical supervision and dealing with violence and aggression, and more broadly in psychiatric nursing.

J. Paul Fedoroff, M.D. is a Forensic Neuropsychiatrist. He is Director of the Sexual Behaviours Clinic at the Royal Ottawa Mental Health Center (ROMHC) and the Integrated Forensic Program (ROMHC). He is Vice-Chair of the ROMHC's Research Ethics Committee, and Director of the Forensic Research Unit of the Integrated Mental Health Research Unit. He is Chair of the American Academy of Psychiatry and the Law's (AAPL) Committee on Sex Offenders. He is also Head of the Forensic Division of the Department of Psychiatry at the University of Ottawa. Currently he is President of the Canadian Association of Psychiatry and the Law. His clinical and research interests include the assessment and treatment of problematic sexual behaviours including the paraphilias. He has a special interest in the neuropsychiatric and ethical implications of these issues, including those related to people with intellectual and developmental disabilities. He has published and lectured nationally and internationally in the areas of neuropsychiatry and paraphilias, and has received grant support from multiple sources including: the Ontario Mental Health Foundation, the Canadian Institute of Health Research, the University of Ottawa Medical Research Fund, and USA Department of Justice.

Thomas Foth, PhD is Assistant Professor in the School of Nursing, Faculty of Health Sciences, at the University of Ottawa, Canada. He has worked on many research projects in the fields of: interdisciplinary cooperation between nurses and physicians, nursing professionalization in Germany as well as in the field of psychiatry. As a nurse, he has worked in different specialties of the profession. He also taught nursing schools in Germany before he moved to Canada. His doctoral research project explores the participation of nurses in the killing of more than 200,000 sick persons during the Nazi regime. He received financial support from the Robert Bosch Stiftung Foundation (Germany) and from the AMS Nursing History Research Unit at the University of Ottawa (Canada). Foth's fields of interest include history of nursing, critical analysis of nursing practice, nursing theories, epistemology, ethics, nursing care provided to marginalized populations, technologies and nursing practice, power relationships between health care professionals and patients and finally gender issues in nursing. Most of his work is influenced by the works of Michel Foucault and Judith Butler. His research is also influenced by actor-network theory and the "newer" critical theory movement in Germany.

Adam Gerace is a postdoctoral research fellow in the School of Nursing & Midwifery at Flinders University, South Australia. His research is focused on conflict and containment in acute psychiatric care, including restraint and absconding, and how empathic processes and responses operate between professionals and consumers in health settings. Adam's background is in social and forensic psychology, in particular prison rehabilitation program evaluation, and his work on empathy was recognized with a national award in 2010.

David Healy, MD is an internationally respected psychiatrist, psychopharmacologist, scientist, and author. A Professor of psychiatry at Cardiff University School of Medicine, Wales, Professor Healy studied medicine in Dublin, and at Cambridge University. He is a former Secretary of the British Association for

Psychopharmacology, and has authored more than 150 peer-reviewed articles, 200 other pieces, and 20 books, including *The Antidepressant Era* and *The Creation of Psychopharmacology* from Harvard University Press, *The Psychopharmacologists Volumes 1–3* and *Let Them Eat Prozac* from New York University Press, and *Mania* from Johns Hopkins University Press. David's main areas of research are clinical trials in psychopharmacology, the history of psychopharmacology, and the impact of both trials and psychotropic drugs on our culture. He has been involved as an expert witness in homicide and suicide trials involving psychotropic drugs, and in bringing problems with these drugs to the attention of American and British regulators, as well raising awareness of how pharmaceutical companies sell drugs by marketing diseases and co-opting academic opinion-leaders, ghost-writing their articles. David's latest book, *Pharmageddon*, documents the riveting and terrifying story of how pharmaceutical companies have hijacked healthcare in America and the life-threatening results. David is a founder and Chief Executive Officer of Data Based Medicine Limited, which operates through its website RxISK.org, dedicated to making medicines safer through online direct patient reporting of drug effects.

Dave Holmes, RN, PhD is Professor, Director (School of Nursing), Associate Dean (Faculty of Health Sciences) and University Research Chair in Forensic Nursing at the University of Ottawa, Canada. After completing his BSc (Ottawa, 1991), MSc (Montreal, 1998) and PhD (Montreal, 2002) in Nursing, Professor Holmes completed a CIHR post-doctoral fellowship in Health Care, Technology and Place at the University of Toronto (2003). To date, Professor Holmes received funding, as principal investigator, from CIHR and SSHRC, to conduct his research program on risk management in the fields of Public Health and Forensic Nursing. Most of his work, comments, essays, analyses and research are based on the poststructuralist works of Deleuze and Guattari and Michel Foucault. His works have been published in top-tier journals in nursing, criminology, sociology and medicine. Professor Holmes has published over 110 articles in peer reviewed journals and 35 book chapters. He is co-editor of *Critical Interventions in the Ethics of Health Care* (Ashgate, 2009), *Abjectly Boundless: Boundaries, Bodies and Health Care* (Ashgate, 2010), and *(Re)Thinking Violence in Health Care Settings: A Critical Approach* (Ashgate, 2012). Hi is the Editor-in-Chief for *Aporia—The Nursing Journal*. He has presented at numerous national and international conferences and has been appointed as Honorary Visiting Professor in Australia, Indonesia, the United States and the United Kingdom.

Jean Daniel Jacob, RN, PhD is an Associate Professor in the School of Nursing, Faculty of Health Sciences, at the University of Ottawa, Canada. His research explores nursing practice in forensic psychiatry, and more precisely how fear influences nurse-patient interactions in this environment. His research has been supported by the Social Sciences and Humanities Research Council (SSHRC). His research interests are situated within the field of psychiatry/forensic psychiatry and include topics such as the violence, risk, ethics and the socio-political aspects of nursing practice.

David Jacobs, PhD is a licensed clinical psychologist in private practice in La Jolla, California, and an independent scholar and critic of contemporary psychiatry. He has published numerous articles on the torturous machinations required to produce "positive" psychiatric drug treatment trials, the under investigation and under reporting of adverse psychiatric drug effects, the conceptual and empirical difficulties involved in distinguishing between therapeutic drug effects and certain forms of toxic drug effects, and the fiction of distinct psychiatric clinical entities that enable biological research as to cause, randomized placebo controlled trials as to efficacy, and FDA approval of new psychiatric drugs. Over the course of the years he has been impressed with the futility of criticism to disrupt the hegemony and growth of bio-psychiatry and drug treatment. David Jacobs therefore has come to feel tremendous inner pressure to come up with at least relatively unused lines of criticism to undermine the medicalization-drug treatment leviathan.

Matthew Johnston, MA is a PhD student and SSHRC Canada Graduate Scholar in the Department of Sociology at the University of Victoria. In addition to his work on social institutions and hegemonic masculinity, Matthew is interested in exploring how some former prisoners who identity as transgender construct and negotiate their gender identities and statuses during their involvement in the criminal justice system.

Jennifer Kilty, PhD is Assistant Professor in the Department of Criminology and the Social Science of Health at the University of Ottawa, Canada. Situated within a critical and feminist framework, her research primarily focuses on gender and different aspects of criminalization, including the social construction of dangerous girls and women, the medicalization/psychiatrization of criminalized women, self-harming behaviours, drug use, and more recently the criminalization of HIV nondisclosure.

Natasha M. Knack received her B.A. (Honours) in Criminology and Criminal Justice, with a concentration in Psychology, from Carleton University, Canada. During the course of her studies she completed an undergraduate thesis examining the effect of stereotypes on eyewitness testimony. She was also accepted into the competitive Criminology Field Placement Program, which she completed in the Sexual Behaviours Clinic (SBC) at the Royal Ottawa Mental Health Center. Shortly after graduating, she began working as a Research Assistant, both in the Forensic Research Unit at the Institute of Mental Health Research, as well as for the University of Ottawa's School of Nursing. She continues to be actively involved in the SBC as a volunteer co-facilitator in four weekly psychotherapy groups for men who have sexually offended, or who have problematic sexual interests.

Rachel Jane Liebert obtained her Master's Degree from the University of Auckland, Aotearoa, New Zealand, and is currently a doctoral candidate in Critical Psychology at the City University of New York, United States. With the support of Fulbright, Bright Futures New Zealand, and The American Association of University Women, she explores how, and with what implications, psychiatric diagnoses and treatments circulate with/in US politics of discipline and terror. Her research has been published in Social Science & Medicine, Women's Studies Quarterly, and The Journal of Theoretical and Philosophical Psychology, among others, as well as mobilized for creative, collaborative activism against the privatization and policing of psyches and bodies with/in medicine and education. Previous projects have included critical analyses of SSRI-induced violence, the rise in Bipolar Disorder diagnoses, and the "cosmetogynecology" industry, and she is currently drawing from critical feminist, race, and security studies to map the discursive and affective logics of "risk" within the criminal justice and public education systems. She is committed to participatory, performative, and non-imperialist epistemologies; interested ultimately in how to nourish spaces for dissent, imagination, and change. At this time Rachel is also co-editing a Special Feature for Feminism & Psychology on/by/with "Young Feminists", and co-curating a fringe art campaign in Aotearoa, New Zealand to challenge misogyny and racism in porn. She is an Adjunct Instructor in Sociology and Interdisciplinary Studies at John Jay College of Criminal Justice.

Joanna Le Noury, PhD is Senior Research Scientist in the North Wales Department of Psychological Medicine. She trained as a biological psychologist and has previously been involved in the development of an international programme aimed at improving health and nutrition in young children, which has since been implemented across several European countries and the US. More recently her research interest has focussed on looking at the incidence and prevalence of serious mental illness, along with comorbidity and mortality rates associated with psychiatric disorders. In addition she has analysed several large pharmaceutical databases in the course of litigation cases.

Jem Masters, RN, PhD(cand) has been a registered nurse for nearly 30 years, with hospital based qualifications in general, paediatrics and mental health nursing. He has tertiary qualifications, which have had a focus within health care management arena. He is currently a part-time clinical nurse specialist working in the psychiatric emergency. He has extensive experience across the health care system in various roles (RN, Clinical Nurse Consultant, CNS and Director of Operations Mental Health). Jem has worked within the academic environment and taught under-graduate, post- graduate and pre-registration students. His main areas of educational interests are mental health/psychiatry, psychological care of patients within the general system, health care management and quality management within the health care system. His PhD study focuses around the impact of people with mental health issues on the emergency department nurse. Jem has presented his work at National and International Conference.

Dave Mercer, RN, PhD is Senior Lecturer in the Directorate of Nursing at the University of Liverpool, United Kingdom. A mental health nurse, his career spans clinical practice, teaching and research, with a particular interest in the care and treatment of the mentally disordered offender. His chapter is based on the findings of doctoral research, and reflects an ongoing interest in therapeutic approaches to male sexual violence. The greater part of his professional life has been devoted to recognizing and developing the forensic nurse role as a specialist area of practice. Undergraduate and postgraduate degrees in sociology and criminology have informed a critical engagement with the concept of medicalized offending and healthcare practice at the interface of criminal justice and psychiatry. He is co-author and co-editor of three books on forensic mental health practice, has published extensively in peer reviewed professional and academic journals, and contributed to national television programmes in the UK. His contribution to the promotion of quality care in secure settings has resulted in invited keynote presentations at international conferences in Australia (2002) and New Zealand (2003, 2004). In Canada (2000) he received an Achievement Award from the International Association of Forensic Nurses in recognition of "advancement of the scientific practice of forensic nursing through research and publications".

Eimear Muir-Cochrane, RN, PhD is Professor of Nursing (Mental Health) in School of Nursing and Midwifery, Faculty of Health Sciences, at Flinders University, Australia, and Chair of the Academic Senate. Eimear is recognized as a national and international expert in research into and policy development around restraint, seclusion, locked doors and absconding. Eimear has been involved in multiple national and international funded research studies attracting over $4 million. Eimear also has a strong educational background having published one book, monographs, over 50 articles and eight book chapters since 2002. Eimear is involved as a national and international expert in mental health research and education and is the Australasian Editor of The Journal of Psychiatric and Mental Health Nursing. Pr Muir-Cochrane serves on three international journal Editorial Boards.

Stuart J. Murray, PhD is Associate Professor and Canada Research Chair in Rhetoric & Ethics in the Department of English Language and Literature at Carleton University in Ottawa, Canada. He is also Director of the Carleton University Rhetoric & Ethics Research Lab. He holds a concurrent appointment as Associate Professor of Social and Behavioural Health Science in the Dalla Lana School of Public Health at the University of Toronto. His work is concerned with the constitution of human subjectivity and the links between the rhetoric and ethics of "life", in the multiple ways in which this term is deployed. Current SSHRC- and CIHR-funded research involves a study of ethics in forensic psychiatry settings (prisons) as well as a phenomenological study on the ethics of seclusion in mental health. He has published numerous essays and book chapters, as well as a collected volume edited with Dave Holmes, titled, *Critical Interventions in the*

Ethics of Healthcare (Ashgate, 2009). He is working on a book-length project on the rhetorical dimensions of biopolitics and bioethics after Foucault, tentatively titled, *Thanatopolitics: The Living From The Dead.*

Amélie Perron, RN, PhD is Associate Professor in the School of Nursing, Faculty of Health Sciences, at the University of Ottawa, Canada. Besides her doctoral research on psychiatric nursing care in a correctional setting, she has worked on many research projects in the fields of psychiatry and forensic psychiatry in Australia, Canada and France. She received financial support from the Canadian Institutes of Health Research for her doctoral work. She also completed a postdoctoral fellowship at the University of Sydney, Australia. Her fields of interest include nursing care provided to captive and marginalized populations, psychiatric nursing, forensic psychiatry, power relationships between health care professionals and patients, as well as issues of discourse, risk, gender and ethics. She also writes on issues relating to the state of nursing knowledge and epistemology. Her clinical practice is grounded in community psychiatry and crisis intervention. She has published many articles in peer-reviewed journals and is the Receiving Editor for *Aporia—The Nursing Journal.*

Sanaz Riahi, RN, MSc is the Director of Professional Practice at Ontario Shores Centre for Mental Health Sciences. She also holds an Adjunct Professor position in the Faculty of Health Sciences at the University of Ontario Institute of Technology. Sanaz's clinical background is in nursing, having completed her Bachelor of Science in Nursing and Master of Science in Nursing. She is currently pursuing her PhD studies exploring nursing sensitive outcomes related to suicide. Her current research involvement and interests are in clinical aggression, restraint minimization, nursing sensitive outcomes, and suicide, to further contribute to the extant empirical evidence within mental health. In her current role she works collaboratively with internal and external stakeholders to support, promote and advance quality interprofessional practice environment to optimize outcomes for patients, staff and the organization.

Thomas Szasz, M.D., D.Sc. (Hon.), L.H.D. (Hon.), Professor Emeritus of Psychiatry, State University of New York Upstate Medical University, Syracuse, New York, is the author of 36 books, among them the classic: *The Myth of Mental Illness* (Harper/Collins, 1961). Widely recognized as a the world's foremost critic of psychiatric coercions and excuses, he maintains that just as we reject theological assertions about people's unwanted religious condition (heresy) as justification for according them special legal status and treatment, we ought to reject psychiatric assertions about people's mental condition (mental illness) as justification for according them special legal status and treatment. Dr Szasz has received many awards for his defence of individual liberty and responsibility threatened by the "therapeutic state", a modern form of totalitarianism masquerading as medicine. A frequent and popular lecturer, he has addressed professional and lay groups, and has appeared on radio and television, in North, Central, and South America as well as in Australia, Europe, Japan, and South Africa. His most recent work is titled *Suicide Prohibition: The Shame of Medicine* (Syracuse University Press, 2010). His books have been translated into every major language.

Sandra West, RN, PhD is an Associate Professor of Nursing at the University of Sydney, Australia. She is a registered nurse with specialisations in emergency and intensive care nursing. She has a degree in Biology and a PhD in Physiology from Macquarie University, Sydney. She has experience has experience in the management of postgraduate coursework and doctoral programs and as head of the department of clinical nursing at the University of Sydney. Her research focuses on the effects of common shift work schedules for women and the organisation of nursing work within clinical environments. She is especially interested in social understandings of the nurses work at night and how the nursing workplace is constituted within current health care contexts.

Foreword

The social and political power of medicine in general and of psychiatry in particular, is above all, definitional. That we should choose to describe what troubles us in medico-psychiatric terms is a commanding reminder of the power of the psychiatric apparatus in Western society. "I've been feeling depressed lately," "I've always thought he was ADD" and "Oh my God, that's psycho!" are examples of how the idiom of psychiatry is anchored in the banality of every day as a powerful authority to explain and justify our experiences.

However, as this volume makes entirely clear, the psychiatric apparatus encompasses a vast field of complex contention, interests and perspectives. Diagnosis is a powerful example. The point at which a disorder gets cemented by its institutional recognition as a diagnosis is also the point at which debates are silenced and particular voices privileged. For example, sexual desire or its absence, shyness, hyperactivity and sadness become confirmed as problems external to the social situations which engender them. This is not to say that people don't suffer from illness and distress, or that psychiatry cannot bring legitimate succor to people with illness, it is simply to underline how, as Ian Hacking wrote, "the idea of nature has served as a way to disguise ideology, to appear to be perfectly neutral. No study of classification can escape the obligation to examine the roots of this idea … no study of the word 'natural' can fail to touch on that other great ideological word, 'real'" (2001: 7).

Every diagnosis once reified not only conceals its social origins in debate, contest and consensus; it enables a social consequence. The delicate relationship between diagnosis and treatment, and the not-as-amiable link between diagnosis and stigma remind us of the important role psychiatry plays in structuring and reinforcing our social experiences of normalcy and deviance.

Psychiatry has the surveillance of the fuzzy boundaries between normal and deviance under its purview. It arbitrates whether the responsibility for deviant actions fits within the rubric of personal responsibility, or alternatively, of biophysiological dysfunction. While these are fuzzy social boundaries, the psychiatric project of diagnostic classification is, as Jacob, Perron, and Holmes write in the introduction to this book, "the very concretization of psychiatry's claim-making activities." Crisp, clean lines of demarcation drive each revision of the DSM, every insurance code, every disability claim.

This collection edited by Holmes, Jacob and Perron brings into relief important critical observations which, while issued from the professions of law, medicine, nursing, and departments of social sciences and critical theory, are of direct relevance to the clinical practitioner. Critical distance is vital to the progression of a field, and to the progress of psychiatry. However, it is extremely difficult for the practitioner to stand back and see the value content for his or her routine activities. As Mary Douglas asked: "How can an individual [in the grip of iron hard categories] turn round his [sic] own thought-process and contemplate its limitations?" (1966: 16). Critical social theory provides just this: a position from which to examine psychiatry and its episteme, to reflect upon how it can be made more robust, and where it fails to achieve its goals.

While psychiatry may have endured greater shifts than other branches of medicine, and may congratulate itself upon its self-reflexivity, it lacks nonetheless, from within its own frameworks, a mechanism to perceive the apparatus, its construction, workings and impact. The social, legal, gender, biopolitical and ethical arguments made within these pages propose a bold set of questions that no practitioner or recipient of psychiatric services should ignore. They should be unsettling and should niggle at the reader's sense of what psychiatry is, even while presenting a picture which resonates in some way or another with his or her sense of what psychiatry should be.

Annemarie Goldstein Jutel
July 2013, New Zealand

References

Hacking, I. 2001. Inaugural lecture: Chair of philosophy and history of scientific concepts at the Collège de France, *Economy and Society*. 31(1), 1–14.

Douglas, M. 1966. *Purity and Danger*. London: Routledge and Kegan Paul.

Acknowledgements

Dave Holmes, Jean Daniel Jacob, and Amélie Perron would like to acknowledge the financial support of the Faculty of Health Sciences at the University of Ottawa. Thanks to Myriam Kaszap, graduate student, whose patient work at various stages of the manuscript has been indispensable. Thanks to Dr Jayne Elliott for her diligent revision of chapters. Special thanks to Diana Thorneycroft for authorizing the use of her work for the book cover. Finally, we would like to thank Neil Jordan at Ashgate for his precious support.

Introduction
Unmasking the Psychiatric Apparatus

Jean Daniel Jacob, Amélie Perron and Dave Holmes

Introduction

This collection is the product of ongoing reflections and analyses that have coloured our professional experiences in the psychiatric domain. We have worked in psychiatric settings (hospital, forensic, and community settings) as clinicians, educators, researchers, and administrators for many years. We have come to realize that psychiatry is a complex field of health care that has so far failed, in most cases, to live up to its promises, despite continuously expanding its scope of interventions. After many years of practice in various capacities we are forced to acknowledge that psychiatry is made up of a dense and intense web of (power) relations that characterizes what Foucault called the apparatus (*dispositif*). Psychiatry is not a mere medical science: it is an intensely political system of interrelated practices, discourses, and institutions.

This book is not a textbook on psychiatry meant for undergraduate students. It is a collection of the most radical essays (inspired by classical texts) that turn psychiatry on its head. More specifically, the purpose of this collection is to critically examine taken for granted past and current psychiatric practices as well as the purported promises of scientific and technological advances. The exceptional list of authors brought together in this important collection makes no excuses for this highly political undertaking. Sensitive topics in the realm of psychiatry are therefore (re)conceptualized in order to give precedence to discourses that have been discarded within and by the psychiatric apparatus. The collection seeks to provide numerous theoretical tools to address issues related to psychiatric power, discipline, and control and theorize their workings in creative and critical ways.

Psychiatry as Social Control: A Brief History

In *Madness and Civilization: A History of Insanity in the Age of Reason*, Foucault engaged in what he calls a "genealogy" of the asylum and its corollary, mental illness. Foucault (2006) argued that in fifteenth-century Europe, madness instilled a collective fascination and fear because it sparked harrowing images of depravity, violence, monstrosity, and the end of the world. During this period, the Ship of Fools represented a way in which society dealt with its mad denizens. Exiled to the sea, the "lunatics" would travel an uncharted path in their quest for reason, but more importantly, this voyage symbolized the use of exclusionary practices to ensure social order. By the mid-seventeenth century, the *Hôpital Général de Paris* was founded by the bourgeois and monarchical orders, signalling a new era in the management of the mad but also the sick, the poor, the vagrant, and the invalid (Foucault 2006, Russ 1979). Confinement, rather than exile, became the modus operandi as a way to administer those who did not fit the prevailing social order. At that time, the mad were seen as embodying all forms of violence and deviance, falling outside of the definition of crime and the scope of judicial authorities (Foucault 1996). Confinement, designed to isolate individuals whose behaviour was qualified as dangerous or disturbing, became a strategy of choice to preserve social order and morality (Geller and Harris 1994, Laplante 1997, Russ 1979).

During the seventeenth century, madness took on animal characteristics and embodied a strange and frightening creature (Russ 1979). From the concrete to the fictitious, the projected image of madness took on new forms of monstrosity – a product arising from the connection between man and creature (Federman, Holmes, and Jacob 2009). This esoteric understanding of madness led to the development of an animalistic model guiding social representation of the time; animals did not partake in the rational order of human nature and as their counterpart, mentally ill persons were treated accordingly. The use of physical restraints to chain the mentally ill to beds or walls was accompanied by extreme living conditions, a reality that fit within the prevailing myth that the mentally ill, as not quite human, were insensible to such things as temperature, comfort, and hygiene (Foucault 2006).

During the time of the French Revolution and under the ensuing *Declaration of the Rights of Man and of the Citizen*, however, arbitrary confinement was no longer an acceptable way of managing mentally ill persons (Garrido and Cayley 1876). References to sub-human criteria as the basis for the development of a descriptive and explanatory model for insanity were replaced by a discourse focused on physical systems, situating mental illness within the body and its dysfunctions. For example, mental illness was, in part, described as a "disease of the nerves" (Foucault 2006: 139). Consequently, a new field opened up, one that would soon form the clinical realm: consolidation, cold baths, showers, and purification techniques became forms of treatment (Foucault 2006). Two doctors of the time, Tenon and Cabanis, imagined and reconceptualized confinement as a kind of restricted and structured freedom rather than the plain elimination of liberty and social exclusion – a "caged freedom" with therapeutic advantages (Foucault 2006). The therapeutic foundation of the asylum was thus established.

Tenon and Cabanis' vision remained a theoretical exercise for the most part, and it is not until the late eighteenth century and the beginning of the nineteenth century that Pinel realized their ambitious project. Foucault (2006) argued that it is through Pinel's work that the modern asylum was born, as it transformed into a clinical territory. Madness came out of a social framework and was re-inscribed in a medical framework (Foucault 2006), whereby the doctor personified the sole legitimate authority capable of identifying, diagnosing, and treating madness. He became a specialist whose expertise governed the institutional (and to a larger extent, social) management of the mentally ill. Many claim that Pinel and those who followed him gave way to the humanization of what would become psychiatric institutions. Gauchet and Swain (1980), for instance, argue that psychiatry was no longer about exclusion and repression; rather, it positioned the mentally ill within the realm of humanity. The nineteenth century bore witness to the emergence of the sciences of Man: psychiatry, psychology, psychoanalysis, sociology. Within the obscurity of insanity, clinical experts uncovered a human subject fit for moral and therapeutic transformation through dialogue and human relationships.

> What the classical age of reason (the period from Descartes to Kant) had recognized as a space of exclusion and correction had, by the 19th century, exchanged its language of punishment for a discourse of scientific truth, where the question of individual liberty and the need for personal restriction dictated mechanism of both cure and conformity. (Federman et al. 2009: 53)

In light of this progression, Foucault believed that Modernity was characterized by new regimes of power/knowledge (Fraser 1989) that differ from previous regimes through the unleashing of new forms of social and political control. The asylum is the logical instrument of deterministic processes of social control carried out by administrative and clinical technicians. Along with Foucault, we argue that, from the onset, psychiatry yearned for an impossible objective. Without detracting from Pinel's intentions towards the mentally ill, we need to recognize that the creation of the modern asylum has led to insidious, even violent, outcomes through the institution and legitimation of subtle, yet more definitive, forms of confinement and control. Foucault perceived the asylum as the crystallization of a rational project that validated prescribed forms of domination. The domination of reason does not constitute a neutral and apolitical event; rather, it signals the advent of justifiable institutional brutality. Instead of a true dialogue between reason and madness, the undeniable ascendancy of the former over the latter would quickly constitute the leitmotif of modern psychiatry (Foucault 2006).

Pinel, and his English counterpart Tuke, did not unwind the ancient practices of confinement; they, in fact, intensified their workings within the institution by tightening the grasp of its technologies of care/cure on the individual and collective body (Russ 1979). In the asylum, the unrelenting gaze of clinical agents seized the mentally ill person from every angle. Every gesture, from the most peculiar to the most commonplace, was recorded and used to build a case – an array of disciplinary technologies deployed into a complex system of micro-penalties and rewards meant to regulate time, activities, bodies, sexualities, and so on (Dreyfus and Rabinow 1984). Discipline served to reinstate social standards through the use of various strategies, such as behaviour modification techniques, privileges, restriction of movements, and later, pharmacological treatment (Castel 1976). The purpose of this new *governmentality* was precisely to seize the whole body of the detainee and to transform it towards a new morality. It is obvious, then, that "[t]he science of mental disease, as it would develop in the asylum, would always be only of the order of observation and classification. It would not be a dialogue" (Foucault 2006: 250).

It is clear that over the course of history, the management of the mentally ill became intertwined with the administration of society's other undesirables, including the unemployed, vagrants, criminals, alcoholics, and, in many regards, women. "Social and moral crises" associated with these fringe groups became widespread following industrialization of the Western world. Populations grew massively, economic growth and opportunities attracted throngs of employment seekers and their families from the countryside, immigrant workers arrived in great numbers, cities expanded, and slums began to appear (Iredale 2000). Unemployment and poverty, alcoholism, violence, prostitution, panhandling, crime, and diseases of all sorts (e.g. tuberculosis, syphilis, smallpox) caught the attention of governing officials and intellectuals of the time who argued that deficient elements of society would contribute to its decline and needed to be controlled (Iredale 2000). In particular, concerns grew as society questioned the threat posed by the offspring of "unfit" citizens and advocated for the need to intervene in their reproduction (Castel, Castel, and Lovell 1982).

In the United States, but spreading rapidly to Europe, mental illness was reframed as a "regenerating" disease, one that could be passed on from generation to generation. A new meaning for psychic deficiency emerged as knowledge in regard to heredity reinforced the idea of mental illness as an incurable disease (Waller 2002). Indeed, in 1914, like many other intellectuals and politicians at the time, the president of the American Medico-Psychological Association (later renamed the American Psychiatric Association) effectively linked social problems and mental "defects":

> That a radical cure of the evils incident to the dependent mentally defective classes would be effected if every feeble-minded person, every incurably insane or epileptic person, every imbecile, every habitual criminal, every manifestly weak-minded person, and every confirmed inebriate were sterilized, is a self-evident proposition. By this means we could practically, if not absolutely, arrest, in a decade or two, the reproduction of mentally defective persons. (MacDonald 1914: 9)

In its most brutal and radical form, social control of "deviant" individuals was achieved through widespread negative eugenic practices (namely social and sexual segregation, forced sterilization and castration, as well as euthanasia), based on new discoveries pertaining to genetics and heredity that were made at the turn of the twentieth century (Iredale 2000, Waller 2002). While the eugenics movement appears to be an extreme event from a distant past, it is important to note that eugenic theory lives on in the shape of forced sterilization in many parts of the world, as well as in other forms of medical interventions such as prenatal screening and genetic counselling (Diekema 2003, Iredale 2000).

Psychiatry was thus able to expand its scope of influence well outside the walls of the asylum (MacLennan 1987). Prisons, for instance, were identified early on as a locus of intervention to modify inmates' behaviours and put them on the path to social rehabilitation (Foucault 1995). Mental disorders provided ways of constructing social deviance, such that individuals behaving outside the accepted norms were not only criminalized but medicalized as well (Gosden 1997), thus blurring the line between behaviours falling under the purview of psychiatry and medicine, and those under the jurisdiction of other authoritative bodies (e.g. courts). In addition, the early twentieth century was also marked by the mental hygiene movement, which repositioned mental illness as a disease rooted in social factors but also introduced the promotion of mental health for the enrichment of human life (MacLennan 1987). While eugenics theories were officially rejected after World War II (though they did not disappear, as seen earlier), psychiatry secured a new domain of influence with the institution of social welfare policies that prevailed during this era, and which gave rise to what Castel and colleagues (1982) refer to as the *advanced psychiatric society*.

The Perpetual Deployment of the Advanced Psychiatric Society

During the post-war period, a new preventive discourse emerged, one that secured access to a growing number of social spheres (Castel, Castel, and Lovell 1982). Risk became the driving force of health and social policies (Lupton 1999), which inevitably led to the need to screen and prevent the development of mental disorders in individuals. Risk-thinking involved an amalgamation of complex, abstract factors acting on the *probability* that an adverse event (or behaviour) would occur (Castel 1991). It produced labels such as "at-risk individuals", "vulnerable populations", and "persons in precarious situations", thus giving rise to an array of surveillance structures (e.g. epidemiology studies, statistical reports). The individual gave way to a "profile" arising out of a speculated interaction between particular risk factors. Castel (1991) argues that in the post-war period, public policy in the Western world shifted from prevention of danger and harm to risk surveillance and management, thereby opening up a whole new field of social and health interventionism: "In the name of this myth of absolute eradication of risk, [modern ideologies] construct a mass of new risks which constitute so many new targets for preventive intervention" (p. 289). Modern psychiatry's imperative would from this point on be focused on developing these preventive interventions that only reinforce its capacity to manage personal and social relations (Federman et al. 2009).

Psychologists, social workers, case workers, child welfare specialists, and nurses were deployed in communities to identify and assist those individuals struggling with various issues ranging from personal crises, lack of maternal skills, and behavioural problems in children, to domestic violence, juvenile delinquency, and the care of invalids. Preventive measures were implemented and assistance was provided in the form of government services, community programs, and medical/psychiatric treatment (Castel et al. 1982). In other words, individuals judged abnormal or at risk of being abnormal were now being identified and pathologized in their natural environment, be it at work, at home, or at school. Children in particular became targets of surveillance, identification, and monitoring measures in order to halt as soon as possible the progression of problems. As a result, individual behaviours were not the sole component of scrutiny; it also included the examination of children's families, their school, their social environment, and other factors that could contribute to functional problems (Donzelot 1979). In this sense, childhood was no longer parents' and teachers' area of expertise: it also became the clinical territory of professionals who "specialize in suspicion" (Castel et al. 1982: 202) and who deployed stringent strategies for (child and parent) behaviour control.

Through the expansion of everyday pathologization, unlabelled citizens and their children have thus become potential candidates for psychiatric intervention: "there is now a self-conscious attempt being made to persuade more and more women (and men) to think of themselves as 'at risk' from illness, and therefore to seek help at the first opportunity" (Lee 2006: 48). In other words, this movement brings people to realize their differences or their "risks" of becoming "troubled" and seek medical attention to confirm or re-establish their normalcy, and, in doing so, cultivate the need to consume psychiatric services and products.

It can be argued that psychiatry – as a discourse, a discipline, a field of inquiry, an economic activity, and a political tool – relies on a powerful web of power relations that forms an integral part of Foucault's definition of the "apparatus" (*dispositif*), a fundamental definition which underpins this collection:

> A thoroughly heterogeneous ensemble consisting of discourses, institutions, architectural forms, regulatory decisions, laws, administrative measures, scientific statements, philosophical, moral and philanthropic propositions – in short, the said as much as the unsaid. Such are the elements of the apparatus. The apparatus itself is the system of relations that can be established between these elements … The apparatus thus has a dominant strategic function. (Foucault 1980: 194–195).

The purpose of the *apparatus* is to create those dispositions needed to influence and enable a broad range of actions in a normative way (Raffnsøe 2008). While the apparatus is firstly instituted in response to a particular crisis, such as a growing social or moral concern, its pertinence and its power rest on the fact that it

> survives the very intentionality and the vision that marked its implementation … the *dispositif* is re-mobilized in order to manage the effects that it, itself, has produced … the Foucauldian *dispositif* has often appeared as a place of technical inscription for a total social project, working through constraint, and seeking to control both the body and the soul. (Beuscart and Peerbaye, 2006: 5; our translation)

The concept of the *apparatus*, then, also allows us to segue into the work of Castel and engage with his notion of the advanced psychiatric society (Castel et al. 1982), a kind of society which, we argue, rests precisely on the deployment of a psychiatric *apparatus*.

Castel and colleagues (1982) argue that the *advanced psychiatric society* (*Société psychiatrique avancée*) is modelled after the American system, where psychiatry "no longer simply censures or represses. It actually *produces* a form of relations delineating a geography of everyday life" (p. xii, italics in original). The advanced psychiatric society designates a thoroughly Modern, sophisticated arrangement of those institutions, policies, laws, experts, and discourses that make up the psychiatric domain in the Western world. Each entity presents with a specific history, plays a specific role, embodies a specific ideology, relies on specific technologies (e.g. research institutes, taxonomies, clinical guidelines, jargon, etc.) to carry out its mandate. Over time, however, there has been an undeniable overlapping of jurisdictions and blurred accountability. This is especially so since there has been a clear departure from repressive practices and an engagement with therapeutic ones in the management of problematic behaviours (Foucault 1995). For example, police officers started to be trained in the humanities in order to relate their practice to some general framework of human experience (Lankes 1970). Recently, police and mental health workers across Canada have come together to form specially designed intervention teams in order to access marginalized groups and manage crises in a more humane/therapeutic fashion. Psychiatric hospitals now house criminals in secured units while mental health units are being set up within penitentiaries – a reality that forces the challenging coexistence of agents of care and peace officers (Holmes 2005, Holmes and Murray 2011, Jacob and Holmes 2011, Perron and Holmes 2011). Treatment rather than punishment seems to be part of new rehabilitation measures that position therapeutic rationales in all aspects of social interventions.

The expansion of therapeutic rationales further illustrates the intersecting and the morphing of various entities that make up the psychiatric domain. For instance, patients become therapists themselves in peer support groups (Simpson and House 2002); community settings have become places of segregation, discipline and surveillance that are reminiscent of the old asylums as forms of social control (Mulvey, Geller, and Roth 1987, Watts and Priebe 2002). Further obscuring occurs at the (malleable) demarcation between "normal" and "pathological" behaviours. Over the years, the notion of deviance has expanded to explain why human beings fail to situate themselves within social norms, as evidenced for instance by their inability to maintain an optimal bodily appearance (e.g. obesity), to achieve intellectual standards (e.g. learning disorders), to control their emotions (e.g. anger, premenstrual dysphoric disorder), and to demonstrate "healthy" sexual practices (e.g. sexual dysfunctions), to name just a few. As psychiatry expanded, it is clear that it no longer forced itself onto people but also through them as "subjects of power", whereby the on-going production of knowledge and discourses regarding psychiatry, mental illness, and mental health, influenced practices and shaped psychiatry-related identities (Mason 1999) so much so, that psychiatry is now being demanded by those who were led to believe that they suffered from a particular emotional ailment in need of attention (Castel et al. 1982).

New claims regarding the benefits of awareness, meaningful presence, interpersonal relationships, liberation, healing, and self-discovery and actualization have become prevalent and suggest a new kind of relationship one ought to develop with oneself and others – the sooner the better, as a mode of prevention of serious emotional ailment. While professional clinicians and corporations were not necessarily involved in the creation of new therapeutic approaches derived from an evolving social need for normalcy, psychology-infused discourses pertaining to crises, distress, health, adaptation, therapy, and recovery remain and perpetuate the belief that anyone could fall "ill" and get better. Alternative services such as sex therapy, Gestalt therapy, family therapy, and the like also preserve the mindset that one must monitor oneself closely in order to know oneself better and take action when signs of dis-ease surface, leading to a new kind of (self) discipline and management that, in our view, differs little in principle with psychiatric approaches. Much like Castel and colleagues (1982: 257) have argued, we concur that "the methods are now so flexible that nothing further stands in the way of their unlimited proliferation", thereby leading to the unrelenting "colonization of social life".

Progressively, the psychiatric enterprise has become a service offered for the greater good of society, one that has produced new forms of treatments dedicated to restoring normalcy. Here, Castel and colleagues (1982) speak of a "post-psychoanalytic" era where symptoms are no longer the signs of specific pathologies but the signs of "dis-ease" with daily life: "now that we have reached the point of 'therapy of the normal', virtually all of social space has been opened up to new techniques of psychological manipulation" (p.174).

The psychiatric domain is characterized by overlapping and fluid categories: normal-pathological, autonomy-discipline, therapist-patient, active-passive, institution-community, etc. Paradoxically perhaps, this blurring of the lines is such that the organization of psychiatry appears to be rational, streamlined and scientifically sound – in a word, advanced. It is no coincidence that psychiatry endures the continuous salvos of criticisms and lawsuits that should have precipitated its downfall. As a social and political entity, psychiatry thrives because it has developed an astonishing ability to both absorb and control counter-discourses about mental health (e.g. women, gay, and patient rights movements) that dispute its activities and legitimacy. It absorbs those very initiatives (e.g. women's groups, self-help initiatives, psychiatric survivors networks, holistic approaches) that aim to depart from its oppressive and normative function, thus producing a seemingly new, adaptable, versatile, modernized, and responsive model of intervention: "The best way to enlarge the scope of the system is to welcome whatever looms up on its boundaries, translating each innovation, as far as possible, into the idiom of the system" (Castel et al. 1982: 254).

Treating mental disorders remains, to this day, the primary objective of psychiatry. Given the shift in psychiatric thinking, whereby everyone is at risk of descending into some sort of psychological affliction, there will always be more people in need of treatment than people being treated. As such, the expansion of psychiatry into the "capillaries" of society ensures that the demand for psychiatric "commodities" exceeds services, thereby justifying the staying power of a "clinico-therapeutic" system (MacLennan 1987). Hence the defining feature of the advanced psychiatric society is

> an organization of everyday life in which manipulative techniques … become coextensive with all aspects of social life. No longer the manifestation of naked power exerted directly to repress social and political differences; but rather diffuse pressures of many kinds, which invalidates such differences by interpreting them as so many symptoms to be treated … a padded world watched over night and day by squads of skilled specialists, many of them well-meaning. Skilled at what? At manipulating people to accept the constraints of society. (Castel et al. 1982: 320)

Psychiatry remains, first and foremost, a normative pursuit, one that relies on disciplinary techniques that need to be developed, experimented with, and refined through complex political/psychiatric apparatuses (Dreyfus and Rabinow 1984). In order to achieve these monumental gains, tools and networks had to be developed, which worked to strengthen psychiatry's hold on most, if not all, aspects of life.

The Politics of Psychiatric "Science"

On the Advent of the DSM and Biopsychiatry

The origins of mental disorders have never been clearly articulated (Caine 2003) and remain, to this day, arbitrarily interpreted and treated by members of the psychiatric enterprise (and therefore disputed) (Kirk and Kutchins 1992). Medicine has historically differentiated madness from sanity by generating classification schemes that labelled any and all kinds of behaviour sane/normal or insane/pathological, based on the "scientific" research available at the time (Federman, Jacob and Holmes 2007). Foucault (2006) argued that the psychiatric enterprise is mainly based on the process of naming, labelling, and classifying mental disorders. Therefore, the nosographic system of modern psychiatry relies heavily on the subjective assessment and description of what is and is not normal social behaviour (Szasz 2003). Where madness intersects with the average man, there is the inevitable presence of moral judgment (Canguilhem 1962).

The labelling and classification process described by Foucault culminated in the 1950s with the publication of the *Diagnostic and Statistical Manual of Mental Disorders (DSM)* by the American Psychiatric Association. The *DSM* was heralded as a major paradigmatic shift in psychiatry (First and Tasman 2004), one that bridged the gap between the ambitions of psychiatry and scientific evidence.

The making of the *DSM* was described as the conventional triumph of science over the mysteries of nature, a sort of revolution and transformation of American psychiatry (Mayes and Horwtiz 2005, Wilson 1993). Yet the psychiatric diagnosis process itself remains largely unquestioned, as do the circumstances leading to this revolution in psychiatric thought (Kirk and Kutchins 1992).

The *DSM* is generally recognized as the standard taxonomic tool used by clinical practitioners in the Western world to diagnose and treat individuals with mental disorders. It is considered to reflect (although imperfectly) natural entities signified as mental disorders (Schmidt et al. 2004). According to First and Tasman (2004), the most important goal of the taxonomic manual of modern psychiatry is to allow researchers and clinicians to communicate effectively. In other words, the classification system of mental disorders serves as a tool to effectively convey "expert" observations and ensure that the labels used to diagnose each individual are congruent with specific clusters of symptoms associated with a particular disorder.

In our view, the *DSM* is used for a purpose that surpasses the simple classification of disease entities and is therefore nothing less than a taxonomic illusion that forms part of the psychiatric apparatus. It is the very concretization of psychiatry's claim-making activities. The *DSM* facilitates the construction of disease entities and the identification of individuals as sick based on the alleged expertise of diagnosing mental disorders and the advances in treating biochemical imbalances with "science" (Lachter 2001). Although it is not the main objective of this collection, there is a pressing need to continue exploring the foundations and justifications for incorporating this taxonomic tool into modern psychiatry, as the rationale for its existence and expansion cannot be found in science but in the need to find "cures" to social ills. Homosexuality is a classic example of such a "social problem" and of a psychiatric label that has targeted specific groups. This "social sorting" was based on a social construction of sexual deviance, despite the lack of evidence for the validity of this assessment (see McDonald 1990). Interestingly, the absence of homosexuality in more recent editions of the *DSM* is not the result of scientific refinement in psychiatry or psychology research. According to Mendelson (2003), the modification of psychiatric nosology had nothing to do with science, but everything to do with the "concatenation of social forces, including political pressure from homosexual organizations, involvement of the wider human rights movement, and the epidemiological data that questioned the 'scientific' basis for considering homosexuality ... a mental disorder" (p.683). In other words, the inclusion of homosexuality as a psychiatric disorder appears to be as arbitrary and culturally/politically determined as its subsequent withdrawal from the *DSM*.

Historically, the field of psychiatry had been relegated to the margins of medical sciences because of its precarious scientific foundations (Mayes and Horwitz 2005). By the 1970s, the psychiatric apparatus was faced with a growing critique of its unscientific taxonomic classifications of mental disorders and its inability to explain their etiologies (First and Tasman 2004). In order to reposition themselves within the realm of "real" medicine, psychiatrists (predominantly from the United States) transitioned in the late 1980s to the development of a biological framework that would shift toward "the search for physiological, genetics, and chemical bases for mental disorders and the development and the use of psychopharmacological agents for treatment" (Kirk and Kutchins 1992: 10). This empirical move was marked by the publication of the third edition of the *DSM* and the adoption of a factual/objective reconfiguration of the classification system. For members of the psychiatric enterprise, a biological interpretation of mental disorders (biopsychiatry) appeared promising since it was compatible with mainstream medicine. The production of the *DSM-III* moved away from a Freudian perspective towards an approach that was deeply influenced by the works of Emil Kraeplin, a German researcher who attempted throughout his career to classify, categorize, and describe psychiatric disorders (First and Tasman 2004).

This transition symbolized the marginalization of theory-derived psychiatric practices and the emergence of rigorous scientific applications to the diagnosis and treatment of mental disorders (Wilson and Guze 1995). However, one is forced to question what is factual about the third (and subsequent) versions of the *DSM*, since it offered no new knowledge to the field of psychiatry but merely a new way to classify mental disorders (Mayes and Horwitz 2005). Furthermore, since the inception of the *DSM*, new, powerful players have entered the psychiatric arena and are moulding the face of modern psychiatry.

The Corporate Link

While producers of the *DSM* argue that psychiatric diagnoses are real entities (*taxon*), they are vague and abstract constructs that lack conceptual boundaries and remain heavily influenced by socio-political realities (Federman et al. 2007). Consequently, it can be argued that the *DSM* as a "scientific" instrument is an oxymoron: "the *DSM* has little to do with science, its content is determined primarily by the gatekeeping efforts of the small number of influential psychiatrists who have the directive to decide which disorders will be allowed to appear and which will not" (Curra 2000: 179). In fact, it is the product of individuals who chair committees and who vote on the inclusion or exclusion of certain diagnostic groups (Kaplan and Sadock 1995, Mendelson 2003). According to Kirk and Kutchins (1992), "to a great extent psychiatric nosology has been a product of committee meetings and smiling faces" (p.29), where psychiatric nosology is not so much about addressing construct validity as it is seeking to address face validity: professional consensus. It is also important to highlight that strong financial ties currently bind the developers of the *DSM* with pharmaceutical and other companies who are powerful drivers of the psychiatric system (Cosgrove, Krimsky, Vijayaraghavan, and Schneider 2006).

Since the publication of the *DSM-III*, biopsychiatry has become an essential determinant of the way research and clinical practices are developed around the notion of "mental disorder". The construction of mental illness is now largely based on the assumptions that physiological, genetic, and/or chemical abnormalities are at the roots of behavioural deviance (Breggin 2006). The hypothetical association between mental illness and the lack or excess of neurotransmitters justifies the need to develop molecules meant to restore balance in individuals' brains (Kaplan and Sadock 1995). In other words, the multiple sites of therapeutic action in the brain are at the heart of modern psychiatry (Breggin 2003). However, the biological classification of mental disorders serves purposes other than clinical. A significant outcome of the *DSM-III* is the growing association between its classification scheme of mental disorders, insurance coverage of mental "care" (Kutchins and Kirk 1997, Mayes and Horwitz 2005), and the rising numbers of chemical compounds produced by pharmaceutical companies – a phenomenon that remains controversial in light of the fifth edition of the *DSM*. These relationships form a dense web, a medical-industrial complex whose members have much to gain financially from additional diagnostic categories. The decision-making process through which behavioural problems are identified and crystallized in the *DSM* is at the very heart of the politics of constructing mental disorders (Kutchins and Kirk 1997). The rise of biopsychiatry and the concomitant expansion of classification schemes are of great interest to pharmaceutical corporations whose business objective lies in the production of drugs that target neurotransmitters' functions in the brain. Pharmaceutical companies are pivotal funding agencies in the promotion, development, and dissemination of (bio)psychiatric research. They therefore constitute powerful instigators (and beneficiaries) of the fabrication of new psychiatric labels (Moncrieff, Hopker and Thomas 2005). Along with Kutchins and Kirk (1997), we therefore contend that the unlabelled masses of individuals in today's societies represent an untapped resource for the economic growth of corporations, such as pharmaceutical industries, who are heavily involved in the "psychiatric business".

It is important to note that the current development of biopsychiatry positions clinicians within an uneven consumer-provider relationship. In effect, psychiatry differs from other forms of enterprises where providers typically respond to a social need by creating a service or product. Psychiatry not only provides its own branch of services and products but it also controls the perception of the social need regarding mental "care". And while there has been a clear shift in the way mentally ill persons are referred to (from *patient* and *sufferer*, to *client* and *consumer*), which should symbolize a purported shift in power relationships between mentally ill persons and the psychiatric system, this change is rather deceptive because, firstly, choices that are made by the former are first developed, sorted, governed, and prescribed by the latter, and secondly, compliance remains an enduring determinant of their relationship (Perron, Rudge, and Holmes 2010).

As a result, despite the apparent dynamic and responsive nature of psychiatric discourse and practice, one cannot help but note that power gradients between providers and consumers of psychiatric products and services remain virtually unchanged, and that discourses of empowerment, emancipation, and citizenship fare little in light of the ongoing discipline, control, and reduction in autonomous thought endured by mentally ill persons (Perron et al. 2010). In fact, the biomedicalization of everyday problems offers newly diagnosed individuals an organic cause for their problematic behaviours. As sufferers of a psychiatric disease, individuals are no longer "responsible" for their problem and rely on the expert knowledge of clinicians (Goffman 1998). Under medical expertise, individuals become passive adherents to a pathologic state rather than active agents in society (Goffman 1998). As such, "the medicalization of social and personal problems … is testimony to the power of psychiatry to create subjectivities" (Moncrieff et al. 2005: 84).

Psychiatry (Re)defined: Repression-Transformation-Assistance

In his outstanding piece of contemporary sociology, Goffman (1998) exposes the inner workings of the psychiatric apparatus. Based on the works of Castel (1976, 1991), Goffman (1998) and Foucault (2006) we believe that psychiatry is positioned on a repression-assistance-transformation continuum that has (perhaps) inadvertently enabled the conceptualization of modern forms of power relations in that medical field. The critique of the psychiatric apparatus offered by this collection is largely influenced by Goffman's perspective and the works of critical theorists, notably Michel Foucault and Robert Castel. Drawing together the latest research and reflections from Australia, Canada, the UK, and the US, the book is organized according to each component of the repression (coercion) – transformation (discipline) – assistance (therapy) continuum. The sections are interconnected to the extent that they not only all engage in a critical analysis of past and current psychiatric practices but also help turn psychiatry upside down. In the first section of the book, repression, the authors set the stage by overtly addressing coercive practices in psychiatry and forcing readers to contextualize these practices within wider legal and ethical frameworks. The second section of the book, transformation, proves to be an extension of the first section by addressing the effects and progression of the psychiatric apparatus in modern society. Finally, the third section of the book, assistance, embraces a broad understanding of assistance in order to go beyond the altruistic and well-intentioned rhetoric of mental health to problematize how the therapeutic apparatus is operationalized in practice.

Therefore, this collection opens with a controversial piece from Professor Thomas Szasz, who passed away six weeks after authorizing the reprint of his last published paper (2013), reproduced here. He was thrilled to be part of this collection and we are forever grateful for his contribution – a radical critique of the psychiatric apparatus. In this (eye) opening chapter, Szasz provides a critique of modern objections to diverse psychiatric practices, focusing on the critics' neglect of the core problematic issue – the psychiatrist's role in depriving innocent persons of liberty. In Chapter 2, both senses of "censoring violence" are exposed by Holmes and Murray. In the most obvious sense, they speak of the violence of censorship in general, including the violence of the censor who works to silence or to undermine the results of research and, often, the integrity of the researchers themselves. Linked to these explicit activities there is a second sense of "censoring violence", one that works implicitly. By this, Holmes and Murray point to the tacit violence of forensic psychiatry itself – a "professional" or "vocational" violence that is self-censored, covered up from within at the institutional level. Thus, research that exposes the constitutive and structural violence of forensic psychiatric settings will find itself face to face with both forms of censoring violence: such research will be met with violent censorship, yes, but more insidiously, it must take place in a milieu in which structural and symbolic violence have regulated in advance the kinds of research that can be conducted, the kinds of questions that can be asked, and ultimately, what can be known, disseminated, hoped for, and done.

Bernheim's contribution in Chapter 3 unpacks how the evolution of civil law around equal rights to integrity and self-determination has taken concrete form in the establishment of an internment mechanism with a completely judiciarized substantive and procedural framework. In this context, the courts are the primary mechanism for protecting and implementing rights. Yet, various organizations, both governmental and non-governmental, denounce the systematic violation of psychiatric patients' rights, which seems to be explained by social, medical, and legal dynamics: the survival of a moral discourse on normal behaviour that justifies both demands for intervention by civil society and the triggering of medical and legal mechanisms; the *psychiatrization* phenomenon in which any situation that is considered abnormal is re-interpreted as a manifestation of mental illness, which turns the debate into a discussion among experts and undermines patients' credibility; and finally, the *instrumentalization* of justice, though it does not have the means necessary to fulfil its mandate.

In Chapter 4, Johnston and Kilty, departing from Johnston's lived experience as a private security guard at a psychiatric facility, examine how the performance of masculinity shapes and contributes to the coercive ways in which hospital guards manage, control, and interact with involuntary mental health patients. Empirical data are analysed using Connell's theoretical concept of "hegemonic masculinity", as well as the available literature on gender and masculinity within security, prison, police, and military institutions. The authors find that the struggle for power is gendered and alpha masculine status entangles the relations, discourses, and associated practices of psychiatric ward nurses, patients, and guards – the outcome of which is ward reliance on punitive mechanisms of control. More specifically, the psychiatric setting fosters the reproduction of masculinity either through physical/chemical force, punishment, intimidation, or repeated expressions of ambivalence towards feminized displays of compassion, sympathy, and concern for the care of patients.

Following on the topic of punitive measures pervasive in many psychiatric settings, Muir-Cochrane and Gerace look at how the use of physical restraint and seclusion by mental health professionals has received increased and sustained scrutiny internationally to reduce such practice. Despite calls from governments and consumer organizations to eliminate or reduce restraint and seclusion, usage has increased in settings such as emergency departments, ambulances, and general hospital wards. This chapter looks at international research literature on the uses of restraint and seclusion in a range of hospital settings and the context in which they occur. Legal, ethical, and clinical perspectives are examined to explore why, in a climate of "least restrictive treatment" environment- and consumer-focussed philosophies, the use of containment practices is increasing, particularly in settings where such practices only recently came into existence .

In Chapter 6, Healy and LeNoury look at how in the past years bipolar disorder in children has been diagnosed with rapidly increasing frequency in North America, despite a century of psychiatric consensus that manic-depressive illness rarely had its onset before adolescence. This emergence has happened against a background of vigorous pharmaceutical company marketing of bipolar disorder in adults. In the absence of a license demonstrating efficacy for their compound for bipolar disorder in children, however, companies cannot actively market paediatric bipolar disorder. This chapter explores some mechanisms that play a part in spreading the recognition of a disorder in populations for which pharmaceutical companies do not have a license. These include the role of academic experts, parent pressure groups, measurement technologies, and the availability of possible remedies even if not licensed.

In Chapter 7, Murray and Burgess provide a thought provoking examination of the forensic psychiatric treatment of patient-prisoners caught between care and incarceration. While the Mental Health Act in most jurisdictions stipulates equal access to health care for all citizens, including prisoners, the neoliberal and biopolitical regulations that govern correctional institutions supervene prisoners' "right" to health. Using Foucault's concept of biopolitics as a theoretical lens, this chapter offers a critical examination of two events: the case of a child being born in captivity to an incarcerated mother (Julie Bilotta), and the case of a young woman (Ashley Smith) committing suicide in her cell. In both cases, correctional officers watched (and in Smith's case, filmed the event) from outside the cell, refusing to intervene and failing to provide even basic medical care. While these cases represent specific failures in the penal system vis-à-vis mental health, in a broader context they are also occasions to reflect on how forensic psychiatry itself often operates as a "correctional service" informed by juridical and biopolitical discourses.

Based on their empirical research, Jacob, Perron, and Corneau explore in Chapter 8 the nursing management of violent patients in an emergency psychiatric unit. Guided by individual accounts from both providers of mental health services (nurses) and recipients of care (patients), the results of this research highlight the multiple contextual factors that inadvertently give therapeutic significance to controlling interventions. Drawing on the works of Rose, Foucault, and Goffman, their analysis will draw attention to the tensions that exist between nursing care and the micro-politics involved in its place of practice, thus positioning the psychiatric emergency unit as an anomaly in the emergency department and as a key factor in the way patients are conceptualized and subsequently treated.

Chapter 9 accounts for Paula Caplan's tense interactions with the American Psychiatric Association regarding the (mis)use of psychiatric diagnosis. According to Caplan, thorough documentation of the unscientific nature of psychiatric diagnosis, its failure to improve outcomes in the effort to help reduce human suffering, and the many risks of harm that it carries has done little to get this information through to the public and professionals or to stop the skyrocketing use of psychiatric labels. Most importantly, little or nothing has been done to gather information about the harm or to redress any of it. In a groundbreaking initiative, nine complaints were filed in 2012 with the American Psychiatric Association, which publishes and profits from the *Diagnostic and Statistical Manual of Mental Disorders*, naming as respondents a large number of APA members who had responsibilities of various sorts with regard to the *DSM*. Caplan created a template to help enable other people who were harmed by psychiatric diagnosis to file complaints as well, and other initiatives are described in this very engaged and engaging chapter.

In Chapter 10, Jem Masters suggest that over the past decades, *mainstreaming* of mental health care has occurred with the closure of the asylums and the development of integrated health care systems. This has meant non-mental health professionals have been expected to provide initial assessments and care with minimal knowledge and skills, especially in emergency departments/rooms. This chapter reflects on the issues associated with *mainstreaming* and the attitudes of general health care professionals who may not perceive psychiatric/mental health patients as "sick".

Following Masters' argument regarding psychiatric care by non-mental health professionals, Chandler's chapter looks at sentencing convicted criminal offenders, where Canadian courts often receive forensic psychiatric testimony from the prosecution and defense about the prospects for rehabilitating the offender. The courts do not, however, specify the treatments in their disposition orders. Instead, they commonly order an offender to follow the treatment recommended by their physicians. Thereafter, the courts have essentially no knowledge or oversight of what treatment is recommended and applied. This makes sense given judicial lack of medical expertise, as well as the remoteness of judges from issues of resource availability and the evolution over time of an offender's condition. However, the splitting of the roles allows physicians and judges to avoid discomforting questions about the coercive aspects of the system. The courts do not order specific treatments, and so are unaware of the concrete results of their orders. Physicians are not responsible for the legal coercion that may drive an offender's consent to the treatments they recommend, and so may regard that coercion as part of the context within which the offender must make his or her own "autonomous" decision. It is hard to know whether doctors are being turned into an arm of the state in its programs of social control or the courts are being turned into an arm of a paternalistic medical enterprise. Indeed, "biopolitics" predicts this pattern in suggesting that power will be dispersed and pervasive such that no one institution controls the other or can be said to be responsible. Instead, they work together in a web of interconnected ideas and practices.

From Rachel Liebert follows the intriguing and cutting-edge Chapter 12. Liebert reports that in November 2012, Adam Lanza walked into Sandy Hook Elementary School in Connecticut, USA, and shot 27 people. Described on National Public Radio as "to schools like 9/11 was to airports", this shooting has triggered another call for increased surveillance and security within schools. And following a long (contested, and politically convenient) tradition of making individuals' psyches accountable for violence, psychiatric diagnoses and interventions have become central to these practices. The ghosts of Sandy Hook have materialized into the Obama administration pushing a large-scale package of reforms to identify and intervene on people "at-risk" of madness. This attention resonates with the December call by Dr Oz on CNN's Piers Morgan Tonight Show that "We need a Homeland Security approach to mental illness". In her chapter, Liebert examines these burgeoning borderlands of psychiatry and security by critically mapping the knowledge(s), practices, and bodies moving through intensifying efforts to "capture" the risk of becoming mad. Drawing predominantly on critical race and critical security studies – the legacies of Franz Fanon and Michel Foucault – she traces the affective and discursive logic of this movement as it spirals through uneasy social imaginaries of responsibility, Otherness, insecurity, and protest. She pays particular attention to the tendency for risk to be ricocheted into the "irrational" flesh of we who are brown, black, poor, queer, and/or "alien", despite that violence – whether school shootings, colonization, "domestic" violence, or corporate brutality – typically emerges from maelstroms of privilege and rationality. Her analysis more broadly explores how, and with what implications for whom, psychiatric diagnoses circulate with/in the politics of discipline and terror that have come to dominate the post-9/11 U.S. context, and in turn, why and how we might resist and reimagine a "Homeland security approach to mental illness".

A new security approach for suicidal persons is what Cutcliffe and Riahi discuss in Chapter 13. According to them, even the most cursory review of the relevant literature will indicate that Mental Health (MH) nurses have a long history of providing care to suicidal people. This may not be entirely surprising given that, for many, there is an almost automatic conflation of suicide with (or as a) mental health problem(s). Yet, if one holds in abeyance preconceived and taken for granted "truths" about suicide and "madness", then an argument can be constructed that posits much of contemporary mental health care for suicidal people as "Snake Oil" salesmanship. Once we begin to deconstruct alleged isomorphic relationships between suicide and mental health problems (most commonly "depression"), then the corresponding so-called treatment and practices can be viewed as the proverbial "House of Cards". Accordingly, this chapter focuses on several areas/issues of care of the suicidal person, and in so doing, critiques the extant literature, such as it is. This critique shows that there is a disconcerting lack of empirically induced evidence to guide or support much of our contemporary care for suicidal people. It illustrates the counter-intuitive nature of and often unquestioning adherence to antiquated, ill-thought out ideas about how best to help suicidal people. Given that we are now operating in the epoch of "evidence-based" (or evidence-informed) care and have embraced and endorsed a "recovery-focused" national mental health policy position, this chapter argues that it is disingenuous at best to camouflage containment-driven, defensive practices for "treating" suicidal people as either "recovery-focused" or "evidence-based" and that a radical re-think in our practice is long overdue.

In Chapter 14, David Mercer draws on discursive and ethnographic data from a research project that explored the language of mental health nurses and detained patients in relation to "talk" about the treatment of sexual offenders in one forensic hospital. In contrast to a body of literature that understands the fashionable status of "relapse prevention" in terms of risk management and assessment as a pseudo-scientific enterprise and measurement tool, the content adopts a critical analysis of collusive relations that defined patient-professional interactions at the subterranean level of a high-security organizational structure. Drawing on the intellectual contribution of Goffman, Szasz and Foucault, attention is given to the micro-power relations, struggles, and resistance strategies that characterize everyday relations within *carceral* institutions – settings where the inmate is "hostage to therapy". The function of modularized SOT programmes are discussed as a symbolic ritual in the process of gaining self-knowledge and presenting particular versions of the self through acts of contrition and confession. Here, engagement is as much a part of the disciplinary and institutional apparatus of detention as are high walls, barred windows, and locked doors, where treatment is a "game" and adherence is the "rule". Forensic psychiatric nurses take on an evangelical role in promoting and policing patient attendance at group therapy sessions, while sharing a dismissive discourse about maintaining control in the hospital and manufacturing a marketable commodity for less secure services.

In Chapter 15 comes an analysis of psychiatric practice under the Nazi regime 1933–1945. According to Foth, psychiatric practice was characterized by the interplay of different technologies that aimed to influence patients' conduct. Nurses, as the delegated representatives of psychiatrists' power, were strategically positioned to govern patients' behaviours using a broad range of political technologies. An in-depth qualitative analysis of medical records gathered at a famous Hamburg asylum highlights the different shock therapies in use and shows that these therapies were primarily deployed for disciplinary purposes in order to correct "bad" behaviours. These forms of treatment also led to patients' deaths. This chapter aims at discussing the results of this historical analysis based in Germany in light of international discussions regarding shock therapies during WW2.

In Chapter 16, David Jacobs, a respected clinician, reports that a symptoms-only approach to mental health problems, although consistent with medical reasoning, ignores *background* and is thus blind to adversity and to the false positive problem. He argues that recognizing the reality of adversity, which can only be ascertained via dialogue and which ineradicably includes first-person subjective components, cannot be assimilated to either medicine or science. Indeed the psychiatrist-patient encounter, in contrast to the physician-patient encounter, is nothing *but* social interaction, dialogue, and interpretation. The difference is so obvious and dramatic that it is hard to see how the claim that the psychiatrist-patient encounter is a *medical* encounter can be presented seriously. Recognizing the reality of adversity shifts the subject matter from medicine and science to something else entirely – from *Naturwissenshaten* to *Geisteswissenshaten.* He states that the APA's paradigm shift at the end of the 1970s should be understood sociologically, i.e., in terms of the profession's adaptation to external threats and demands that were too powerful to ignore. He concludes by arguing that it is barely possible that the *DSM-5* Task Force's insistence on applying medical reasoning to all aspects of a person's life may have created a backlash among the non-medical mental health professions that could bear on the APA's exclusive ownership of official diagnosis in America.

To conclude the collection, Fedoroff and Knack also criticize forms of assistance, if any, that sex offenders (SOs) are able to receive in correctional settings. In Chapter 18 they argue that controversies concerning the treatability of SOs have arisen because of mistaken beliefs about the causes of sex offenses and the failure to approach SOs from treatment perspectives that match their specific needs. One of the most important areas of controversy is whether incarceration assists or impedes therapy and management. Although some research has found that correctional treatments can lead to a reduction in recidivism, there are multiple ethical and practical issues concerning treatment provided to SOs while in custody. Similar issues arise concerning imposed monitoring via conditions and registries. The chapter focuses on providing a critical analysis of the clinical and ethical issues involved in providing treatment for SOs in community versus correctional (psychiatric) settings. The effectiveness of correctional versus community and mandated versus non-mandated treatments is also examined. A brief discussion of the various treatments and treatment programs that are currently used with SOs and how these have evolved from the types of treatment originally used with this population is included. Comparisons are made between Canada's Dangerous Offender legislation and the Sexually Violent Predator laws in the United States and how these laws relate to treatment.

This rich collection of courageous essays constitutes a radical analysis of the psychiatric apparatus. Critical analyses like the ones presented in this collection provide important insights into how power and psychiatry intersect. Using a wide range of radical perspectives, which are mainly influenced by social sciences theories, allows analyses of discourses, texts, and practices within social relations, and thus our hope is to expose the psychiatric apparatus and produce a more nuanced account of the complexities of psychiatric power in the fabric of society. Such forms of analysis lead to explorations of the world of psychiatry and mental health care and speak to the social structures and discourses that make psychiatry what it is today.

References

Beuscart, J.-S. and Peerbaye, A. 2006. Histoires de dispositifs. *Terrains et travaux*, *11*, 3–15.

Breggin, P. 2006. Politics, practice and breaking news. *Ethical Human Psychology and Psychiatry*, *8*(1), 3–6.

Breggin, P. 2003. Psychopharmacology and human values. *Journal of Humanistic Psychology*, *43*, 34–49.

Caine, E.D. 2003. Determining causation in psychiatry. In K.A. Philips, M.B. First, and H.A. Pincus (Eds). *Advancing DSM. Dilemmas in Psychiatric Diagnosis*. Washington: American Psychiatric Association, 1–22.

Canguilhem, G. 1962. *Le normal et le pathologique*. Paris: Presses Universitaires de France.

Castel, R. 1976. *L'ordre psychiatrique*. Paris: Éditions de Minuit.

Castel, R. 1991. From dangerousness to risk. In G. Burchell, C. Gordon, and P. Miller (Eds). *The Foucault Effect*. Chicago: The University of Chicago Press.

Castel, R., Castel, F., and Lovell, A. 1982. *The Psychiatric Society*. New York: Columbia University Press.

Cosgrove L., Krimsky S., Vijayaraghavan, M., and Schneider, L. 2006. Financial ties between DSM-IV panel members and the pharmaceutical industry. *Psychotherapy and Psychosomatics*, *75*(3), 154–160.

Curra, J. 2000. *The Relativity of Deviance*. Thousand Oaks: Sage Publications.

Diekema, D.S. 2003. Involuntary sterilization of persons with mental retardation: An ethical analysis. *Mental Retardation and Developmental Disabilities Research Reviews*, *9*(1), 21–26.

Donzelot, Js. 1979. *The Policing of Families*. New York: Pantheon Books.

Dreyfus, H. and Rabinow, P. 1984. *Michel Foucault : un parcours philosophique*. Paris: Editions Gallimard.

Federman, C., Jacob, JD., and Holmes, D. 2009. Deconstructing the psychopath. A critical discursive analysis. *Cultural* Critique, *72*, 36–65.

First, M.B. and Tasman, A. 2004. *DSM-IV-TR. Mental Disorders: Diagnostic, Etiology, and Treatment*. Chichester: Wiley.

Foucault, M. 1980. The confession of the flesh. In C. Gordon (Ed.). *Power/Knowledge: Selected Interviews and Other Writings*. New York: Pantheon Books, 194–228.

Foucault, M. 1995. *Discipline & Punish*. New York: Vintage books.

Foucault, M. 2006. *Madness and Civilization*. New York: Random House.

Fraser, N. 1989. *Unruly Practices. Power, Discourse and Gender in Contemporary Social Theory*. Minneapolis: University of Minnesota Press.

Garrido, F. and Cayley, C.B. 1876. *A History of Political and Religious Persecutions*. Nabu Press : Charleston.

Gauchet, M. and Swain, G. 1980. *La pratique de l'esprit humain*. Paris: Gallimard.

Geller, J.L. and Harris, M. 1994. *Women of the Asylum: Voices from Behind the Walls, 1840–1945*. New York: Doubleday.

Goffman, E. 1998. *Asiles. Études sur la condition sociale des maladies mentaux*. Paris: Éditions de Minuit.

Gosden, R. 1997. The medicalisation of deviance. *Social Alternatives*, *16*(2), 58–60.

Holmes, D. 2005. Governing the captives: Forensic psychiatric nursing in corrections. *Perspectives in Psychiatric Care*, *41*(1), 3–13.

Holmes, D. and Murray, S. 2011. Civilizing the barbarian: A critical analysis of behaviour modification programs in forensic psychiatric settings. *Journal of Nursing Management*, *19*(3), 293–301.

Iredale, R. 2000. Eugenics and its relevance to contemporary health care. *Nursing Ethics*, *7*, 205–214.

Jacob, JD. and Holmes, D. 2011. Working under threat: Fear and nurse-patient interactions in a forensic psychiatric setting. *Journal of Forensic Nursing*, *7*(2), 68–77.

Kaplan, H.I. and Sadock, B.J. 1995. *Comprehensive Textbook of Psychiatry*. Baltimore: Williams & Wilkins.

Kirk, S.A. and Kutchins, H. 1992. *The Selling of DSM. The Rhetoric of Science in Psychiatry*. Hawthorne: Aldine de Gruyter.

Kutchins, H. and Kirk, S.A. 1997. *Making Us Crazy*. New York: The Free Press.

Lachter, B. 2001. "Chemical Imbalance": A clinical non sequitur. *Psychiatric Language*, *9*(4), 311–315.

Lankes, G. 1970. How should we educate the police? *The Journal of Criminal Law, Criminology, and Police Science*, *61*(4), 587–592.

Laplante, J. 1997. *Libérer le traitement*. Article non-publié. Communication personnelle.

Lee, E. 2006. Medicalizing motherhood. *Social Science and Modern Society*, *43*(6), 47–50.

Lupton, D. 1999. *Risk*. London: Routledge.

MacDonald, C.F. 1914. Presidential address. *American Journal of Insanity*, *7*, 1–12.

MacLennan, D. 1987. Beyond the asylum: Professionalization and the mental hygiene movement in Canada, 1914–1928. *Canadian Bulletin of Medical History*, *4*, 7–23.

Mason, G. 1999. *The Spectacle of Violence. Homophobia, Gender and Knowledge*. London: Routledge.

Mayes, R. and Horwitz, A.V. 2005. DSM-III and the revolution in the classification of mental-illness. *Journal of History of the Behavioral Sciences*, *41*(3), 249–267.

Mendelson, G. 2003. Homosexuality and psychiatric nosology. *Australian and New Zealand Journal of Psychiatry*, *37*, 678–683.

McDonald, F. 1990. A comment. *The Journal of Politics*, *42*(2), 31–35.

Moncrieff, J., Hopker, S. and Thomas, P. 2005. Psychiatry and the pharmaceutical industry: Who pays the piper? *Psychiatric Bulletin*, *29*, 84–85.

Mulvey, E.P. Geller, J.L. and Roth, L.H. 1987. The promise and perils of involuntary outpatient commitment. *American Psychologist*, *42*, 571–84.

Perron, A., Rudge, T. and Holmes, D. 2010. Citizen minds, citizen bodies: The citizenship experience and the government of mentally ill persons. *Nursing Philosophy*, *11*, 100–111.

Perron, A. and Holmes, D. 2011. Constructing mentally ill inmates: Nurses' discursive practices in corrections. *Nursing Inquiry*, *18*(3), 191–204.

Raffnsøe, S. 2008. Qu'est-ce qu'un dispositif? L'analytique sociale de Michel Foucault, *Symposium (Canadian Journal of Continental Philosophy / Revue canadienne de philosophie continentale)*, *12*(1), Article 5. Retrieved online September 20th 2012 from http://ir.lib.uwo.ca/symposium/vol12/iss1/5.

Russ, J. 1979. *Histoire de la Folie/Michel Foucault*. Paris: Éditions Hatier.

Schmidt, N.B., Kotov, R., and Joiner, T.E. 2004. *Taxometrics*. Washington: American Psychological Association.

Simpson, E.L. and House, A.O. 2002. Involving users in the delivery and evaluation of mental health services: Systematic review. *British Medical Journal*, *325*, 1–5.

Szasz, T. 2003. Psychiatry and the control of dangerousness: On the apotropaic function of the term "mental illness". *Journal of Medical Ethics*, *29*, 227–230.

Waller, J. 2002. The illusion of an explanation: The concept of hereditary disease, 1770–1870. *Journal of the History of Medicine and Allied Sciences*, *57*(4), 410–448.

Wilson, M. 1993. DSM-III and the transformation of American psychiatry: A history. *American Journal of Psychiatry*, *150*, 399–410.

Wilson, M. and Guze, S.B. 1995. The neo-Kraepelinian revolution in psychiatric diagnosis. *European Archives of Psychiatry and Clinical Neuroscience*, *245*, 196–201.

Watts, J. and Priebe, S. 2002. A phenomenological account of users' experiences of assertive community treatment. *Bioethics*, *16*(5), 439–454.

PART I
Repression

Chapter 1
Varieties of Psychiatric Criticism[1]

Thomas Szasz

> The American people have always been anxious to know what they shall do with us. … I have had but one answer from the beginning. Do nothing with us! Your doing with us has already played the mischief with us. … All I ask is, give him a chance to stand on his own legs! Let him alone! … What I ask for the Negro is not benevolence, not pity, not sympathy, but simply justice. (Frederick Douglass 1865)[2]

Introduction

In the eighteenth century, Americans considered the right to liberty – called "unalienable" in the Declaration of Independence – one of their most important moral values and legal protections from despotism. Today, they consider the psychiatrist's right to protect them from being dangerous to themselves (or others) – called civil commitment – one their most important medical values and legal protections from their hard-earned liberties. Incarceration of law-abiding individuals in an insane asylum – ostensibly a form of preventive and therapeutic medical practice – constitutes the backbone of psychiatry.[3] Abolishing psychiatric coercion and the threat of such coercion would spell the end of psychiatry as we have known it in the past and know it today.

Carl Wernicke (1848–1905) – a founder of modern neuropsychiatry – correctly noted that "the medical treatment of [mental] patients begins with the infringement of their personal freedom. … By virtue of his carceral authority, the psychiatrist had become the true guarantor of individual rights and the rule of law" (Engstrom 2003: 251, citing Wernicke 1889). The first task of the psychiatric critic

1 From Szasz, T. (2012). Varieties of Psychiatric Criticism, *History of Psychiatry, vol. 23(3)*, 349–355 Copyright 2012, with permission from Rightslink (Sage).

2 Douglass F (1865) "What the black man wants". Address at the Annual Meeting of the Massachusetts Anti-Slavery Society, Boston, April 1865, delivered within days of the close of the Civil War and the assassination of President Abraham Lincoln. Retrieved (12 Nov. 2011) from: http://www.frederickdouglass.org/speeches/index.html

3 The term "psychiatry" (*Psychiatrie*) was coined in 1808 by the German physician Christian Johann Reil (1759–1813); see Marneros A and Pillmann F (2005) *Das Wort Psychiatrie ... wurde in Halle geboren*. Stuttgart: Schattauer.

worth his salt is to repudiate this psychiatrized politics: he must oppose the use of psychiatric force and fraud, reject the idea of mental illness, eschew psychiatric language and condemn its journalistic and professional use. Most psychiatric critics, past and present, fail miserably to pass this elementary test. Or, more precisely, they regard the principle as benevolent and support the therapeutic state.

By the eighteenth century, the western Zeitgeist had fully embraced the view that madness is a malady properly treated by the incarceration of the mad person in a mad-house managed by a mad- doctor. The belief that the individual identified as "mentally ill and dangerous to himself or others" is justly deprived of liberty is now accepted as not merely lawful but scientific, and dissent is dismissed as "unscientific" and "irrational". Mental health codes form an integral part of the legal systems of all modern nations and of the United Nations. These social developments have had far-reaching consequences, among them the popular and political acceptance of a medicalized- psychiatrized vocabulary.

Because the management of persons identified as "mental patients" is synonymous with their legal control by psychiatrists, objections against the practice arose even before psychiatry was so called. Ironically, the history of psychiatry is thus synonymous not only with the medical justification of psychiatric coercion but also with the criticism of such coercion.

In 1818, in his trend-setting *Lehrbuch der Störungen des Seelenlebens ...* (Textbook of Disturbances of Mental Life, or Disturbances of the Soul and their Treatment), the German physician, Johann Christian Heinroth (1773–1843), explained:

> The complete concept of mental disturbances includes permanent loss of freedom or loss of reason ... which manifests itself as a diseased condition, and which comprises the domains of temperament, diseases of the spirit, and will. ... All these diseases, however much as their external manifestations may differ, have this one feature in common, namely, that not only is there no freedom but not even the capacity to regain freedom ... Thus, individuals in this condition exist no longer in the human domain, which is the domain of freedom, but follow the coercion of internal and external natural necessity. Rather than resembling animals, which are led by a wholesome instinct, they resemble machines. (Heinroth 1818/1975: 21–25)

This idea is as popular today as it was 200 years ago. Michael S. Moore, Professor of Law and Philosophy at the University of San Diego, asserts: "[Mental patients] resemble infants, wild beasts, plants, and stones – none of which are responsible because of the absence of any assumption of rationality". (Moore 1975: 1495).

Eventually, people began to recognize that the mad-doctor's power to deprive innocent persons of liberty poses a threat to everyone's freedom. In late nineteenth-century Germany, the fear of so-called "false commitment" – sane persons being "incorrectly" diagnosed and detained as insane – generated a growing revolt against the practice of involuntary mental hospitalization. The psychiatric profession quickly nipped this opposition in the bud, dismissing it as "*Antipsychiatrie*" ("antipsychiatry") in 1908. A half-century later, a small group of British would-be psychiatric reformers adopted this term as the linguistic emblem of their pseudo-liberatory movement (Szasz 2009).

Viewing the person controlled by his passions rather than his reason as unfree is a classic Graeco-Roman idea. Heinroth used this attribution to define madness: "The man who is fettered by passions deceives himself about external objects and about himself. *This illusion, and the con- sequent error, is called madness*. … In madness the spirit is fettered and man, just as in passion (both being indissolubly linked), is unfree and unhappy". (Heinroth 1818/1975: 16, emphasis added). The early alienists thus conflated psychiatrically imputed loss of internal liberty with legally imposed deprivation of political liberty. Yielding to sexual, pharmacological or monetary temptation is radically different from being deprived of liberty by the action of a human agent, such as a judge, jailer or psychiatrist. A stroke deprives the subject of freedom. But such a person is not, properly speaking, "deprived of political liberty". Nor is he incarcerated by a physician. As mental illness is a metaphorical illness, so the unfreedom attributed to the mental patient is a metaphorical loss of freedom. It becomes a literal loss of freedom only as a result of the actions of psychiatrists (and judges and their deputies).

Heinroth's assertion that the insane lack freedom – "individuals in this condition exist no longer in the human domain, which is the domain of freedom" – is a strategic claim, not a description or an observation. Because the patient is unfree, the psychiatrist is justified in coercing him: medical control is treatment, psychiatric oppression is liberation. For patients for whom there is hope for recovery, Heinroth (1818/1975, Vol. 1: 25) recommended:

> What is needed in such cases is constraint, which is in no way cruelty or inhumanity, but necessary for the reeducation of such patients to the norm of reason. … For as long as such and similar patients have their will, nothing can be done with them. … They [mental disturbances] all have a common starting point, a main principle to which they are subordinated: selfishness.

In contrast, "The doctor of the soul (or psyche) … has overcome selfish interests and treats for purely humanitarian reasons. He influences the patient by virtue of his, one may be permitted to say, holy presence, by the sheer strength of his being, his glance, and his will". (1818/1975: 332). The secret of curing mental illness lies in dominating the patient: "First, be master of the situation; second, be master of the patient. … Unless this superiority is established, all treatment will be in vain" (1818/1975: 332).

Having justified torture as treatment, Heinroth proclaimed the medical profession's monopolistic control over the study and treatment of mental illness: "Since we are speaking of medical art and science, we should think that nobody but a doctor should have a right to make mental disturbance the object of his studies and treatment … It is the duty of the state to care for mentally disturbed persons whenever they are a burden to the community or present a public danger" (1818/1975, Vol. 1: 332). In France similar ideas were advanced by the Jacobins. Pinel's *magnum opus, Traité médico-philosophique sur l'aliénation mentale ou la manie*, was published in 1801 and quickly became enormously influential in both Europe and the USA. In the 1806 English translation, *A Treatise on Insanity, in which are Contained the Principles of a New and More Practical Nosology of Maniacal Disorders than has yet been Offered to the Public, etc.*, we read:

> If [the madman is] met, however, by a force evidently and convincingly superior, he submits without opposition or violence. ... In the preceding cases of insanity, we trace the happy effects of intimidation, without severity; of oppression, without violence. ... For this purpose the strait-waistcoat will generally be found amply sufficient. ... To effect and expedite a permanent cure, *unlimited power* in the choice and adoption of curative measures were given to his medical attendant. (Pinel 1806/1962: 27–60–69; emphasis added)

Ostensibly, the Jacobins revolted against Louis XVI's unlimited political power. In fact, they transferred their trust from royalty blessed by God to medicine blessed by science. Pinel and the Jacobins advocated that society entrust mad-doctors and their attendants with unlimited power, succeeding in the process in transforming psychiatric totalitarianism into curative treatment animated by "living beneficence". Nothing illustrates the central role of coercion in the practice of psychiatry more dramatically than the historical sanctification of Pinel as the "liberator" of the madman.

In the USA, the "credit" for creating the state mental hospital system belongs to Dorothea Lynde Dix (1802–1887). A poor woman trained as a school-teacher, she became a zealous social reformer whose passions meshed with the temper of her times. Growing in numbers and becoming more urbanized, American families and communities wanted to get their troublesome members out of sight and out of mind. Dix offered to satisfy their need: she soothed them with the fiction that her proposed psychiatric plantations would make the slaves healthy and happy (Szasz 1961, 1970, 2009). Ever since, the more self-righteously psychiatric reformers liberated the mental patients, the more firmly enslaved they became. Replacing chains with total institutions was merely a first step in a seemingly endless process of enslavements, culminating in the self-enslavement of today's so-called "service users", "voice hearers" and miscellaneous mental patients on the dole demanding free "professional services" from the very professionals they identify as their victimizers.

From 1945 to the Present

I will skip over the long list of psychiatric liberator-oppressors to consider briefly the post-World War II scene. In the late 1960s, a group of psychiatrists in Britain, led by Ronald D. Laing (1927–1989), began to oppose traditional mental hospital practices and sought to replace them with their own version of asylum care, epitomized by Kingsley Hall. In his autobiography, *Wisdom, Madness and Folly*, Laing defended psychiatric slavery as the natural order of modern society:

> Mental hospitals and psychiatric units admit, routinely, every day of the week, people who are sent "in" for non-criminal conduct, but for conduct which their nearest and dearest relatives, friends, colleagues and neighbours find insufferable. … it is our only way to keep people out of the company that can't stand them. … To say that a locked ward functions as a prison for non-criminal transgressors is not to say it should not be so. Our society may continue to "need" some such prisons for unacceptable persons. As our society functions at present such places are indispensable. This is not the fault of psychiatrists, not necessarily the fault of anyone. (Laing 1985: 5–6)

In 1999 a collection of British psychiatrists organized a group they called the Critical Psychiatry Network (CPN), dedicated to challenging "the stranglehold of a biomedical approach within the psychiatric profession" (Double n.d.). I thought I had done that challenging, and more, a long time ago (Szasz 1961). Not according to Duncan Double, an NHS consultant psychiatrist and one of the leaders of the Network: "Szasz goes too far, to my mind, in arguing that society can manage without any mental health law". (Double n.d.). For thousands of years societies had managed without such laws.

Double (2002) seeks to liberate psychiatry from its anatomical-medical bonds and make it a more explicitly political form of social control:

> Critical psychiatry sees itself as an advance over anti-psychiatry in the sense that it accepts the social role of psychiatric practice. … For example, the Critical Psychiatry Network's concern about the government's proposals for reform of the Mental Health Act are based on ethical reasons and linked to its critique of the explanatory model of mental illness, not a rejection of the need for the Mental Health Act itself. In essence, critical psychiatry argues that psychiatric practice does not have to justify itself by postulating brain pathology as the basis for mental illness.

Pat Bracken, an NHS consultant psychiatrist-CPN leader, and Philip Thomas, a psychiatrist- philosopher, state:

> We are particularly concerned with the implications of critical psychiatry for us as medical practitioners. … [W]e question whether such binary thinking [as Szasz's] is adequate to the lived reality of struggling and suffering human beings. … It is possible to imagine forms of political organization that are not state bureaucracies … such a development would require a move to

> "postpsychiatry". … This would be to move in the opposite direction to Szasz. (Bracken and Thomas 2010)

Members of the CPN, like their American counterparts, criticize the proliferation of psychiatric diagnoses and "excessive" use of psychotropic drugs, but embrace psychiatric coercions. To be sure, opposing the use of psychiatric force – even to the minimal extent of insisting on a clear economic-legal-political separation between private-voluntary and public-involuntary psychiatric interventions – would have incalculable consequences on the lives of mental health professionals as well as on everyone else's. Instead, so-called critics support established psychiatric authority and single out one or another aspect of mental health practice for "reform".

The CPN's position is not psychiatric criticism, it is a plea for prettifying the psychiatric plantations. Psychiatrists either have the right to forcibly molest persons they call "patients" by calling it "medical treatment" or do not have such a right. As long as the psychiatrist is legally empowered to place his own personal interests and professional opinions ahead of those of the coerced citizen, regardless of "safeguards" the "patient" remains powerless vis-à-vis political-psychiatric despotism. In 2007 the UK Government established:

> a shadowy new national anti-terrorist unit to protect VIPs, with the power to detain suspects indefinitely using mental health laws. … The team's psychiatrists and psychologists then have the power to order treatment – including forcibly detaining suspects in secure psychiatric units. Using these powers, the unit can legally detain people for an indefinite period without trial, criminal charges or even evidence of a crime being committed … NHS documents obtained by *The Mail on Sunday* reveal the unit's role "concerns the identification and diversion into psychiatric care of mentally ill people fixated on the prominent". … The centre, which is based at a secret Central London location, has a staff of four police officers, two civilian researchers, a forensic psychiatrist, a forensic psychologist and a forensic community mental health nurse. … Research led to FTAC [the Fixated Threat Assessment Centre] being set up with a £500,000-a-year budget from the Home Office and Department of Health. NHS documents say: "It is a prototype for future joint services". (Anonymous 2007)

At the same time, unlike establishment psychiatrists in the USA, Susan Welsh and Martin P. Deahl, both respected psychiatrists in the UK, emphasize in the pages of *The Lancet* that, "Such power over individuals and its consequent restriction of freedom ("one person cannot coerce another unless he has power over him" [citing Szasz 1987]) will always distinguish psychiatry from other medical specialties". (Welsh and Deahl 2002).

The livelihood of critical psychiatrists and psychologists in Britain depends on the financial support of the National Health Service. Who pays whom for what?

The Contemporary Scene in the USA

What about contemporary American "critical psychiatry"? American objections to mad-doctoring range widely, from old-fashioned protests against false commitment, especially in cases of insanity acquittees, to new-fashioned propaganda for unorthodox chemical-medical treatments, ranging from the practices of so-called orthomolecular psychiatrists to the practices of antipsychiatrists, and a plethora of other so-called "ethical", "empathic", "existential", "cognitive" and other "psychotherapies" (Szasz 2007).

All these quacks claim to treat mental diseases whose existence they acknowledge or deny as suits their economic interests. Some assert that the patients are not ill, just different. Others reject the role of psychiatric critic, call themselves "reformers" and testify under oath in both civil and criminal prosecutions that mental illnesses are caused by psychotropic drugs and exonerate the drug-taker of criminal responsibility for his offences. Others, evasive about what if anything is "wrong" with mental patients, resort to self-promotion by name-calling: competitors' practices are "unethical" and "toxic", their own practices are "ethical" and "therapeutic". None of these parasites of the public psychiatric system support themselves by serving the needs of private persons willing to pay for private help to cope better with their private personal problems.

From a contractarian-libertarian point of view, all contemporary psychiatric criticisms are misdirected. If a person is law-abiding, he and he alone should have the authority and power over his relations with others: no one should be able to do anything for or to him without his consent. Even if the subject has been convicted of lawbreaking, the authorities are not thereby justified in "treating" him against his will for an alleged (non-contagious) illness, a punishment judges nowadays routinely authorize and impose.

Conventional and critical psychiatrists alike rely on state agencies to validate the "therapeutic benefits" of their interventions. Psychiatric critics make a fatal mistake playing doctor, trusting the coercive power of the totalitarian-therapeutic state rather than peaceful contract with clients to define which psychiatric practices to permit and which to prohibit. Unfortunately, most mental health professionals approach their work imbued with the deeply ingrained left-socialist disposition characteristic of the professional aids worker. Not satisfied with helping his beneficiary help himself, as the beneficiary defines help, the self-appointed benefactor seeks to enlighten his ward, forcibly if necessary, to choose the "right" path. With respect to such practices as the use of drugs, electroconvulsive therapy and surgery, the advocate – ostensibly an "investigator" or "researcher", but in effect a prohibitionist – seeks the help of the state to make the practices he loathes illegal. The result is the criminalization of various psychiatric acts between consenting adults.

The historical evidence compels us to conclude that, after more than 200 years of psychiatric criticism, we have made no progress in unshackling the psychiatric slave from his psychiatric master. So-called psychiatric critics are largely responsible for this situation: instead of focusing on the timeless task of enlarging the sphere of human liberty by seeking the abolition of psychiatric slavery, they choose to pursue fleeting popularity by the self-righteous denunciation of one or another psychiatric treatment of a non-disease, and/or converting inpatient insane asylum slavery into outpatient medical disability-dependency.

Let us not fool ourselves. Mental patients and mental health practitioners are more securely attached to the coercive apparatus of the therapeutic state than they have ever been. And let us not lose sight of the falsehoods psychiatric leaders tell politicians, the press and their fellow psychiatrists. Thomas Insel, MD, Director of the National Institute of Mental Health, explains:

> It's time to fundamentally rethink mental illness. ... Psychiatric research today promises to produce a true science of the brain ... Mental disorders are brain disorders. ... What is emerging today is a picture of mental illness as the result of a pathophysiological chain from genes to cells to distributive systems within the brain, based on a patient's unique genetic variation. ... With a true science of mental illness – from genes, to cells, to brain circuits, to behavior – psychiatrists will be able to better predict who is likely to develop a mental disorder and to intervene earlier. Once that happens, we will be in a different world. (Moran 2011)

Armed with "a true science of mental illness", the scientific psychiatrist "intervenes early". He possesses power and imposes "help". If we are serious in our opposition to psychiatric slavery, our goal must be to dispossess the despot of his power. This is not mere theorizing. In the 1970s, we witnessed gay Americans doing just that.

The psychiatric critic's primary duty is, and has always been, to reject the legal-political legitimacy of the use of psychiatric force and fraud. Employed as "mental health professionals" or coopted as "mental health users", psychiatric slaves have been unwilling to bite the hand that feeds them: they have failed, and continue to fail, to renounce and denounce psychiatric despotism.

The diverse problems that occupy the attention of psychiatric critics originate from a single source: psychiatric power. As long as so-called psychiatric services may be imposed on individuals against their will, efforts to "reform" psychiatry distract from what must be our task, the abolition of every kind of involuntary psychiatric intervention. Being inseparable from coercion, psychiatry cannot be reformed. It must be abolished.

Paraphrasing Douglass, quoted at the start, what I ask and have always asked for the "mental patient" (as if "he" were a valid abstraction or category) is not benevolence, not pity, not sympathy, assuredly not better or more "psychiatric services", but simply justice.

References

Anonymous. 2007. Revealed: Blair's secret stalker squad. *London Evening Standard* (27 May 27). [Online], Available at: http://www.thisislondon.co.uk/news/article-23398188-details/Blair's+secret+stalker+squad/ article.do. [accessed: 12 November 2011].

Bracken, P. and Thomas, P. 2010 From Szasz to Foucault: On the role of critical psychiatry. *Philosophy, Psychiatry & Psychology*, *17*(Sep.), 219–228.

Double, D. n.d. The acceptable limits of psychiatry. [Online], Available at: http://www.soteria. freeuk.com/176_26-27.pdf. [accessed: 12 November 2011].

Double, D. 2002. Education and debate: the limits of psychiatry. *British Medical Journal* [Online], 324 (13), 900–904. Available at: http://www.bmj.com/content/324/7342/900 [accessed 12 November 2011].

Engstrom, E.J. 2003. *Clinical Psychiatry in Imperial Germany: A History of Psychiatric Practice*. Ithaca, NY: Cornell University Press.

Heinroth, J.C. 1975. *Textbook of Disturbances of Mental Life, or Disturbances of the Soul and Their Treatment*, translated by J Schmorak, 2 vols. Baltimore: Johns Hopkins University Press; originally published in German in 1818.

Laing, R.D. 1985. *Wisdom, Madness, and Folly*. London: Macmillan.

Moore, M.S. 1975. Some myths about "mental illness". *Archives of General Psychiatry*, *32*, 1483–1497.

Moran, M. 2011. Brain, gene discoveries drive new concept of mental illness. *Psychiatric News*, *46* (17 June), 1.

Pinel, P. 1962. *A Treatise on Insanity*, translated by DD Davis [facsimile of 1806 edition]. New York: Hafner Publishing Company; originally published in French in 1801.

Szasz, T. 1961. *The Myth of Mental Illness: Foundations of a Theory of Personal Conduct*. Later Editions. New York: HarperCollins.

Szasz, T. 1970. *The Manufacture of Madness: A Comparative Study of the Inquisition and the Mental Health Movement*. New York: HarperCollins.

Szasz, T.S. 1987. *Insanity: The Idea and its Consequences*. New York: Wiley.

Szasz, T.S. 2002. *Liberation by Oppression: A Comparative Study of Slavery and Psychiatry*. New Brunswick, NJ: Transaction Publishers.

Szasz, T.S. 2007. *Coercion as Cure: A Critical History of Psychiatry*. New Brunswick, NJ: Transaction Publishers.

Szasz, T.S. 2009. *Antipsychiatry: Quackery Squared*. Syracuse: Syracuse University Press.

Welsh, S. and Deahl, M.P. 2002. Modern psychiatric ethics. *Lancet*, *359*, 253–255.

Wernicke, C. 1889. Zweck und Ziel der Psychiatrischen Kliniken. *Klinisches Jahrbuch*, *1*, 218–223.

Chapter 2

Censoring Violence: Censorship and Critical Research in Forensic Psychiatry

Dave Holmes and Stuart J. Murray

> The spectacle is essentially tautological, for the simple reason that its means and its ends are identical. It is the sun that never sets on the empire of modern passivity. (Debord [1967] 1995: 15)

Introduction

That representatives of "total" institutions (see Goffman 1998 for details) such as prisons and psychiatric hospitals often react violently is hardly surprising; their reactions exist simultaneously within the realms of the spectacle and the non-event, what Debord calls the "*materialization* of ideology" ([1967] 1995: 150). Approximately two years ago, one of our studies was the target of a virulent ideological attack not only on the credibility, but on the very existence, of both its data and analysis by two experienced researchers (Holmes and Murray 2011). Despite the fact that the editor of the scientific journal that published our findings had access to the entirety of our raw data and confirmed the wealth of information on which our analysis was based, representatives of a specific total institution, headed by an individual psychiatrist, attempted without success to minimize, indeed discredit, our critical analysis of a still widespread but scientifically obsolete psychiatric practice: behavior modification plans.

But why expend so much energy challenging our data, our analysis, and our choice of theoretical framework rather than engaging in a thorough and productive academic debate about a treatment method we consider simply anachronistic and ineffective, in addition to unethical? The answer to this question lies, in part, in the psychiatric-penal apparatus's inability to receive and respond appropriately to criticism, as well as in some of its representatives' capacity for unrestrained violence and, even more worrisome, in the disturbing and always possible association, however dangerous, between medicine and corrections (where one comes to the aid of the other), a connection that we had yet to encounter in 12 years of research and 25 years of clinical practice in forensic psychiatry in Canada and in France.

In order to silence us, our adversaries, for they cannot be considered colleagues, employed violent strategies ranging from the devious to the direct; every effort was made to censor the counter-discourse put forward. The violence of those in power, which we criticize in our text (Holmes and Murray 2011), is total, regardless of who dares challenge them: patients (subjected to behavior modification plans), personnel (required to follow behavior modification plans whether they believe in them or not), and researchers (subjected to false accusations concerning the existence of data and the quality of analysis). However, although our story made headlines in a highly conservative national newspaper, it is unlikely to be unusual enough to attract anyone else's interest—quite the opposite, in fact. The public is well aware of the correctional system's capacity for violence in the face of anyone who opposes it, at least in Canada.

In this chapter, we suggest that the phrase, "censoring violence," must be understood in two senses. First, there are those instances in which violence is more or less straightforwardly exercised by individual agents in the act of censoring, silencing, or actively discrediting opposing points of view. But alongside violence that censors through such repressive measures, a second form of violence is frequently at play. Violence of this sort is much less easy to discern because the agents of this violence are difficult—sometimes impossible—to identify. We qualify this second form of violence as structural, institutional, and essentially ideological violence. Its vectors of power and agency are diffuse; it is systemic and its hierarchies and chains of command are complex. Effectively, this second form of violence is committed by "no one," we might say; it is a "non-event" and it is "recommended" or it operates in the name of the complex system itself. It hides behind a public spectacle of care, justice, and the rule of law, permitting or even vindicating what is essentially abusive, unjust, and illegal. Individual agents—what we might once have called the subjects and objects of this violence—soon become instances, nodes, or switch-points in the operation of an anonymous apparatus. Total institutions function according to these inscrutable mechanisms: we might think here of the crimes committed in Abu Ghraib prison, the indefinite detention and treatment of detainees at Guantanamo Bay, or similarly, the fate of particular mental health patients treated in Canadian penal institutions. These are systems in which "nobody" acts and "nobody" appears to be responsible. Indeed, our ethical critique of behavior modification plans (Holmes and Murray 2011) sought to expose the violence of just such a system, and so the violent reaction that our discussion provoked is in some respects unsurprising and further evidences the kinds of systemic violence at play.

Prisons, Power, and Spectacle

Our general research program is concerned with the activities of nursing staff involved in the double duty of social control/nursing care, in ethical relationships with incarcerated psychiatric patients and institutional personnel, and, finally, in the prison setting and concrete organizations that constitute what is understood as "prison." We have always believed it important to describe and understand the mechanisms involved in practicing nursing in the forensic psychiatric context. We continue to believe that studying this phenomenon of interest is a fundamental step in understanding the daily experience of nurses working in forensic psychiatric settings (Murray and Holmes 2013). For Senior (1998), exploring and understanding this issue is of vital importance for all health professionals, "because of the nature of interpersonal interactions within a custodial setting" (p. 235).

According to Rostaing (1997), studies describing "prison culture" are now out of date and no longer offer an understanding of "prison society" as a whole. "Social relations" between prisoners and correctional personnel merit researchers' renewed attention. Such research would allow a better understanding of certain specific phenomena that are part of daily life in penal environments (whether by studying those who watch or those who are watched). The particular *carceral* relations between inmates and prison personnel are the product of a contradiction that exists between prison rule and the normal rules of the everyday, free civil society (Rostaing 1997) in which nursing is embedded (Holmes and Jacob 2012). Psychiatric nursing in correctional environments and its specific *carceral* relations must be situated within the contradictory framework defined by the prison's functions (custody, public protection, correction, discipline, control, security maintenance, successful social reintegration, etc.) and the socio-professional expectations of the nurses who work there (Holmes 2005, Holmes, Perron, Michaud, Montuclard, and Hervé 2005, Holmes, Perron, and Michaud 2007, Jacob and Holmes 2011, Perron and Holmes 2011, Holmes and Jacob 2012). It is therefore imperative to study this issue from macro and micro perspectives simultaneously in order to both examine psychiatric nursing practice in the prison setting while including this practice in the larger framework in which our contemporary societies' psychiatric and penal apparatus play a part.

The work of many researchers has shown that correctional environments produce the components necessary for the anatomo- and bio-political management of psychiatric patients, and that these correctional components clearly disrupt nursing practice. Years of research have produced a consensus stating that nursing practice is threatened not only by prison culture but also by the violence to which nurses are often subject.

Between 2006 and 2009, we conducted research with the expectation that, for nursing staff, being hired by a hospital rather than a prison would create enough distance to keep the experience of psychiatric nursing care somewhat intact, albeit with full knowledge of the extreme environment in which care would be provided. Instead, our results (2006–2009) show that behavior modification plans were implemented as a primary "therapeutic" approach despite research showing that forensic psychiatric settings should oppose, as much as possible, the inclusion in nursing practice of political technologies specific to the prison model (Holmes 2005, Mason and Mercer 1998). In fact, nurses' use of behavior modification plans only serves to exacerbate the paradoxical (double) mandates of nursing practice in a correctional environment (punishment/nursing care), with unsurprising consequences: feelings of estrangement and alienation, distancing from health care activities in favor of correctional activities, and a transformation in the representations of those under their care (amplification of delinquent characteristics). In short, the result is the integration of punitive elements into nursing practice and total cognitive dissonance relative to nursing work.

Despite the violence to which we ourselves have been subjected, the goal of our intervention (Holmes and Murray 2011) was and remains the exposure of unethical professional practices whose violence affects both patients and nurses. We believe that this violence affects nursing staff through the medical prescriptions that force them to incorporate into their practice activities whose effectiveness and legitimacy they openly question. Although all of our previous research reveals the polarization of care and incarceration in correctional psychiatry, the study in question (Holmes and Murray 2011) instead reveals a co-optation of (para) medical practices with correctional ones. For us, this is the context into which nursing staff are incorporated. Ethical considerations are required to counter this trend, and criticizing the use of behavior modification plans is one of the necessary steps in the process.

At the macro level, it is important to bear in mind the wider social, political, and institutional context within which our study took place and our research was accepted for publication on 20 October 2010. This will permit a better understanding of the ways the psychiatric-penal apparatus pre-emptively censors and discredits critical research, exercising a seemingly anonymous form of violence that is structural, institutional, and essentially ideological in nature. At the time of our study, Corrections Canada was managing a public relations disaster with the high-profile case of Ashley Smith, a 19-year-old woman who in 2007 strangled herself to death in her cell while correctional officers watched and filmed the event. Three front-line staff and one correctional manager were charged with criminal negligence causing death, but unsurprisingly, these charges were soon dropped. On 20 June 2008, Howard Sapers, the Correctional Investigator of Canada, published his report on Ashley Smith, entitled *A Preventable Death* (http://www.oci-bec.gc.ca/cnt/rpt/pdf/oth-aut/oth-aut20080620-eng.pdf). The 33-page report details the "inhumane" conditions of Ms Smith's custody and the systemic failures and abuses of Canada's correctional facilities, particularly vis-à-vis mentally ill prisoners and the medical care they receive. Among a long list of horrors, Ms Smith was "assaulted" by Correctional Services staff, subject to the inappropriate use of force (both chemical and physical), and denied her right to basic hygiene, such as toilet paper and sufficient sanitary products during her menstrual cycle. It also soon came to light that Ms Smith was transferred 17 times during custody, which effectively re-set the clock on her solitary confinement, bypassing strict legal limits for the length of time it can be used. "The attempts that were made to obtain a full psychological assessment were thwarted in part by the Correctional Service's decisions to constantly transfer Ms. Smith from one institution to another" (Sapers 2008: 6). Consequently, despite years in custody, much of it in seclusion, no full psychological assessment was completed and no comprehensive treatment plan was put into place. After a two-year legal battle with Corrections Canada, and two weeks after our article was accepted for publication, CBC's *The Fifth Estate* broadcast on 12 November 2010 a special investigative report on the life and death of Ashley Smith, entitled "Behind the Wall" (http://www.cbc.ca/fifth/2010–2011/behindthewall/). The documentary aired the shocking video of Ashley's Smith's death in its entirety as filmed by correctional officers. At the time of writing this chapter, the Coroner's Inquest into the death of Ashley Smith is still underway, but what has emerged is a system that is patently abusive, unjust, and illegal.

Amidst this public relations disaster and mounting public outrage, as if by coincidence, *The Globe and Mail* on 21 January 2011 published a "Photo Gallery" or photo essay containing seven images, with captions, called the "St. Lawrence Valley Correctional and Treatment Centre" (http://www.theglobeandmail.com/news/national/st-lawrence-valley-correctional-and-treatment-centre/article631320/). Flipping through these images and reading the captions is a lesson in what Guy Debord calls the "totalitarian bureaucracy" ([1967] 1995: 9) of the spectacle, an institutionally integrated, systemic, and systematic fantasy. Captions inform the reader that this prison "has none of the grim trappings normally associated with one" and that the facility is "ground-breaking" in its treatment of inmates with "mental problems." "Floors are carpeted and there is an abundance of natural light and soothing music. Most of the 100 'residents' saunter between their roomy cells and common areas." There are photographs of a smiling prison psychiatrist speaking with a patient in his room, artwork laid out on his bed. And there is an image of an inmate strumming a guitar on his bed.

A typical reader might not question this *mise-en-scène* or wonder whether it is a calculated response to all the bad press surrounding the Ashley Smith case. Nor would a typical reader know that guitars are rarely, if ever, permitted in prisons or in psychiatric facilities, for obvious reasons of security. As pointed out by Mason and Mercer (1999: 95–96), "in a surreal approximation of life outside, the deception of life inside is intensified … the in-vogue 'hotel-ization' produces gardens and gadgets invoking images of Eden with surreal statues, rolling rockeries, and fashionable fountains … Today it is merely the fashion to create fashionable forensic fads." The photo essay in the *Globe and Mail* is pure spectacle. As Debord writes, the spectacle "erases the dividing line between true and false, repressing all directly lived truth beneath the *real presence* of the falsehood maintained by the organization of appearances" ([1967] 1995: 153). In the same way that many federal penitentiaries colluded and collaborated in the many transfers of Ashley Smith, correctional staff, psychiatrists, and even inmates themselves are co-opted to put a beneficent face on the penal-psychiatric apparatus (care, justice, and the rule of law) for public consumption through the use (and arguably, abuse) of a national newspaper. This is just a very small snapshot of the kinds of coordinated forces that serve to censor in advance critical points of view, and to discredit research that would expose the spectacle as a lie which itself may seem harmless enough, but which nonetheless is a condition within which violence—too often to the point of death—continues behind the scenes.

The Psychiatric-Penal Apparatus: Conformation, Violence, and Censorship

At the micro level, in the prisons themselves, analysis of data collected during our years of research reveals that many nurses share a common fear. Indeed, conflict resulting from the antagonism between various components of care and prison rules leads nursing staff to fear the loss of their professional identity. In our opinion, the phenomenon of obvious "moral contamination" (Goffman 1998) seen in a majority of nurses attests to a basic social process stemming from the coexistence, in a single work environment, of divergent cultural paradigms imposing their respective jurisdictions on a single clientele: the incarcerated patients. According to our analysis of symbolic issues discussed by participants, in our various research over years, the dominant (prison) ideology modifies the provision of nursing care and even affects nurses' representations of their own professional practice. It is therefore unsurprising that a large portion of nursing staff acknowledge having internalized the primacy of security concerns over patient care. Several nurses also mentioned the constant challenges involved in performing their duties, since each professional act must, in order to conform to expectations, strike a balance between care, security, control, and punishment.

The results of years of research we performed in correctional psychiatric environments bring to light a *conformation* process to prison mores that reveals the hold various forces have over nursing staff. Nurses see their professional practice, as in the case of behavior modification plans (BMP) to use this example, modeled by the powers that be, even when they do not believe in what is being asked of them. These ideological forces (carceral and medical) impose themselves on the nurses who find themselves co-opted by the correctional paradigm and recruited as impersonal agents in the deployment of political (punishment) technologies (BMP being just one example). This ideological modeling seeks, in our opinion, to transform nurses' representations of their socio-professional identity through daily interaction with patients, interactions themselves determined in part by the combined effects of political technologies involved in the process of conformation to prison system norms.

Some of our participants adopted a deferential attitude not only toward prison rule but also, and even more so, toward the doctors they work with. This attitude is motivated by the assumptions that corrections officers are the leading occupants of the environment and that doctors are the source of expertise. There are also pragmatic reasons for such deference; avoiding conflict with corrections officers and doctors greatly facilitates a nurse's practice, in addition to reducing the risk of conflict at work. Our participants find it difficult to perform their professional duties as they would in a hospital, for example, because external pressures inevitably impose limits on their nursing practice.

In prison environments, nursing staff enjoy far less autonomy regarding care management than in hospitals. According to participants, nursing practice is certainly possible in penal psychiatry, so long as it conforms to the ends, needs, and limits of the penal environment understood as a dense, coherent, and complex microcosm. A number of nurses indicated that they are professionally concerned, even worried, by the constant ideological proximity of the prison mentality's tenets and their subjugation to medical power. This proximity is responsible, according to many participants, for the lack of differentiation between psychiatric nursing practice and the prison culture the health care provider is informally enjoined to espouse.

Our Overall Research Program

In no way does our analytical approach, in all our research, call into question the legitimacy of the security requirements in place in correctional psychiatric environments, and there can be no doubt that the nurses in our study must respect practical security measures in forensic psychiatric settings. That said, the maintenance of a safe distance between prisoners/psychiatric patients and nursing staff is valued by the institution and reinforced by questionable (para)medical practices such as behavior modification plans. Despite the indisputable wisdom of maintaining a secure distance, the internalization of the security discourse itself undoubtedly affects the nature of the therapeutic relationship between nurse and patient. This is particularly true in the case of psychiatric care as understood in nursing science, which assumes the establishment of therapeutic relationships based on confidence and the prisoner's/psychiatric patient's ability to express the existential and behavioral issues faced as a result of his or her condition and treatment. As indicated earlier, our research program is concerned with nursing practice as inscribed within conflicting social relations with the understanding that ideological factors exacerbate nurses' cognitive dissonance.

Most of the nurses interviewed over the years (in various research projects) reported significant tension created by the prescription of ineffective treatment plans (such as behavior modification plans for example) and attempts to conform to them. This tension was said to cause a variety of different kinds of suffering. According to some of our participants' testimonies, the impact of the *conformation* process to prison mores contributes, when pushed to its limits, to the deformation of a nurse's professional identity. In fact, certain participants expressed a feeling of being tarnished by the prison environment. Several nurses feared "moral contamination," that is, spoiling their professional identity as a result of the pressures of security requirements for personnel and patient control to which they must conform in a correctional setting. This is why we criticize, without reservation, the implementation of behavior modification plans in these environments (Holmes and Murray 2011), whatever our adversaries may think. Some participants admit to no longer knowing who they are socio-professionally, while others report the simultaneous development of two socio-professional identities. In July 2010, during data collection for a research project concerning ethical tensions in nursing practice in a correctional psychiatric setting, a number of participants seemed to have entirely integrated these two facets of their identity (nurse and agent of social control) to the extent that they indicated feeling completely comfortable with the antagonistic aspects underlying these two mandates.

Based on the findings of much of our research, and at this point in the discussion, we assert that the *basic social process* that is "conformation to prison mores" is responsible for the various forms of suffering identified and denounced by nurses practicing in correctional psychiatric environments. We believe that the *conformation* process to prison mores is the primary reason nurses accept prison rule, an act whose consequences include manifestations of deference not only toward representatives of the prison system but also toward doctors/psychiatrists who, in the end, control their practice. For the nurses, this troubling situation diminishes the sense of professional autonomy, blurs the boundaries of the health care provider's role, creates moral contamination, and produces psychological distress.

When nurses, as objects of power who constitute a human material, are exposed to the ideological pressures of the correctional psychiatric environment, several aspects of their initial professional identity are molded by formal and informal penitential prescriptions. For some, the *conformation* process to prison mores, with the nurse as its object, also produces feelings of estrangement or dispossession related to their initial identity. The nursing staff's feeling of estrangement appears to be grounded in a constant comparison of the role of health care provider in a hospital *versus* the role played in a correctional psychiatric environment. We can therefore state with authority that the pressures present in the prison setting weaken nurses' initial points of reference and foundational representations of the individual (patient) and of care. We would also like to note, incidentally, that in all of our empirical research, the qualms and doubts expressed by participants regarding the adequacy of care provided attest to a modification of symbolic points of reference and a *distanciation* from certain fundamental representations of the nursing discipline. In light of these observations, how can the implementation of punitive (para)medical practices, such as behavior modification plans that only exacerbate this sense of estrangement, be explained?

Our inductive analysis is based on data highlighting the nature of prescriptions issued by correctional services representatives and certain doctors/psychiatrists. These prescriptions are related, in fact, to ideological vestiges and the prison system's rigid and patriarchal old guard, whose excesses we can only condemn. These prescriptions work counter to the provision of "ethical and respectful" psychiatric nursing care to patients, to the extent that the nursing care provided does not correspond to the concept of the patient as "person," a notion central to the philosophy of care, and exceeds the limits of practical consent to care with regard to incarcerated patients. Furthermore, prescriptions following from penal ideology are partially reiterated and reinforced through punitive approaches such as the "behavior modification plan" approach. The socio-professional and psychological consequences of nursing practice in forensic psychiatry raise issues on many levels: existential, social, professional, and interprofessional, as well as political and ethical. It is important to note here that political and ethical issues directly involve the foundational concept of the patient as "person" in nursing.

Given our results collected from multiple sources, we assert that nursing staff are objects of power, insofar as ideological forces wield power over them and require them to conform to rules herein identified as "correctional." We consider them correctional because political technologies such as behavior modification plans, as reported in this chapter, are informed by a logic of punishment and reward that exists far outside the functions a nurse would normally assume. Indeed, we establish, on the basis of testimonies collected, that nurses are molded in a way that allows them to work toward meeting the penal institution's specific objectives while internalizing the formal correctional and medical prescriptions in effect within this closed space. Our analysis allows us to affirm that nurses are objects of correctional and medical power; however, we also observe that nursing staff take up these powers in their interactions with patients. What can be concluded from this apparently paradoxical result, if not that nurses, as agents of care and social control, are also carriers of the power they exert over the clientele under their care? If nursing staff are objects of power, then the same is true for the researchers who are often unable to publish research findings without having to face multiple forms of threats and violence, including attempts to censor their work.

Conclusion: Détournement

If an institution's current practices merit transformation, they must first be exposed before developing a plan to change them. If its members hide behind false and deceptive accusations against researchers in order to save an institution's reputation, what might they be capable of, on a daily basis, to justify the use of anachronistic therapeutic methods? The diffuse and repressive political technologies that the psychiatric apparatus uses, are more often than not, obscure techniques suddenly converted into therapeutic rules. Institutionalized and elevated to "therapeutic" status, these practices and prescriptions are most often placed above current law and professional codes of ethics. We consider our reflections on current practices (specifically, behavior modification plans) entirely legitimate and emphatically reassert the validity of our analyses based on empirical data gathered over years of research. We believe that a kind of osmosis may be taking place between socio-professional groups of corrections officers and nursing staff and that, more than ever before, a growing number of researchers determined to expose the inner workings of an infernal machine are being subjected to violent attacks.

Our findings demonstrate an ethical and ideological disconnect between care and corrections, as these affect the socio-professional identity of nursing staff and the quality of care they are able to provide. But the forms of institutional violence that operate in this professional setting are not restricted to human relationships "on the inside," whether these are therapeutic, professional, or institutional. As we have discussed, in this case an analogous violence extends to the censorship of our research. Since our research seeks to represent the ethical and professional concerns of nursing staff, the violence effectively disciplines and censors the nurses that our research seeks to represent. And finally, the violence in question is exercised towards the public, and what citizens have a right to know about what goes on inside institutions paid for by public funds. Who will control the representation of our public institutions and the care that they provide? While our research focuses on the microcosm of violence within the prison's walls, this quickly plays out in the macrocosm of the public sphere, as the integrity of journal articles are contested and as the penal-psychiatric apparatus manages its public face through public spectacle.

The spectacle is, as Debord claims, pernicious. Debord's understanding of the spectacle is undoubtedly Marxist: the spectacle prevents us from engaging in the critique of ideology, producing ideological forms as yet another commodity to be consumed, and masking the material conditions—the violence—of their production. "The spectacle is not a collection of images," he writes; "rather, it is a social relationship between people that is mediated by images" ([1967] 1995: 12). It is a question, then, of managing social relationships or human capital, whether this is understood as the labor of nursing staff, the bodies of inmates, or the body politic. So what, then, is the necessary work of critical researchers, investigative journalists, coroners' inquests, and the like? In Debord's terms, it is *détournement*. The word *détournement* remains untranslated in *Society of the Spectacle.* Among other things, in French the word can mean a change of course or direction, a deviation or detour, a renunciation, an abduction, the seduction of a minor, or even the embezzlement of funds. It means a twisting or a turning away; it is "the fluid language of anti-ideology," a language that "mobilizes an action capable of disturbing or overthrowing an existing order" ([1967] 1995: 146). In brief, it is an insurrectionary force that relies not on the autonomy of individual agents acting in isolation, but on a movement, in the style of a discourse. Debord writes:

> *Détournement* is the antithesis of quotation [*le contraire de la citation*], of a theoretical authority invariably tainted if only because it has become quotable, because it is now a fragment torn away from its context, from its own movement, and ultimately from the overall frame of reference of its period [*son époque*] and from the precise option that it constituted within that framework [*à l'option precise qu'elle était à l'intérieur de cette référence, exactement réconnue ou erronée*].

The *détournement* is essentially critical in style, turning against ideologies that have become "commonsense," "true," and infinitely quotable—against the stuff of everyday chatter, and against the violence of "theoretical authority," such as the spectacle of care, justice, and the rule of law that that we found deployed in *The Globe and Mail* photo essay, or that nursing staff experience within the penal-psychiatric apparatus, or that critical researchers experience when their work is censored, silenced, and discredited. *Détournement* involves the critical work of analysis, much as we try to do when we analyze interviews with nursing staff. *Détournement* is the effort to re-contextualize, re-historicize, and to understand the implicit and underlying social, professional, political, institutional vectors of power—to expose how power functions to produce discourses of "truth" and "commonsense," and how violence operates in these settings.

References

Debord, G. [1967] 1992. *The Society of the Spectacle*. New York: Zone.

Goffman, E. 1998. *Asiles : études sur la condition sociale des malades mentaux*. Paris: Éditions de Minuit.

Holmes, D. 2005. Governing the captives: Forensic psychiatric nursing in corrections. *Perspectives in Psychiatric Care*, *41*(1), 3–13.

Holmes, D. and Jacob, JD. 2012. Entre soin et punition: la difficile coexistence entre le soin infirmier et la culture carcérale. *Recherche en soins infirmiers*, *111*, 57–66.

Holmes, D. and Murray, S. 2011. Civilizing the *barbarian*: A critical analysis of behaviour modification programs in forensic psychiatric settings. *Journal of Nursing Management*, *19*(3), 293–301.

Holmes, D., Perron, A., and Michaud, G. 2007. Nursing in corrections: Lessons from France. *Journal of Forensic Nursing*, *3*, 126–131.

Holmes, D., Perron, A., Michaud, G., Montuclard, L., and Hervé, C. 2005. Scission entre le sanitaire et le pénitentiaire : réflexion critique sur les (im) possibilités du soin infirmier au Canada et en France. *Journal de réadaptation médicale*, *25*(3), 131–140.

Jacob, JD. and Holmes, D. 2011. Working under threat: Fear and nurse-patient interactions in a forensic psychiatric setting. *Journal of Forensic Nursing*, *7*, 68–77.

Mason, T. and Mercer, D. 1998. *Critical Perspectives in Forensic Care: Inside Out*. London: Macmillan.

Mason, T. and Mercer, D. 1999. *The Sociology of the Mentally Disordered Offender*. London: Routledge.

Murray, S.J. and Holmes, D. 2013. Toward a critical ethical reflexivity: Phenomenology and language in Maurice Merleau-Ponty. *Bioethics*. doi:10.1111/bioe.12031.

Perron, A. and Holmes, D. 2011. Constructing mentally ill inmates: Nurses' discursive practices in corrections. *Nursing Inquiry*, *18*(3), 191–204.

Sapers, H. 2008. *A Preventable Death*. [Online]. Available at: http://www.oci-bec.gc.ca/cnt/rpt/oth-aut/oth-aut20080620-eng.aspx. [accessed: August 1, 2013].

Chapter 3
The "Rhetoric of Rights" in Mental Health: Between Equality, Responsibility and Solidarity[1]

Emmanuelle Bernheim

Introduction

The question of solidarity has always been at the heart of the social problem of insanity. Because it represents a disparity between formal and informal norms of collective life (Goffman 1980), a gap between the normal and the abnormal (Foucault 2004, Canguilhem 1991), and a "social offense" (Goffman 1959), insanity constitutes a form of social status (Foucault 1976). Throughout different periods in history, including that of the "great lockup" (the *grand renfermement*, as described by Foucault) (Foucault 1965), the era of deinstitutionalization, the witch hunts, the years of lobotomies or shock therapies, the constant challenge of all of these practices was to ensure the stability and cohesiveness of the social fabric. Whether through concealing the existence of the insane, imposing sanctions on them, or reforming and then reinserting them into society, the objective has always been to uphold the strength of the social bond by marginalizing them, on the one hand, or attempting to integrate them through socialization, on the other (Goffman 1963). Our present era of the "rhetoric of rights" (Scheingold 2004) is no different.

For some, the development of normative rhetoric is nothing more than the symptom or the manifestation of the social model as defined by Michel Foucault (2003): societal norms are defined by a transmutation of power, from that enforced from top to bottom to that enforced through a chain of individuals linked to each

1 This chapter was inspired by research done for a PhD: Emmanuelle BERNHEIM, *Les décisions d'hospitalisation et de soins psychiatriques sans le consentement des patients dans des contextes clinique et judiciaire: une étude du pluralisme normatif appliqué*, thesis submitted to the Faculté des études supérieures et postdoctorales de l'Université de Montréal and to the École doctorale sciences pratiques de l'École normale supérieure de Cachan, March 2011. This research was funded by the Social Sciences and Humanities Research Council of Canada (SSHRC). I would like to thank my research directors, Professors Pierre Noreau and Jacques Commaille, for their substantial contributions to this project. I would also like to thank Annie Rochette for her valuable comments on an earlier version of this chapter.

other, in a disciplinary rather than an authoritarian fashion (Elias 1982, 2012). Social control is thus transmitted through the integration of social norms – the various "rhetorics" – by the individual and by the standardization of behaviours through individual responsibility and accountability (Martuccelli 2005).

A global repositioning of the status of citizenship and of the political role now places the individual at the centre of the democratic process and social structure. The State and civil society are indivisible, each acknowledging the power, rights, and legitimacy of the other. The social and the political are subordinated to the law (Bumiller 1988) and citizens must participate actively in the formation of this egalitarian society. If the "rights revolution" (Commaille 2010: 151) happens only in a civil society that is engaged and mobilized, then the phenomena of marginality and exclusion are depoliticized and are seen tied to individual responsibility rather than to a systemic social dynamic. Substantive equality, which calls forth the social dimension of state action and tends to give equal weight to all by establishing objective priorities (Dworkin 2000) cannot, in this context, arise in law. A strictly formal recognition of rights thus constitutes a *de facto* transfer of responsibility to the individual as a personal freedom. The aim is not to protect society against the negative consequences of social inequalities but rather to ensure the formal recognition of the rights of those people faced with the individual consequences of those inequalities. In this social model, any expression of solidarity is skewed or even impossible to attain (Supiot 2010). This perspective forms the main argument of this paper, which is based on the results of my doctoral research.

My initial doctoral research questions (Bernheim 2011a) did not relate to the mechanisms of social responsibility and solidarity, but the results compelled me to develop an analysis of them. I had originally decided to study the ways in which judges and psychiatrists mobilize norms, especially legal norms, in the context of confinement and psychiatric care. Indeed, in the last twenty years in Quebec civil law, this context has drawn from two distinct legal regimes to find exceptions to the fundamental principles of the rights to physical integrity, to inviolability, and to self-determination. The first regime, "confinement in an institution", constitutes only a time-out technique that allows for people whose mental state represents a danger for themselves or for others to be confined against their will within a health facility; however, this mechanism should never be used as a means to coerce a person into treatment. The link between the danger the person represents and his or her mental state must be proved by the health institution with two psychiatric reports. In the second regime, the "authorization for treatment" allows the health institution to impose a precise treatment for a set period of time, providing the person is considered to be lacking the mental capacity to consent to treatment and that this treatment is required by his or her health condition. The health institution must then prove, with a psychiatric report, both the inability to consent to treatment and the need for it. In both cases, the person is entitled to legal representation by a lawyer and to a full answer and defence. During this entire process, procedural rules and safeguards ensure that psychiatric patients' rights are protected, and these rules include strict timelines, the obligation of the courts to interrogate the defendants, appeal *pleno jure*, etc. (*Civil Code of Québec, Code of Civil Procedure, Act respecting the Protection of persons whose mental state presents a danger to themselves or to others*).

We first conducted interviews with judges and psychiatrists and then observed proceedings at the Palais de justice de Montréal. These hearings are held in closed sessions on the day the applications are presented (these are urgent applications) and the judge on the bench then renders his or her decision immediately. Our observations confirmed what some governmental and non-governmental organizations have been decrying for many years (Quebec 2011, Quebec Ombudsman 2011, Action autonomie 2012, 2009, Association des groupes d'intervention en défense des droits en santé mentale du Québec 2009): while timelines are well-defined, they are regularly exceeded; psychiatric reports are often incomplete; in many instances, the right to information and to informed consent to care are not respected; the criteria of danger and incapacity remain unclear and their interpretation varies; and in many cases, defendants are not present during their hearing in court.

This systematic rights violation is a direct consequence of the rhetoric of rights at the start of which is a chain of interrelated elements: 1) the disengagement of the political sphere; 2) the illusion created with regard to the tangibility of equality; 3) the fact that responsibility devolves to the individual and 4) the erosion of solidarity and the social pact, and the transfer of responsibility. These elements are organized in the following manner:

1. Entrusting the courts with these decisions is considered by politicians as a sure bet in preventing past abuses in psychiatry and as a result, they have disengaged themselves from these issues both financially and through public policies. Care conditions are now considered in terms of rights and the courts must ensure their implementation, especially in terms of confinement and mandatory care. An important advocacy movement for the recognition of rights, especially the right to equality, stems from a plurality of social groups, and we thus notice the development of a rhetoric of rights in the field of psychiatry;
2. A rhetoric of health is also emerging parallel to the rhetoric of rights movement. Considering that in theory all patients have equal rights, it is up to each of them to know what these rights are, to exercise them and to require access to health and social services, which are also considered rights. In this framework, exercising rights and maintaining one's good health become individual citizen obligations;
3. The failure of legal claims (either through failing to exercise one's rights or having one's arguments rejected) and the failure to remain in good health are considered opportunities lost and rest entirely on the shoulders of the person then considered deficient; and
4. These failures warrant the transfer of responsibility to the medical establishment through a legal decision. This transfer does not, however,

translate into the implementation of rights but rather constitutes a form of social sanction, accompanied by a mechanism of resocialization. This process stems from the erosion of solidarity and the breach of the social pact.

The Rhetoric of Rights: Magical Thinking, Political Disengagement and Civic Responsibility

The history of psychiatric law speaks to a constant tension between the objectives of social and moral protection on one hand, and the implementation of rights and freedoms on the other. While confinement was long considered the only intervention method in this area, the discovery and development of psychiatric medication coincides with the recognition of universal human rights and the dissemination of the rhetoric of rights. The possibility of maintaining psychiatric patients within the community and favouring freedom of action and decision while offering adapted care focused on access to care and a person's right to integrity, has completely changed the perspective on coercive measures in psychiatry.

This change of paradigm becomes very clear in the discourse of Quebec legislators from the 1960s onwards. Psychiatric patients who until then had been kept in asylums by the thousands (sometimes on simple denunciations), and lost their civil rights, began to be progressively recognized as citizens (Bernheim 2011b). This recognition fits within the larger pattern of a rights revolution and a democratization of the law. Indeed, the right to equality – a rallying point for various marginalized groups – is officially recognized for all citizens and access to public services and to justice becomes one of the core issues of public policies. Reforms to psychiatric law in the 1970s and the 1990s are adopted in the context of this social movement and thus have as common denominator the strong prevalence of individualistic and egalitarian mechanisms. Just as in civil and medical law, the bases of psychiatric law rest on the responsibility of patients to use available services and exercise their rights (Conrad 2007, Knowles 1977). It is not so much a question of the State providing services and ensuring that rights are respected as it is the responsibility of citizens to use them and to speak out against irregularities.

An analysis of parliamentary debates (Quebec 1997) shows that recourse to the courts is presented as a guarantee for the application of procedural mechanisms formalizing the exceptional character of confinement to an institution and authorization for treatment measures, and for their "legal" necessity. The fact that doctors no longer have the power to make these decisions would thus constitute a true protection against abuse providing the benevolent dimension characterizing clinical decisions was evacuated. By not having the obligation to follow psychiatric reports presented by various health institutions, the courts could, in theory, call upon a variety of experts. However, in practice, the fact that doctors are the only ones who have the competence to diagnose and prescribe strongly reduces the appeal of psychosocial or psychological expertise.

Courts are presented as guardians of rights and, for the patients, as the ultimate means of individual responsibility and empowerment. Resorting to the courts thus appears as the sine qua non condition for social equality, again the responsibility of the individual (Solomon 2011). In this context, however, equality can only be formal: all patients will be treated in the same manner despite the existence of unequal physical, socioeconomic, or cultural factors. During these hearings, health institutions are systematically represented by lawyers, whereas defendants are rarely present or represented. In the vast majority of cases, they are ill-prepared and are shown in an unfavourable light in front of the court, especially because of their lack of knowledge of judicial rituals: specific and hermetic language, the pre-established format of the proceedings, translation of issues at stake into legal issues, etc. ... The noticeable disparity of legal forces clearly has strong detrimental consequences for the people subjected to these proceedings, where applications are authorized in more than 95 per cent of cases (Action Autonomie 2009). These statistics directly challenge the efficiency of the judicial process and of its effects. Judicial formalism seems to bring forth the consequence that, even when treated in the same manner, people in different situations will be confronted with different legal effects (Dworkin 2000). While the law should act as a protection mechanism for psychiatric patients, it appears rather as a means for perpetuating a relationship based on power (Bourdieu 1986).

The use of the rhetoric of rights in the political discourse inevitably helps to depoliticize the issues and to allow the State to discharge itself of any responsibility. Resorting to the law and the courts appears as an almost magical solution: the law is the ultimate instrument for equal treatment, and the courts, independent, impartial and trusted by the public, naturally represent competent legal interpreters. As a result, courts are directly involved in the interpretation and the shaping of public health policies. Indeed, case law establishes the criteria and conditions to determine cases justifying psychiatric interventions and their modalities.

The Rhetoric of Mental Health: Formal Equality and Opportunities

The rhetoric of health is based on the same premises of dynamism and responsibility as the rhetoric of rights. A constant increase in phenomena considered as strictly medical denotes an evolution in the social relationship to health, perfect health having become a sort of substitution ideology (Conrad 2007) filling the void left by the loss of moral references. The rhetoric of health puts health at the centre of shared values, thus justifying preventive public health policies and the dissemination of medical knowledge by numerous agents. In fact, the State, through multiple policies including large-scale prevention campaigns, promotes health education based on the premise that individuals will then take responsibility for their own health. Each is then presumed to have the same capacity to understand information related to health and to implement it.

The aim of these policies is to reinstate desirable behaviours in those who, through their lifestyles, had moved away from them. This type of intervention is based on individual responsibility as each person, having the necessary information, then becomes the only manager of her or his daily health (Foucault 1994). The objective is prevention rather than treatment (Richter 2006, Gabe 1995), to transform and normalize rather than to treat (Foucault 2004). A collective recommendation becomes a "personalised injunction" (Knowles 1977), materializing an obligation to heal oneself instead of being treated. Good health is now a moral obligation or a norm from which deviation becomes suspect or even reprehensible.

However, the premises of the rhetoric of health are in practice contradictory to those of the rhetoric of rights. If individuals can, in theory, participate in the elaboration of their health care plan and make their own therapeutic choices, including that of refusing the treatments proposed, these rights are nevertheless exercised within the framework of medical rhetoric (Gori and Del Volgo 2008). In this context, it is an obligation to be healthy; individuals are not only responsible for their health but also have the moral and the legal obligations to preserve and restore it. Can anyone refuse treatment after having been informed of the risk and potential consequences? Would the choice to take such a risk, even if it is legally possible to do so, be perceived as unreasonable, especially in a context of health education and information?

In psychiatry, this paradox is exacerbated because of the objective of the discipline itself: classifying and treating behaviours and abnormal social functioning (Conrad and Schneider 1980, Lane 2007, Szazs 1991). While the paradigm of biopsychiatry establishes a relationship between abnormal behaviours and a dysfunctional biological process, the emergence of the concept of "mental health", described by Alain Ehrenberg (2005) as a "great reversal", has widened the scope of psychiatry. The constant increase in the number of psychiatric diagnoses (Horwitz 2002, Houts 2002) and reliance on psychotropic medication (Quebec 2009), including its prescription to children and adolescents – and this despite side effects (Horvitz 2010, Whitaker 2002) – only serves to reinforce this interpretation. The notion of mental health is so vague that it transforms the usual divide between normal and abnormal into a continuum, going from the more normal to the less normal, allowing for the psychiatric diagnosis and treatment of a wider range of behaviours. The definition of mental health proposed by the World Health Organization (WHO 2013) serves in fact as the ideal illustration:

> Mental health is not just the absence of mental disorder. It is defined as a state of well-being in which every individual realizes his or her own potential, can cope with the normal stresses of life, can work productively and fruitfully, and is able to make a contribution to her or his community.

Not only does this definition not propose any criteria for evaluation, it represents an explicitly normalizing discourse: work, productivity, contribution to civil society. Mental health would thus simply correspond to the model of vibrant and egalitarian citizenship. In our social context, mental disorder is thus considered a deficit in one's responsibility towards one's health and rights, in other words, a form of social dysfunction.

This rhetoric of mental health can only foster intolerance towards difference. Interventions under this rhetoric aim for normalization and conformity of behaviours (Foucault 1965, Goffman 1963). The implicit end of psychiatric treatment measures, especially institutional confinement and authorization for treatment measures, is a patient's return to society as a functioning member of it. "Reintegration", "rehabilitation", and "resocialization": confinement and psychiatric treatment are designed as experiences of learning for citizenship, as "opportunities" to influence the course of one's life (Astier 2007).

Individual Responsibility, Resocialization and Vulnerability: Rhetoric within Legal and Psychiatric Discourse and Practice

During our field work, the question of responsibility arose spontaneously in interviews and during observations of judges and psychiatrists. This question arises in three phases. First, there is the responsibility of psychiatric patients with regard to their personal situation; secondly, there is the responsibility of resocialization, which should allow them to come out of this situation; and finally, responsibility arises out of the paradoxical reasoning that considers psychiatric patients simultaneously as vulnerable and as incapable of making decisions for themselves.

The observations carried out speak to the existence of a typical profile for people for whom an application for confinement or authorization for treatment is requested. While mental illness can affect all strata of society without distinction – a notion integral to the paradigm of biopsychiatry – the vast majority of those people are poor, live on the street, in low-income housing, or in notably precarious conditions. This is not surprising since the relationship between socio-economic conditions and health has often been established. Living in a precarious environment, being stigmatized, facing anxiety and stress are all recognized as factors in the development of mental disorders (WHO 2010).

Many psychiatrists have observed this specific socio-economic profile in their patients, explaining that economic hardship is often accompanied by social isolation and a deficit of "cultural capital". However, when asked about this situation, many judges said they had never noticed it. Those who had thought about it did not provide a systemic or social analysis of the situation, claiming, for example, that homelessness is a choice or a freedom. Issues frequently brought forth during hearings, especially with regard to institutional confinement, are those of education, employability, and social relationships, but drug or alcohol consumption habits, sexuality, and financial situations were also frequently raised.

Individual responsibility thus also determines living conditions, pointing to the initiatives that individuals could not or did not wish to take: not only are they responsible for what they do or don't do – studying, working, taking drugs, getting angry – but also for what happens to them – failing school, losing a job, divorcing. In this perspective, and despite the intentions voiced by judges, hearings look more like the "trials" of the choices and the lifestyle of psychiatric patients than opportunities for them to be heard on an equal basis. The adjudication process, which pits parties against each other on the model of classic civil cases, exacerbates this situation.

This trial of the choices and lifestyles of psychiatric patients is, in fact, an appreciation of "normality", interpreted as the capacity to function in a given society according to the parameters set by the rhetoric of mental health. Because of their vulnerable material situation, some participants seem to consider confinement to an institution or authorization for treatment as a "service" rendered to psychiatric patients by the State. In this perspective, opposing confinement or treatment is considered an aberration according to the following line of reasoning: between living on the street or in precarious conditions and being hospitalized, how can someone choose the former? Furthermore, why and especially how can one refuse the help offered by psychiatrists who have both the knowledge and the means to help?

For the judges and psychiatrists we talked to, measures of confinement and authorization for treatment are opportunities for individuals to re-enter a normal life and to rehabilitate themselves. They claim that they must take advantage of these opportunities to "give responsibility back to individuals", and to make them self-sufficient so that they may then better function within society without recourse to special socialization measures. Ironically, to justify the implementation of such supportive measures, many informants claim that though most psychiatric patients are, for the most part, legally competent, they are, in fact, incapable of making decisions for themselves and are "vulnerable". Thus, despite the historic recognition of human rights and of specific rights for psychiatric patients, most of our participants (both judges and psychiatrists) do not consider the purpose of legal mechanisms for confinement and authorization for treatment as being one of protecting rights, but rather as one of protecting vulnerable people. Fundamental rights are thus not really dealt with, other than the opportunity to be heard and the obligation to explain to these patients that protective measures for "vulnerable" people are being applied to them. Judges and psychiatrists thus substitute themselves for the consent of psychiatric patients who are considered unable to act in their own best interest. Confinement and authorization for treatment appear as paternalistic mechanisms formalizing a transfer of responsibility from the deficient individual to health and justice authorities. In this context, decisions are made "from the heart", without regard to the will expressed by the people themselves. Imposing a confinement or an authorization for treatment is justified by what psychiatrists and judges consider as being in the best interest of psychiatric patients in accordance to their own interpretation of the situation (Brown and Murphy 2000). A lifestyle not adapted to the rhetoric of mental health thus justifies violations of legal protections under the guise of the rhetoric of rights whose egalitarian premises ironically act as justification for these violations.

Rhetoric of Rights, Erosion of Solidarity, and Violation of the Social Pact

Two types of citizens thus come before the courts: those for whom the legal process allows, even ensures, the recognition and the implementation of their rights, and the others. In itself, this observation is nothing new: difficulties related to access to justice, such as, for example, the abuse of procedures for strategic purposes, the disproportionate costs of the justice system, or the drastic increase in non-represented parties, have been amply documented by researchers in social law. However, our research sheds light on an application of the law, based on the particular circumstances of each case and on behavioural parameters set by the rhetoric of the health framework, not unlike a hijacking of the judicial process for the purpose of normalization. The result of this hijacking is the invisibility and the disentitlement of individuals' rights and freedoms, informed by the confiscation of citizenship's attributes (Goffman 1963). The erosion of solidarity is manifested through this disentitlement.

The erosion of solidarity is a phenomenon through which the welfare state's typical social functioning, and the citizenship model associated with it – where citizens contribute to society according to their ability and for which they receive a type of redistributive insurance – are replaced by a direct and uniform individual involvement in the construction of society. Individual responsibility to society comes before collective responsibility towards individuals (Astier 2007) and social integration is realized mainly through the exercise of individual rights. Beyond situations of proven discrimination, exclusion stems directly from this citizenship model through which are played out tensions between three dimensions of social dynamics: 1) contractual exchanges between individual rights and obligations, 2) freedom as the structure for civil society and 3) equality and democracy as cornerstones of the political process (Silver 1994).

The rhetoric of rights appears as a symptom not only of the individuation of issues which had, up till now, been taken care of collectively – work, education, illness, etc. – but also of the profound change in the foundations of the social contract (Rosanvallon 2000, Ewald 1985). Whereas the philosophical premise of the social contract (Rousseau 2010) is the reciprocal involvement of each individual and his or her rights for the benefit of the collective good, personal fulfilment and empowerment now constitute the basis of any social relationship. This paradigm not only hides power relationships, which are reduced to individual will or the lack thereof, but it also allows for sidestepping fundamental social questions integral to collective life, and ignoring alarming observations such as those which our research brings to the forefront. Why and how in a society as rich as ours and where fundamental rights have been recognized for all equally, can there be citizens living on the street, hungry and abandoned? Which social offence could, in 2013, justify the systematic violation of fundamental rights? How can we explain, in the context of the rhetoric of rights, the social objectives of socialization and normalization? Through a rhetorical trick, in the words of our participants, these questions are reduced to a compendium of similar stories labelled as socially problematic, that all have in common individuals' deficiency, responsibility, and freedom. The absence of any structural and contextual analysis eliminates any substantive debate; the rhetoric of rights is a fiction through which situations are examined, interpreted, and understood, but mostly straightened out and lustred (Bumiller 1988). The law, and individual rights, are ironically hollowed out of a large part of their substance: while we talk about them at length and while they serve to justify any action at the outset, in some situations and for some individuals, they have little application.

It is thus not accepted that some citizens may need medium and long-term support, unless they are legally incompetent. As a full and competent subject of the law, the individual must take responsibility even when he or she does not have the financial, intellectual, or social means to do so (Castel 2003). Should the situation uncontrollably deteriorate or worse, should it become inconvenient, individual responsibility is then transferred to psychiatrists who are called upon to come up with a solution, and then to judges who must justify this transfer of responsibility by law. It is not a mechanism of social solidarity but rather a form of paternalistic assistance through which social control is exercised. To that end, the central role played by psychiatric institutions in the erosion of solidarity is at least partly attributable to their inclusion in a coherent body of policies through which positive opportunities for the poor and the marginalized are proposed (Thomas 2010: 75).

We have also observed a considerable discrepancy between what is expected of psychiatry and psychiatrists politically and socially on the one hand, and their daily reality on the other. This discrepancy takes shape in two ways: the first one deals with the status of psychiatrists as the sole recognized experts in mental illness; the second concerns the nonmedical nature of the emergency measures they have to decide upon. First, many psychiatrists expressed a discomfort with the status of experts in mental illness attributed to them by the judicial process. Legal criteria and the procedural framework of the hearings force them to render a definitive judgment: "This man is dangerous", "This woman is incapable". Not only is this evaluation difficult, but the situation also keeps evolving. Furthermore, this judgment will then be considered by judges and lawyers as the truth despite the established difficulty of evaluating the reliability of experts' testimonies, especially with regard to methodology (Haack 2004, Skurka and Renzella 1998). Some psychiatrists thus mentioned the subjectivity of their evaluations and the limits of possible prognostics. As for the second question, almost all the psychiatrists we met spoke of interventions with patients who were brought to them by police or ambulance services, who suffered from no clear mental illness. All agreed that the problems of homelessness, poverty, prostitution, and drug use might be, and maybe should have been, resolved differently. However, had they not acted, those patients would have had no other support.

This situation is problematic and worrisome on at least two levels. Firstly, in addition to contributing directly to the psychiatrization of social issues, the absence of policies with regard to social solidarity justifies and legitimizes the hijacking of legal mechanisms and institutions. Furthermore, replacing mechanisms of social solidarity by clinical and legal interventions as substitutes for the ineffectiveness or the absence of political will justifies the absence of systemic public action. The situation in the past decades has, however, demonstrated the limits of the rhetoric of rights social model, and the necessity of taking positive actions to improve the substantive equality of psychiatric patients (Dworkin 2000). To that end, we outline the advantages of a human rights-based approach to health (Dudley, Silove and Gale 2012, Gruskin, Mills and Tarantola 2007, Gruskin 2006), which establishes a relationship between civil rights and social and economic rights in a collective perspective that considers rights as a whole with the aim of attaining established and clear social objectives (Meier and Fox 2010, Bhatia 2010).

Concrete existence of fundamental rights, over and above formalist discourses, should be measured by the yardstick of social solidarity. As long as certain groups do not benefit from the material, social, legal, and other advantages of our societies, how will we be able to speak truly of the "rule of law" without resorting yet again to rhetoric?

References

Act respecting the Protection of persons whose mental state presents a danger to themselves or to others, RSQ, c P-38.001.

Action Autonomie – Le Collectif pour la défense des droits en santé mentale. 2009. *Nos libertés fondamentales ... Dix ans de droits bafoués!* Montreal.

Action Autonomie – Le Collectif pour la défense des droits en santé mentale. 2012. *Les usages des autorisations judiciaires de traitement psychiatrique à Montréal: entre thérapeutique, contrôle et gestion de la vulnérabilité sociale.* Montreal.

Association des groupes d'intervention en défense des droits en santé mentale du Québec. 2009. *La garde en établissement: Une loi de protection ... une pratique d'oppression.* Montreal.

Astier, I. 2007. *Les nouvelles règles du social.* Paris: PUF.

Bernheim, E. 2011a. *Les décisions d'hospitalisation et de soins psychiatriques sans le consentement des patients dans des contextes clinique et judiciaire : une étude du pluralisme normatif appliqué.* Thèse déposée à la Faculté des études supérieures et postdoctorales de l'Université de Montréal et à l'École doctorale sciences pratiques de l'École normale supérieure de Cachan.

Bernheim, E. 2011b. *Garde en établissement et autorisation de soins: quel droit pour quelle société?* Cowansville: Yvon Blais.

Bhatia, V. 2010. Social rights, civil rights and health reform in Canada. *Governance*, *23*(1), 37–58.

Bourdieu, P. 1986. La force du droit. *Actes de la recherche sciences sociales*, *64*, 3–19.

Brown, K. and Murphy, E. 2000. Falling through the cracks: The Quebec mental health system. *McGill Law Review*, 45, 1037–1079.

Bumiller, K. 1988. *The Civil Rights Society – The Social Construction of Victims*. Baltimore: Johns Hopkins University Press.

Canguilhem, G. 1991. *The Normal and the Pathological*. New York: Zone Books.

Castel, R. 2003. *From Manual Workers to Wage Laborers: Transformation of the Social Question*. London: Transaction publishers.

Civil Code of Québec, LRQ, c C-1991.

Code of Civil Procedure, RSQ, c C-25.

Commaille, J. 2010. La justice et la transformation des sociétés contemporaines. Quelles politiques de justice? In P. Noreau (Ed.). *Révolutionner la justice. Constats, mutations et perspectives*. Montréal: Thémis, 141–154.

Conrad, P. 2007. *The Medicalization of Society*. Baltimore: Johns Hopkins University Press.

Conrad, P., Schneider, J. 1980. *Deviance and Medicalization: From Badness to Sickness*. St. Louis: The C.V. Mosby Company.

Dudley, M., Silove, D. and Gale F. 2012. *Mental Health and Human Rights – Visions, Praxis and Courage*. Oxford: Oxford University Press.

Dworkin, R. 2000. *Sovereign Virtue: The Theory and Practice of Equality*. Harvard: University Press.

Elias, N. 1982. *Power and Civility: The Civilizing Process*. New York: Pantheon Books.

Elias, N. 2012. *On the Process of Civilisation: Sociogenetic and Psychogenetic Investigations*. Dublin: UCD Press.

Ewald, F. 1985. A concept of social law. In G. Teubner (Ed.). *Dilemmas of Law in the Welfare State*. Berlin: Walter de Gruyter, 40–75.

Foucault, M. 1965. *Madness and Civilization: A History of Insanity in the Age of Reason*. London: Tavistock.

Foucault, M. 1976. *Mental Illness and Psychology*. New York: Harper and Row.

Foucault, M. 1994. *The Birth of the Clinic: An Archaeology of Medical Perception*. New York: Vintage Book Edition.

Foucault, M. 2003. *Society Must be Defended : Lectures at the Collège de France, 19751976*. New York: Picador.

Foucault, M. 2004. *Abnormal: Lectures at the Collège de France*, 1974–1975. New York: Picador.

Gabe, J. 1995. *Medicine, Health and Risk: Sociological Approaches*. Oxford: Blackwell Publishers.

Goffman, E. 1959. *The Presentation of Self in Everyday Life*. New York: Anchor Books.

Goffman, E. 1960. La folie de "position". In F. Basaglia and F. Basaglia (Eds). *Les criminels de paix*. Paris: PUF, 269–318.

Goffman, E. 1963. *Stigma: Notes on the Management of Spoiled Identity*. Upper Saddle River: Prentice-Hall.

Gori, R., and Del Volgo, M.-J. 2008. *Exilés de l'intime – La médecine et la psychiatrie au service du nouvel ordre économique*. Paris: Denoël.

Gruskin, S. 2006. Rights-based approach to health: something for everyone. *Health and Human Rights Journal*, *9*(2), 5–9.

Gruskin, S. Mills, E. J., and Tarantola, D. 2007. History, principles, and practice of health and human rights. *The Lancet*, *370*, 449–455.

Haack, S. 2004. Truth and justice, inquiry and advocacy, science and law. *Ratio Juris*, *17*(1), 15–26.

Horvitz, A. V. 2002. *Creating Mental Illness*. Chicago: University of Chicago Press.

Horvitz, A. V. 2010. Pharmaceuticals and the medicalisation of social life. In D.W. Light (Ed.). *The Risk of Prescription Drugs*. New York: Colombia University Press.

Houts, A. C. 2002. Discovery, invention, and the expansion of the modern Diagnostic and Statistical Manual of mental disorders. In L.E. Beutler and M.L. Malik (Eds). *Rethinking the DSM – A psychological perspective*. Washington: American Psychological Association.

Knowles, J.H. 1977. The responsibility of the individual. *Daedalus*, *106*, 57–80.

Lane, C. 2007. *Shyness – How Normal Behavior Became a Sickness*. New Haven and London: Yale University Press.

Martuccelli, D. 2005. Critique de l'individu psychologique. *Cahiers de recherche sociologique*, *41–42*, 43–64.

Meier, M. and Fox, A.M. 2010. International obligations through collective rights: moving from foreign health to global health governance. *Health and Human Rights Journal*, *12*(1), 61–72.

Noreau, P. 1993. *Droit préventif: le droit au-delà de la loi*. Montréal: Thémis.

Québec, Ministère de la Santé et des Services sociaux, Direction de la santé mentale. 2011. *Rapport d'enquête sur les difficultés d'application de la Loi sur la protection des personnes dont l'état mental présente un danger pour elles-mêmes ou pour autrui*. Québec.

Québec, Institut de la statistique du Québec. 2009. *Utilisation de services et consommation de médicaments liés aux problèmes de santé mentale chez les adultes québécois*. Montréal.

Quebec, National Assembly, Committee on Social Affairs. 1997. Étude détaillée du projet de loi no 39 – Loi sur la protection des personnes atteintes de maladie mentale et modifiant diverses dispositions législatives (2). In *Journal des débats (Hansard) of the Committee on Social Affairs*, 35(100) (december 5).

Quebec Ombudsman. 2011. *Problems with the Application of the Act Respecting the Protection of Persons whose Mental State Presents a Danger to Themselves or to Others* (R.S.Q., c.P-38.001). Quebec.

Richter, I.K., Berking, S., and Müller-Schmid, R. 2006. *Risk Society and the Culture of Precaution*. New York: Palgrave-Macmillan.

Rosanvallon, P. 2000. *The New Social Question: Rethinking the Welfare State*. Princeton: Princeton University Press.

Rousseau, J.-J. 2010. *The Social Contract: Or Principles of Political Right*. Whitefish: Kessinger Publishing.

Scheingold, S. 2004. *The Politics of Rights: Lawyers, Public Policy, and Political Change*. Ann Arbor: University of Michigan Press.

Silver, H. 1994. Social exclusion and social solidarity: Three paradigms. *International Labour Review*, *133*(5–6), 531–578.

Skurka, S. and Renzella, E. 1998. Misplaced trust: The courts' reliance on the behavioural sciences. *Canadian Criminal Law Review*, *3*, 269–284.

Solomon, J.M. 2011. Civil recourse as social equality. *Florida State University Law Review*, *39*, 243–272.

Supiot, A. 2010. *L'esprit de Philadelphie – La justice sociale face au marché global*. Paris: Seuil.

Szasz, T. 1991. *Ideology and Insanity: Essays on the Psychiatric Dehumanization of Man*. New York: Syracuse University Press.

Thomas, H. 2010. *Les vulnérables. La démocratie contre les pauvres*. Broissieux: Éditions du Croquant.

Whitaker, R. 2002. *Mad in America*. Cambridge: Perseus Publishing.

World Health Organization. 2010. *Mental Health and Development: Targeting People with Mental Health Conditions as a Vulnerable Group*. Genève.

World Health Organization, *What is mental health?* [Online]. Available at: <http://www.who.int/features/qa/62/en/index.html> [accessed: 20 march 2013].

Chapter 4

Power, Control and Coercion: Exploring Hyper-Masculine Performativity by Private Guards in a Psychiatric Ward Setting

Matthew S. Johnston and Jennifer M. Kilty

My Last Day on the Job

04:00hrs. Approximately. A tired officer, exhausted from another night of machismo, exaggerated anecdotes of sexual encounters, and routine chemical injections. I keep telling myself "this is the last night". The last night since the nineteen-year-old kid got punched three times, thrown down bleeding with his wrist placed in a lock and crying, reminding you of the spanked three-year-old you see in the supermarket every few months. The nurses call. It goes something like this: "Hello, security speaking". "We need a med-assist!" "We're on-route". The phone slams down.

And the three of us waddle over to the elevator. I don't remember who was there. One guard recalls the girl he fucked, yes "fucked" two nights ago. He met her on an online dating site. Clearly he doesn't sleep like the rest of us on our downtime. Another guard comments how hot he thinks one of the psych-patients is on the E-Wing. I'm less turned on from their stories, and more nervous about how the call will turn out. I don't perform the absence of fear as well as they do. I don't want to get my ass kicked anymore. I've survived these sterile, blood-covered walls. But how? I'm not like them … I was still wondering who to blame.

We get to the unit. Our IDs give us clearance. There are gentle "hellos" and "how are yous" exchanged with the nurses. The same nurses my buddy just told me in the elevator he wants to fuck. "Thanks for coming guys! It's at the end of the hallway". One of the nurses orders us. Yes, orders. "Oh no problem, how did your exam go?" one of the guys ask. "We'll see I guess!" And the two of them laugh. Next, the latex gloves go on. This is routine. We pick a fresh pair even though we all know we always keep an extra set in our pocket. Just in case. Just in case some crack addict attacks us in the tunnels. According to my trainer, this happens.

We confront her, "the patient", at the end of the hallway. It isn't hard because she is just standing there talking to the nurses about how she doesn't like being in her room. We talk to her, pleasantly. Meanwhile, the nurses prepare a sedative. I keep thinking what a pleasant girl she is. She has a British accent and tanned skin. She mentions that she is pregnant. It's the first thing she makes clear to us. She must have seen this before, or gone through it. The nurse takes one of the other guards and me aside. She tells us, quickly: "She's been known to be aggressive. We told her to go to her room". "Can she take it orally?" someone usually asks. "No, we've been there before. She's not co-operative". "Right, let's get this done". And we corner the woman. "Ma'am, we need you to come to your room please". She looks up at us. "Why, what are you giving me?"

"Come on, we'll talk about this in your room". There are eight of us in total: four nurses, three security guards, and a back-up personal care assistant "just in case". Most of the guys think they're pathetic. But the more the merrier as the adage goes. The curtain around her bed is pulled open. We first ask her to lie on the bed stomach-down. Then we demand that she lie on the bed stomach-down. This is to facilitate the exposure of her buttocks in the cold, sterile room. Routine.

She fights for a while. She doesn't kick, punch, or yell. Just fights for a little while like most of them do. There are voices in the midst of the struggle: "you can't have my necklace, it's my religion". "Let's cut the necklace, she might choke herself", the nurses say. "No!" I hear. The necklace is cut off. She doesn't kick, punch, or yell. Then another voice: "Turn over on your stomach please". By now, everyone has said it. Time passes. And there is the final image in a collection of images I have of bottoms. I count four limbs in total: two legs and two arms. Each is pressed on firmly as the needle goes in. The patient manages to mutter one thing in the middle of all this. It is quiet. I have to listen so I can hear it: "I've never been so sexually assaulted in my life". I release my grip and leave the unit. I never come back. Because I realized just being there was enough.

On March 08, 2010, after sixteen months of intensive emotional and ideological struggle, the first author resigned from his position as a private security guard at a local hospital in Canada. The reason for his departure is best summarized in a passage from the resignation letter he wrote to the institution's Board of Governors the same night he laid to rest his uniform, military boots, protection vest, and tactical belt:

> I could no longer withstand the moral conflict I was experiencing as a result of my exposure to the hospital security department and mental health system. To summarize a description of the hospital's security team, management and psychiatric system, I would use the words broken and unjust. Each and every day, both voluntary and involuntary patients residing in [the hospital] encounter gross, neglectful violations of rights that are guaranteed to them under the Ontario Mental Health Act. Having developed a close personal relationship with a number of the security staff over this past year, I can assure you that I am not the only individual who is aware of this claim.

Indeed, his resignation signalled an intrinsic shift in attitude toward patients whom he was professionally required to surveil, restrain, seclude, punish, and certainly at times, hurt; the same persons he was mandated to protect and assist. Old feelings of indifference metamorphosed into regret, anger, and frustration, but most of all a new and shared vision (Ashcraft and Anthony 2008, Barton, Johnson, and Price 2009,

Cleary, Hunt, and Walter 2010, Fairman and Happ 1998, Holmes, Rudge, Perron, and St-Pierre 2012, Jones 1984, Mason 2006) for the ways in which healthcare facilities provide care, compassion, cooperation, trust, respect, integrity, and empathy to persons we come to define as sick and unwell – the noted mission statements of several hospitals in Ontario (Lakeridge Health 2011, McGill University Health Centre 2012, University Health Network 2008, The Scarborough Hospital 2012),Canada more broadly (St. Paul's Hospital Saskatoon 2012, Victoria General Hospital 2003), as well as other hospitals across the globe (McLean Hospital Harvard 2012, National Health Service UK 2012, The Wesley Hospital Australia 2012).[1]

Departing from the first author's traumatic lived experiences as a hospital guard, this chapter engages in a qualitative analysis of how eight hospital private security guards construct and perform masculinity and how these performatives affect and intersect with the ways they assess security risks and threats and use force or other coercive security tactics on involuntarily committed mental health patients. The narratives are framed by Raewyn Connell's (1987, 2009) theoretical notion of hegemonic masculinity, as well as the available literature on gender and masculinity within security, police, prison, and military institutions. Ultimately, these findings urge psychiatric facilities to critically examine the necessity of restraint and seclusion-based practices. We argue that the reliance on punitive and hyper-masculine mechanisms of control as a primary feature of "care", in conjunction with the gendered relationships that exist between predominantly male security officers, predominantly female nurses, and patients, fosters the carceral-like practices of force, restraint, and chemical injections over other and potentially more humane methods of care and control. We suggest that revising hospital management discourses that privilege staff safety and ward control (Allen, Lowe, Brophy, and Moore 2009, Crocker, Stargatt, and Denton 2010, Delaney 2006, Doeselaar, Sleegers, and Hutschemaekers 2008, Gillespie, Gates, Miller, and Howard 2010, Liberman 2006, Moylan 2009), sometimes at the peril of the legal and human rights of patients (Federman 2012), may help to reduce (Donat 2003) the "all too frequent" patient deaths and injuries that occur under psychiatric "care" (Hem, Steen and Opjordsmoen 2001, Mason-Whitehead and Mason 2012: 224).

Now that we have reflected on the events and politics that shape the critical epistemology steering this research, we turn to a discussion of the discursive and gendered power structures that preserve hegemonic masculinity and its "dangerous" (Connell 2009: 143) accomplices – power, control, and violence.

Hegemonic Masculinity, Power, Control, and Violence

Bio-medical thinking positions psychiatry as a gateway to uncovering the "truths" of the mind and thus of human emotion, providing psychiatrists and other hospital

1 These institutions were not studied for this project and do not have any affiliation with this research.

agents who adopt and practice its discourse with the authority to define notions of sickness and health, madness and sanity (Leifer 1990). Power is conceptualized discursively in the Foucauldian tradition (1977, 2003), and as Holmes and Federman (2006) argue, psy-power in its discursive form elicits control strategies by influencing the discourses and associated practices of those employed in forensic psychiatric settings:

> Control over captive populations within some forensic psychiatric settings still rely on old-fashioned techniques of control, the manipulation of caring professionals, the use of pacification techniques to obtain docility, and the outright use of power and fear to tame potentially recalcitrant populations ... On the contrary, inquiry into the role of nurses reveals just how "capillary" power is. It comes from all sides of the prison hospital complex [emphasis added]. It resides not in one institution or within one regulatory scheme, but attaches itself to bodies throughout the organization. Power infects everyone in forensic psychiatric settings. (p. 17)

This research holds that hegemonic masculinity, which we see materialized in the hyper-masculine performatives of hospital security officers, is one axis of the "capillary" power infecting psychiatric facilities. As discovered in the literature on prisons (Acker 1992, Bandyopadhyay 2006, Bosworth, and Carrabine 2001, Donaldson 2001, Evans and Wallace 2008, Jewkes 2005), policing (Fletcher 1996, Herbert 2001, Prokos and Padavic 2002, Rabe-Hemp 2007), private security (Micucci 1998, Monaghan 2002, Rigakos 2002, Walby 2009), and military work (Albuquerque and Paes-Machado 2004, Duncanson 2009, Johnson 2010, Shefer and Mankayi 2007), institutional discourses and associated practices mean that some hospital agents (i.e. male security officers and nurses) are rewarded for their physicality and authority to punish and control "captive populations", while others (i.e. patients and female guards) are subordinated and pacified by their gendered status. As Hearn (2004) notes, the widespread presence, growth, and delivery of men's power ultimately appears in many, if not all dimensions of our lives:

> [P]ower is a very significant, pervasive aspect of men's social relations, actions and experiences ... Men's power and dominance can be structural and interpersonal, public and/or private, accepted and taken-for-granted and/or recognized and resisted, obvious or subtle. It also includes violations and violences [sic] of all the various kinds. (p. 51)

Drawing on Gramsci (1971), Connell (1987) argues that the extensive social practice of masculinity is hegemonic, that is to say, actors engage in a process of domination, control, and subordination of others through their "essentialized" (West and Zimmerman 1987) definitions of gender, social situations, phenomena, and interactions. Hegemonic masculinity refers to the idea that patriarchal power relations are sustained through the consent of men and, in a different way, by some women (Connell 1987). Not only do men actively reproduce their tacit consent of this hierarchical gender structure, but also the dominant construction of women's consent to it as well (Hearn 2004: 52). Our "seamless" gender identities then, or what Butler (1988) calls the "appearance of substance" (p. 520), are not assembled subjectively, but are rather a product of an overarching gendered structure.

Of course, this structure is inextricably linked to the ways we "do gender", that is, how we organize and produce social interactions, performatives, and activities in a way that expresses gender and which help us construct the actions of others as conditioned by gender (West and Zimmerman 1987). Achieved in and through human interaction, gender is discursively produced and practiced through the collective meanings we inscribe onto bodies (Fenstermaker and West 2002). Building on the notion of hegemony, and West and Zimmerman's (1987) "doing gender" framework, Connell (2009) specifically asserts that the embodied experience of doing gender is attached to the essentialist, patriarchal, and "most important … heterosexual" (Connell 1987: 186) differences we construct between what is thought of as masculine and feminine. Constituting the backbone of the patriarchal system of gender-power relations (Carrigan, Connell, and Lee 1985, Connell 1985), gender differences formulate the widespread practice of hegemonic masculinity, which subordinates (rather than eliminates) femininities and less dominant and subversive masculinities. Femininities, on the other hand, are constructed only in relation to masculinity and women's power only in relation to men's, which indeed highlights the "asymmetrical position of masculinities and femininities in a patriarchal gender order" (Connell and Messerschmidt 2005: 848). Undoubtedly problematic, Connell (2009) cautions us against the "dangerous" repercussions that such routinized, oppressive, homophobic, heteronormative gender performatives have on our social, institutional, and interpersonal relationships:

> Contemporary hegemonic masculinity, to take the most striking case, is dangerous, regardless of patriarchal dividend. It is dangerous because it provides a cultural rationale for inter-personal violence … It is harmful to men themselves; the masculinity reformers were on strong ground when they argued that men would be safer not fighting, would be healthier without competitive stress, and would have a better life with improved relations with women and children. (p. 143)

While hegemonic masculinity is not necessarily preserved by physical or social force, it can threaten the stability and peacefulness of our social interactions, cultures, and institutions whose primary mission is to provide compassionate and empathetic care to persons we have come to define as sick, needy, and vulnerable. As this study and others demonstrate, hyper-masculinity can: romanticize and materialize an agent's desire to engage in physical aggression/dominance (Herbert 2001, Micucci 1998, Monaghan 2002, Prokos and Padavic 2002, Rigakos 2002); trigger a discursive ambivalence towards feminism and the feminine (Acker 1990, Dell,

Filmore, and Kilty 2009, Evans and Wallace 2008, Fletcher 1996, Kilty 2012, Prokos and Padavic 2002, Rabe-Hemp 2007, Simpson 2004) and towards homosexuality (Herbert 2001, Miller, Forest, and Jurik 2003, Walby 2009); contribute to heteronormative and patriarchal beliefs about and cultural practices of sexuality such as the perpetration of sexual harassment or assault (Carlson 2009, Eigenberg 2000); and may lure hospital guards into perpetuating the quasi-militant, alpha-masculine practices of intimidation, demeaning surveillance, deception, and authority (Albuquerque and Paes-Machado 2004, Duncanson 2009, Johnson 2010, Monaghan 2002, Shefer and Mankayi 2007) over "captive populations".

This research fills a gap in the topical and theoretical literature on hegemonic masculinity within institutions of social control by unearthing tensions in local security officers' hyper-masculine practices. Our findings contend that local hospital security guards must maintain the explicitly sexist and often physically brutal, homophobic, anti-feminine, authoritative, and hierarchal codes of behaviour while interacting with nursing staff, patients, and each other. These demonstrations of power and control, which are often depicted as facilitating patient-care and integration in hospital/healthcare settings (Holmes and Murray 2011, 2012: 27), are in tension with contrasting health discourses that promote acts of compassion, understanding, forgiveness, sympathy, nurturance, and freedom – the coined performatives of emphasized femininity (Korobov 2011).

Methodological Framework

Our research is driven and shaped by a call for justice, that is, a critical epistemological lens that shapes our "varying degrees of social actions, from the overturning of specific unjust practices to radical transformation of entire societies" (Guba and Lincoln 2005: 268). We take the position that human experience is produced by social, political, cultural, economic, racial/ethnic, and most important to this research, gendered forces, all of which inform our understandings of, and places within the world. Through critique, reflexivity, and voice, the goal of this research is to stimulate social and internal transformation of the widely reproduced gender hegemonies and systems of patriarchy (Wickramasinghe 2006: 607) that infect our collective conscience as well as our institutions of social control. Thus the knowledge produced here presumes gender as epistemology with regard to the ways in which we as critical feminist researchers employ gender to forward our political aspirations and theoretical constructs, as well as to mediate the enactment of ontological reality (Wickramasinghe 2006: 609). Put bluntly, we seek to empower ourselves, and activists, scholars, nurses, criminologists, biomedical professionals and students alike to challenge the gendered nature of capillary and structural power relations that are manifest within the institutional discourses and associated practices that oversee psychiatric facilities.

After obtaining ethics clearance from the university REB, eight in-depth, semi-structured interviews were conducted with male guards who currently work or formerly worked at local hospitals.[2] The interviews were conducted over the span of six months and in one session for each participant; the interviews lasted between one and two and one half hours exclusive of taking short breaks. Every interview was held outside hospital grounds in order to help the guards become more comfortable discussing the sensitive, violent, and disturbing aspects of their work (Dickson-Swift, James, Kippen, and Liamputtong 2009). Each participant was allowed to choose the location of the interview, which consisted of public coffee shops, a mall lobby area, the participants' homes, and a fast-food restaurant. Due to the time constraints of this research, the principle researcher could only recruit male guards between the ages of 23 and 30.[3] Although several women were asked to take part, only one expressed interest and, unfortunately, was unable to participate.[4] While the sample size is small and limited in terms of generalizability and representation, it is our intent to focus on the vivid details and deep nuances of each guard's story, instead of quantifying meaning (Young 2011).

The first section of the analysis and discussion demonstrates how particular signs and symbols of masculinity, such as soldierly uniforms, "SWAT[5]-like" choreography, discourses, and practices of intimidation, and unconditional loyalty to militant authority figures cement the guards' alpha- or hyper-masculine status for the hospital's patients, nurses, and other security staff. The second section explores how these hegemonic masculine performatives interact with the performatives of other agents of the asylum, and consequently, reinforce biomedical discourses that endorse the use of force, restraints, and chemical sedatives to manage a captive patient population.

Ontological Machismo: Protecting the Alpha Self and Taming the Feminine Other

> Jackson: Jerry is like the perfect security guard because I mean you got a guy who can speak calmly … can back it up physically. (…) Big as a fridge so if you did fuck with him he's going to put you down but … at times Jerry would be very like … "Ok Sir I'm going to have to put you in a controlled position man, can you relax?" And he'll put you on the ground. "I'm gonna hold you there gently, if you cannot breathe let me know and we will walk you through it" … as he's kicking your ass.

---

2 Each participant was a former colleague of the first author/principle researcher.

3 We are not sharing any additional demographic information on the participants to ensure that their identity remains anonymous to readers, colleagues, and their organization.

4 We speculate that the lack of communication with recruits who identify as women may be linked to an uneasiness they may have towards speaking with a former male-bodied colleague about the sensitive and gendered nature of their job.

5 SWAT is a common acronym for Special Weapons and Tactics, which are highly specialized enforcement units.

As demonstrated in the above quote from Jackson, the militaristic conditions the aspiring guard must adopt for hospital security work include ongoing demonstrations of physicality and loyalty towards the rules and codes that are established by his superiors (Albuquerque and Paes-Machado 2004, Duncanson 2009, Johnson 2010, Shefer and Mankayi 2007). Performing hegemonic masculinity in the hospital setting requires that the guard yield both to his security superiors and to other agents who hold positions of power within the institution, most notably nurses and doctors. Not only must he submit to and reproduce the institutional hierarchies that are embedded in the relations between guard and nurses, simultaneously, the guard is expected to maintain a steadfast air of confidence and authority through all interactions (Connell 2009, Prokos and Padavic 2002). For example, one participant, Charles, flaunted and rehearsed expressions of his physical prowess and self-control, which he suggests is paramount to ensuring he survives the tough, violent, and even "warlike" conditions of the job (Herbert 2001, Micucci 1998, Monaghan 2002, Rabe-Hemp 2007).

> Charles: A security officer is a drone of the establishment. (…) Ok. They are the grunts. They are the muscle, they are the brute force. They are not the ones to make … you know decisions. They take … what is the norm in our society and enforce it. They're not there to prove a thing, to prove to a judge, they're there to obey their superiors, such as the military … even in an, an, an atmosphere of complete disaster, complete danger. And that's something that most of us don't even believe in.

Charles emphasizes that his participation in public displays of brutality, toughness, rule enforcement, and intimidation are not only part of the job, but exist as the predetermined and unchallenged ways of doing masculinity in an essentialist quasi-military culture. In this case, the alpha-asylum guard parallels state policing agents (Rigakos 2002) who similarly draw on the associated practices of hegemonic masculinity, such as physicality and loyalty to authority (Connell 1987, 2009), to learn and reproduce a determinist and fixed way of communicating with nurses, patients, and colleagues. Just as Holmes and Federman (2006:17) assert, this passage highlights how power in forensic healthcare settings "infects" individuals discursively and from many angles, so as to take full and even "drone-like" possession of their ontology, which drives and shapes their discourse and actions.

With very little autonomy to do gender outside of hegemonic guard discourses, Troy discussed the need to become "compassionless" in order to intimidate patients for the greater good of the institution. In this narrative, Troy asserts that the need to control "unruly" (Monaghan 2002) populations and protect the more vulnerable nursing personnel (Evans and Wallace 2008: 485, Prokos and Padavic 2002, Rabe-Hemp 2007) outweighs the need for guards to illustrate kindness, accommodation, and sympathy – the ironically feminine (Korobov 2011) and at times unpracticed objectives of patient care (Federman 2012, Holmes 2011, 2012, Mason 2006, Mason-Whitehead and Mason 2012: 224).

> Troy: We're the bad guys. We can't be compassionate towards them because then people will walk all over ya … I can't be like "it's ok sir", no I have to defend myself in public with staff around me. I can be compassionate to a point but after, after that point I can't … I just can't do it.
>
> Matthew: Right … what happens when you get a guard who thinks … really compassionately?
>
> Troy: (…) I don't think it's ever happened (laughs).

Fearful that people will "walk all over him", Troy argues that losing a battle with a patient because he resorted to a more nurturing approach would embarrass him in front of the nursing staff and most assuredly, the other male guards. Accordingly, the subordinated or "failed" guard emerges as a kind of failed man, effeminate in his weakness to adequately demonstrate to both the nurses and the guards his capacity to physically overtake a dangerous patient in a potentially violent showdown. As Jackson painfully recalls, the alpha guard's ability to appear intimidating goes beyond what can be performed through loud words, strong muscles, and determination; rather this aspect of the alpha- or hyper-masculine performativity is a product of the guard's assessment by his superiors (West and Zimmerman 1987).

> Jackson: He said to me in no uncertain terms: "Congratulations on getting [a security promotion] … I hope for your sake and the hospital that nobody gets hurt when you're on duty. Because I just don't think you can cut it … I think they made a mistake hiring you … you're a nice guy, you're good at administrative work but … sometimes there's a point when you gotta be physical and you … don't have it".

In this passage, Jackson describes how his superior claimed that he was unable to diffuse situations before they become violent because he lacked the requisite aura of self-assuredness and control. Jackson's failure to mirror the intimidation rituals of other male guards is closely linked to his struggle to subversively transform his gendered identity into a disguised self or "appearance of substance" (Butler 1988: 520) bound by the discourses and practices that constitute hegemonic masculinity. "Confin[ed] to ghettos, to privacy, to unconsciousness" (Connell 1987: 186), the guard who exhibits a subordinated masculinity is chastised for failing to adequately perform as the hyper-masculine hospital guard.

Similar to Jackson, Sean encountered tension with the hyper-masculine presumption that the presence and image of power and authority creates a deterrent to an attack by a patient (Albuquerque and Paes-Machado 2004, Duncanson 2009, Johnson 2010, Rigakos 2005, Shefer and Mankayi 2007). Even though what he terms a "bluff charge" may win most confrontations with "troublesome" patients, Sean warns that mimicking tactical police choreography will panic, repress, and frighten many on-lookers, including patients.

> Sean: Our way of dealing with situations, it's to act macho and to appear really strong … like a bluff charge almost … like for a rhino or an elephant. A majority of the time … it's almost as if we're like riot people. You come in and there's … three people coming at you that are wearing all the same uniform, it's the same tactics as you know, SWAT. They all, walk and step … you know with their shields or whatever. It's like uh a mace, you look a lot bigger than what you are … Things get out of control, everyone wearing the same uniform … wearing the, the vests and walking in (…) You know, it's intimidating. Especially when you have four or five people running for a call that didn't need that, you know? And … people who would be you know, "here come … the cops".

In addition to the fear that is provoked in hospital patients and observers from the SWAT-like onslaught of large, muscular, uniformed men, the guard's drive to tame the "out of control" situation problematically implies a collapse in the patient's will to resist or question institutional authority (Leifer 1990) and in her autonomy to make decisions about her safety, care, and treatment (Federman 2012, Ontario Mental Health Act 1990: S. 1). While some maintain that violent and coercive measures are a necessary strategy to control ward outbursts and protect healthcare staff from unruly patients (Crocker, Stargatt, and Denton 2010, Gillespie, Gates, Miller, and Howard 2010, Monaghan 2002), we cannot ignore the disturbing repercussions such discourses and practices have on patients. As Jackson bravely recalls, the arbitrary and unscientific classification of "dangerousness" (Federman 2012: 297) yields more than a series of restrictions and isolations. At their worst, these management practices reproduce the delivery of sexual embarrassment, physical pain, and punishment.

> Joey: Simple scenario. We go up there … um patient is in the bathroom … one of the RNs … knock on the door, "Come out". No response. "Come on [patient] take your meds". (…) Guy is very aggressive … at the drop of a hat. Open the door … he was butt naked on the toilet taking a shit. Non-responsive to us, he's just sitting there … head down … not talking, not looking at anybody. I'm at the door … kneels down to, to match his eye level while he's on the toilet. Put the hand on his shoulder … "[patient] … we need you to go back to your room. If you don't come with us … we're going to help you". Which is code for "We're going to fucking grab you". So yeah. "We're going to 'assist' you". … Pull him down to the ground bare ass naked. Shit hanging off his ass. He's uh, he's uh a black belt or something. He's really well … trained to hurt people bad. I would say kill. And he's wrestling us; they call a Code White[6] we just … hold him down – the injection happens on the bathroom floor. Right in his ass. Two injections. Another nurse. Two injections. He got a straight shot to the balls – I don't know how he handled it or whatever. Tough enough guy. Got him back to his room, put him in restraints, and he's out for the night.

6 Code White means "aggressive patient". When paged overhead, security and medical staff meet in the area that "requires" emergency assistance.

Here, a patient remaining in the washroom for longer than what is deemed an appropriate period of time is constructed as enacting a deviant plot to avoid taking medication, which is interpreted by hospital staff as a challenge to the nurse's authority. Since this particular patient holds the reputation that he is, as Joey stated, "trained to kill", the guards are able to justify using coercive force on the grounds that the patient may become resistant and thus dangerous while nursing staff restrain, expose, sedate, and humiliate him. This scenario is ideal for the guard in two ways. Since the patient is already constructed as risky and harmful by nursing and other hospital staff members, responding security guards are awarded with notoriety and status for subduing a potentially lethal threat. The patient, who one might argue is in a vulnerable position as he is seated naked on a toilet, represents a relatively easy mission for security given that he is clearly outmatched by the number of guards, supporting medical staff, and sedatives with which he is involuntarily injected.

Indeed, achieving victory in the course of potentially "life-threatening" circumstances, especially during the early stages of one's career, allows the guard to prove, in a heroic fantastical manner (Huey, Ericson, and Haggerty 2005), his physicality and thus worthiness as a member of the security team to a hyper-masculine troupe of men. Symbolically, these encounters also reflect how security officers are competitively driven (Bandyopadhyay 2006) to obtain notoriety and recognition from senior authorities in order to excel and earn promotion into a higher status career in public policing (Rigakos 2002: 30). As the next section illustrates, it is when these "warranted" masculine aggressions, whether in the form of physical punishment, cunning, deception, or intimidation, are perpetuated as a rite of passage into hospital security culture (Prokos and Padavic 2002, Rabe-Hemp 2007) that agents of the institution become influenced by and participate in the reproduction of hegemonic discourses of masculinity.

Reproducing Hegemonic Masculinity through Patient, Guard and Nurse Relations

The Patient's Circumstance

When circumstances deteriorate between the patient and security, guards may sometimes express remorse towards any physical reaction they initiate. For example, even though Troy indicates that restraint practices are necessary emergency measures to subdue aggressive patients (Delaney 2006, Doeselaar, Sleegers, and Hutschemaekers 2008) and prevent staff/patient injury (Allen et al. 2009, Crocker, Stargatt, and Denton 2010, Gillespie, Gates, Miller, and Howard 2010, Lancaster et al. 2008), the sympathies he demonstrated earlier in his career still resonate.

> Matthew: So what's it like then when you do have to get physical with women patients?

> Troy: Um … a lot of them actually break down. Near the end of it … they start crying … It's not easy to take sometimes, and obviously I'll feel bad, I have feelings right? Like sometimes it just has to be done, it's for their own good … If they don't know what they're doing, they're mentally unstable … it's better that they're at least restricted and it's better than them at least hurting themselves right?
>
> Matthew: Right. And you feel that they get help there?
>
> Troy: They do … as bizarre as it may sound … being restrained to the bed is help … at least they can't hurt themselves or somebody else for that matter. Right?

Yet in light of Troy's emotional sympathy towards tearful female patients, we once again witness how the belief in a greater good within the hospital justifies the use of coercive force (Fairman and Happ 1998). Importantly, there are two major assumptions behind his support of this discourse of restriction. The first is that chemical sedatives will in fact lessen the likelihood (even if only temporarily) that patients harm either healthcare staff or themselves (Delaney 2006, Doeselaar, Sleegers, and Hutschemaekers 2008); the second is that security and nursing staff hold the capacity, even without an adequate scientific definition (Federman 2012: 297), to measure and perceive the extent to which patients pose a "dangerous" threat to themselves or others in the event that they are not tranquilized (Mason-Whitehead and Mason 2012: 229).

Further, Troy's statement that female patients often "break down" and cry when confronted with the security force implies the pity he feels for women whom he essentializes as weaker (Evans and Wallace 2008, Fletcher 1996, Prokos and Padavic 2002, Rabe-Hemp 2007), "hysterical", and in need of institutional, or more specifically, paternal protection (Kilty 2012: 164). Women who are able to demonstrate and abide by the alpha guard's definition of emphasized femininity, for example, crying in lieu of physical resistance such as spitting, biting or fighting, are constructed as more deserving of compassion and empathy than the unfeminine woman (Dell, Filmore, and Kilty 2009) who verbally and/or physically resists the intrusive demands and discourses of security/ward staff. As Ed remembers, the intersection of cultural interpretations about the female body, namely that heavier women are unfeminine and thus dangerous, with biomedical discourses that promote chemical incarceration, can impose a grievous impact on overweight female patients who attempt to resist the coercive power of hospital authorities.

> Ed: There was one person who I think their arm did get dislocated. I don't remember the exact details, but I think we were restraining her on the ground, and then with her arm behind the back and I guess it just lynched too far, well … she was wrestling with us. A big girl and I think her arm got dislocated; but other than that I can't think of … any patient that was injured.

Ed's narrative demonstrates two key points. First, patients are suffering grievous bodily injuries and ultimately a violation of their human rights to bodily integrity and security of person at the hands of security guards (Hem, Steen, and Opjordsmoen 2001, Mason-Whitehead and Mason 2012). Second, guards use hegemonic masculine discourses and associated practices of physical restraint to mitigate the effects of violence they anticipate from patients who embody masculine largeness and who physically resist (Herbert 2001, Miller, Forest, and Jurik 2003). At least for some guards, such as Troy in the above quote and Ed in this passage, discursively constituting patients as physical threats is done to manage the emotional stress and toil that results from their use of force against them.

Alternatively, some guards manage and disguise their distrust of patients by presenting themselves as a friend who can offer advice. In so doing, the guard convinces captive patients that docile behaviour will accelerate their release from the hospital, and that breaking the ward's rules will only lead to an extension of their confinement (Holmes and Murray 2011, 2012). By downplaying his authority, that is, playing the "good cop", the security guard uses his knowledge and understanding of the system to encourage patients to be instrumental in their own incarceration (Holmes and Federman 2006). This way, the guard secretly achieves the wants and desires of the establishment – to keep patients inside.

> Troy: I like to … sometimes make the patient believe that I'm on their side … regardless if it is true or not.
>
> Matthew: Mmm hmm. How do you do that?
>
> Troy: Umm … creative ways of saying things. Like … if the patient really wants to leave the hospital I'll tell him what [he has] to do in order to leave … he has to give up at least a one night stay … if someone is on a psych hold they can remove that anytime after the 24 hours.[7] And if he wants to go home, I go, look pal, I understand but you're not helping your case right now acting this way because everything is documented, and if they document that you comply … that is gonna help you maybe get home tomorrow or get more privileges that way … So I make it kind of seem like I'm trying to help him … which I am. But I'm also … being able to get what I want and what the staff wants.
>
> Matthew: Which is?
>
> Troy: Which is for him to stay.[8]

---

7 Normally, patients on a Form-1 are involuntarily held for a minimum period of 72 hours. The attending physician, however, may revoke the Form after 24 hours if s/he deems the patient to be no longer a threat to him/herself or others.

8 During the interview, Troy admitted that he had not read or received any meaningful instruction/training on mental health legislation.

In this way, the guard is able to coerce patients through cunning and manipulation, as well as the medically unwarranted imposition of an infantilizing privilege/reward system (Holmes and Murray 2011, 2012), which are components of the alpha guard's strategy to prove to other hospital agents that he can effortlessly render a patient docile. Underlying Troy's rehearsed exchange is a subtle and even endearing authority, that is, a performed expertise that coaxes the patient into believing he is in control of his situation. This too is "for the patient's own good" (Fairman and Happ 1998) because the written documentation of the consequences for refusing to cooperate are, as Troy explains with precision, determined and confining. Although the patient depicted here does not suffer bodily harm at the hands of security, the "control", "authority", and "danger" (Connell 1987, 2009) of the situation frame and shape the alpha guard's discourse.

Many times, the patient's second encounter with the guard takes place after s/he has been sedated and restrained. Memories of patients who appear unstable are revised once the guard is introduced to the new and improved, often heavily medicated, patient. The patient's "stabilized" appearance reassures the guard that coercion is a necessary step in her recovery (Moylan 2009, Liberman 2006). Interestingly, as Taylor recounts, any hesitance the patient demonstrates to recall the grim details of her encounter with security reinforces to the guard that no hard feelings remain and that the patient understands the necessity of the guard's actions.

> Taylor: They usually remember going back in those restraints again. They usually remember that part. But it's funny because the part they don't remember is when they actually believe in how good they feel.
>
> Matthew: What's it like for you when they get their property back from the office and you know a week ago you had just … been in an intense incident
>
> Taylor: (laughs)
>
> Matthew: – with them.
>
> Taylor: They remember the incident, they don't remember you per se. Or remember exactly what happened. They usually don't bring it up. They don't bring it up. I'll say "You look better than last time I saw you" and they go "Last time you saw me I was in restraints". Something like that.
>
> Matthew: Like joke about it eh?
>
> Taylor: Yeah … sometimes.

Taylor's experience of seeing a previously "unstable" patient leave the hospital looking well and smiling legitimizes for him any confrontation he may have had with the patient as a necessary part of the process of getting well. Saving face, the guard mitigates his participation in coercive practices by deferring to psychiatrized discourses that render his work instrumental in helping these vulnerable members of society to regain their sanity, and thus control/dominance over their actions, words, and gestures (Connell 1987). Unlike the last time they met, the patient is able to convince the guard he is "better" by not acting out verbally or physically when Taylor reminds him of a potentially traumatic incident. Satisfied that the patient is not permanently damaged from being tranquilized and strapped to a bed, often in four-point leather restraints, the alpha guard interprets the patient's gesture of goodbye as a symbol of appreciation towards his authority and medical responsibility to impose pain, punishment, and assault (Carlson 2009, Eigenberg 2000).

Feminine Weaknesses

As we have demonstrated thus far, participants emphasized the value and even necessity for security guards to be physically powerful and large in size and stature; in fact, they claimed that this is a very real reason why security work is better suited to men than to women. This gendered assumption illustrates the degree to which strength and physical power are prioritized in this work, similar to the fields of policing, corrections, and the military that have historically marginalized women's potential to successfully perform these forms of work (Carlson, Anson, and Thomas 2003, Cohn 2000, Crouch 1985, Rabe-Hemp 2007, 2009, Remington 1983). As Taylor discussed, if a petite woman works as a guard she will be targeted and tested by rowdy patients in ways that larger male guards will not be.

> Taylor: People are less likely to … get physical with me right off the bat. I've had patients tell me that "You know what … if it was someone else I may have tried to fight" but "Looking at you … I don't have a chance in hell to beat you so I'm just gonna be nice to you" … I've had it twice in the past couple years. Where you know … people won't even try because I'm a big guy but if … a five foot two female [guard] walks in there. Guess what's gonna happen? They're gonna push their luck because even at five foot four they're still bigger than the security guard.

Implicit in Taylor's narrative, and reflecting the production of hegemonic discourses about masculinity, is the position that the first and potentially the only way security guards are able to communicate with a patient is through making orders that are followed with physically overpowering the recalcitrant patient – something female guards will be hard pressed to do. This narrow view of the role of the security guard is inherently gendered, and dismisses the potential for a more caring or empathic approach to communicating with patients to be woven into the structure of hospital governance. However, not every guard is expected or is able to handle the patient on his own. At times, security guards require a nurse to serve as a sidekick in securing, subduing, and restraining patients. To ensure that physically smaller and weaker healthcare staff members are protected and safe (Fletcher 1996, Prokos and Padavic 2002, Rabe-Hemp 2007, 2009), guards may invite a male nurse to assist them with physical tasks that require a helping hand. As Joey points out, camaraderie between the security officer and the male nurse alleviates any fear that the patient may achieve physical victory and thus success over a key pillar of the guard's masculine appearance and substance – his physical integrity.

> Joey: Yeah, he's, he's actually one of my favourites … Because he doesn't put up with crap … I trust Jeremy. I know that, that if I'm stuck in a situation there … and it got physical I know Jeremy … would come in there and give me a hand … it's happened before where he's helped me out and it's happened before where I've helped him out … He's there. He'll go physical. He'll back me.

Notably, male nurses who meet hegemonic masculinity's standard of physicality and aggression can transcend the gender status of subordinated guards such as Jackson (who was seen to be physically inadequate for the job by his superior), and may subsequently be expected to physically "back" security in the event that a patient attacks or attempts to physically overpower one of the guards. Guards construct male nurses who "go physical" as a hegemonic masculine accomplice rather than leader, but their assistance in these matters does allow them to transcend the stigma of what is often viewed as an effeminate profession (in the same way that policing and security work are viewed as hyper-masculine professions) by successfully engaging in physical confrontations with patients. This sidekick role affords the male nurse admiration and "enhanced leadership/responsibility" (Simpson 2004: 349) from the guards. In this case, hegemonic masculinity, as exhibited by physical power and aggression, overrides other markers of masculinity, such as the gendered nature of one's work or profession (Acker 1990).

The female nurse, on the other hand, is excluded from sidekick candidacy on the grounds that she is a physical liability (Prokos and Padavic 2002, Rabe-Hemp 2007). Fearing that she is too vulnerable and will succumb to her biological inferiority, the hegemonic masculine guard forbids her from engaging with a patient who threatens the sanctity of her body.

> Jackson: I know they'll do what they'll do, but there's obviously a few that I don't expect to come in and that's more than fine. Like if a nurse is pregnant and I'm getting my ass handed to me I don't expect her to come in and give me a hand, she can go back and lock the doors. I'll handle it … then come back in a couple of hours.

This passage establishes how the female nurse's entrusted responsibility and ability to procreate is, as Acker (1990) writes, "suspect, stigmatized, and used as grounds for control and exclusion" (p. 152). Although Jackson appears to be acting chivalrously in his duty to protect the vulnerable nurse (Cohn 2000), Troy asserts that any woman he encounters on the job carries a threat to the guard's sexual integrity on the grounds that she may use her feminine powers of manipulation to gain revenge on her male captors (in the case of female patients) or counterparts (in the case of female guards) by accusing them of sexual harassment. Indeed, the physical and sexual integrity of the guard emerges as the most at risk and exposed component of his masculinity that, if called into question by his colleagues, will shatter the legitimacy of his heterosexual prowess (Connell 1987: 186). To guard against this, Troy uses the female nurse assisting him as a witness in a patient encounter to prevent the suspect patient from challenging his sexual legitimacy.

> Troy: I would never go into a situation with a woman with the door closed. They definitely have more to play on than a man does. Like when it comes to that ... there is stuff that they can say that a man won't say ... if I go to a situation with the door closed she can say something like I, I asked her to do stuff or something right? Like sexual things for example. Just to cover myself I always keep the door open for a woman. And they usually try to have a woman with me ... just to make sure that she can't say anything wrong. At all. And they just, I found that they become more manipulative than men. (...)
>
> Matthew: Just the mental health patient women or women kind of in general?
>
> Troy: Women kind of in general ... even in mental health ... And in general.

Troy's passage clearly references a gendered and already threatened relationship with women, female nurses, and patients alike. In fact, his perspective paints all of the female agents of the hospital – patients, nurses, and guards – as inherently manipulative and untrustworthy characters who pose a biologically predetermined threat to the order and established values of any hegemonic masculine culture (Connell 2009, West and Zimmerman 1987). Since this anti-feminist discourse (Evans and Wallace 2008) reproduces essentialized, patriarchal definitions of femininity that presume women to be driven by a duplicitous sexual scheme, it follows that the alpha guard must always tread lightly around a female figure, treating her with suspicion and caution. Simultaneously, this demonizing construction of women's motives lends itself to the reproduction of hegemonic masculinity and women's perpetual displacement into a subordinated and inferior role (Connell 1987: 186), as women are seen as innately manipulative figures in dire need of a man's supervision and control.[9]

Nurse-guard-patient Relations and Discourses of Blame

Participants in this study spoke at length about their relationships with nurses and how those relationships shaped the work they do. A common narrative in

9 Given this, it is unsurprising that security women experience exclusion and marginalization on the job and hence were hesitant to participate in this study.

the interviews was that nurses and, to a lesser degree, physicians, treat guards as though they are theirs to command – as "tools" to call in to do the dirty work of the institution.

> Charles: A person who you have to obey to … is the uh physician or nurses because they know more of the history … If I could do something to prevent any kind of mistreatment I would, but in the position that I was in as contract security your word is nothing … I've made statements about mistreatment before, and I've always been pushed aside, this is how it goes, because you're, you know … just a tool. That's really what you are.

In this passage, Charles elicits a discourse of blame, suggesting that nurses, the institutional agents in control of ward order, administration, and governance, participate in the mistreatment of patients including via the problematic use and reliance on security to physically engage with and subdue patients. He does not, however, locate the role of guards in challenging abuses of power, and in fact evokes a discourse of his own marginality that emphasizes his lesser status in the hospital governance hierarchy as a way to mitigate his responsibility in mistreating patients.

Perhaps sensing this critical judgement of their authority, nurses do not always trust guards to get the job done. Jackson and Ed, who both demonstrate a weaker physicality in relation to their peers, discussed feeling emasculated by the nurses' expectation that they greet each problematic patient with an army of backup as a security precaution.

> Ed: I think that if you're in that sort of industry, that's something you go through … a nurse will look at you because you're a bit smaller … or they'd say … "I'd rather have him or … you know Jordan or somebody like that".
>
> Matthew: Who's huge.
>
> Ed: He's just massive. But that's gonna be anywhere. That's like if you're … a 160 pound hockey player you're still gonna get looked at differently than someone who's 20 pounds heavier.

Clearly, the guards are not the only hospital agents who understand and reproduce discourses about and the associated practices of hegemonic masculinity. Jackson and Ed demonstrate how different actors within this closed environment (Holmes and Federman 2006: 17) reproduce hegemonic masculinity both discursively and through their actions as an essential component of the guard's makeup. They contend that nurses see physical demonstrations of hegemonic masculinity as a guard's professional responsibility (Rigakos 2002), similar to how police officers and soldiers are summoned by their institutions and public audiences to appear and act tough, strong, aggressive, competitive and, if needed, violent (Albuquerque and Paes-Machado 2004, Johnson 2010, Prokos and Padavic 2002).

Of course, the building tensions, distrust, and gendered demands between guards and nurses can lead to discourses of blame (Holmes and Federman 2003), which are a primary social survival feature of alpha-guard masculinity. By using the professional staff's assumed expertise in medicine and psychiatry as proof of their competence, the guard passes off accountability for healthcare violence onto the nurses, and other medical professionals such as psychiatrists who are responsible for providing a medical assessment of the patient's "dangerousness" and stability. Any concerns the guard has for the wellbeing of the patient are trumped by the loyalty he must demonstrate to his medically licensed superiors (Albuquerque and Paes-Machado 2004, Connell 1987, Duncanson 2009, Johnson 2010, Shefer and Mankayi 2007). Put simply, the security guard's role in using force against a patient is but a minor cog in a grander system of discipline, surveillance, and control.

> Troy: This girl kept just wanting to leave, she was completely like catatonic and … I don't remember at the time if the Mag-locks[10] there were locking so I, and she definitely needed to stay but … I didn't think that she needed restraints … actually when we put her in the restraints we changed her into gowns first, but there was nurses doing it mostly, we were standing by.
>
> Matthew: Just watching her.
>
> Troy: Well not watching her but watching the wall. And her putting her hands up … And uh … then we put her in restraints and she actually started to cry and she was like eighteen. I just didn't … like I don't think that she needed to be put in restraints for that.
>
> Matthew: Mmm hmm. Did you, were you able to tell the nurses?
>
> Troy: No I didn't. I don't want to tell them how to do their jobs it's their call … I didn't want to do it, but I did it. Because that's my job … I have to say to myself I'm not a trained professional. The only person that knows in that room is that nurse or … whatever the doctor has ordered.

10 Patients are restricted from leaving the ward by powerful magnetic locks that secure all exits. As tested in front of the principle researcher by former colleagues, it is unlikely that the lock can be breached by human force. To leave, a nurse, personal-care assistant, security guard, or other staff member who holds the required access level on his or her identity card must scan the patient out. Any escape from the ward that is not verified by hospital staff is referred to security as a "Code Yellow" or "Missing Patient", which then obligates each guard to search for and return the involuntary patient back to the floor. Should the patient escape successfully, security is required by law to inform police that s/he is at large.

Even though the patient, albeit against her will, submits to being forcibly changed into a hospital gown – akin to a uniform that acts as a constant and symbolic reminder that she is ill, mentally unstable, and in need of protection from herself – she is also physically put in restraints as a punishment for her resistance, or what nursing staff conceptualize as a disobedient outburst. While the alpha guard took a hands-off approach when dealing with her, his uniform and wandering panoptic gaze serve as a subtle caution and reminder of his authority and willingness to use coercive force (Bandyopadhyay 2006, Bosworth and Carrabine 2001). While Troy is able to demonstrate his compassion for a helpless patient, his conditions of employment responsibilize him to practice violent restraint when it is "for their own good" (Fairman and Happ 1998).

Quite similarly, Joey discussed his role as a security guard to be one of maintaining order but also one that requires him to be deferential to medical and psychiatric experts and their decisions to use force. Whether or not the security guards wish to follow the orders of nurses and doctors, they believe that doing their job correctly requires them to do so.

> Joey: Well I'm not the medical professional but sometimes you can tell, the person's took the meds, they're cooperating, they agreed to do everything. And a nurse will come in and say "Too bad he acted out – in restraints no matter what. I don't care what's happening now". And we're like "no". Like he's fine … and they're like … "no I'm the medical professional and you are security and you will do what I say". You're … the grunts. You're … the … enforcers. You're the whatever you want to pick … eggheads. We end up doing it. And they just go nuts again.

Here, Joey blames the nurse for aggravating the patient to the point that security is needed, and describes the nurse as reinforcing the construction of security's image as a goon squad by pressuring the guard to take down and restrain patients on their demand. While the expectation that the alpha guard practice an aggressive and tactical police style of engagement with patients as a mechanism to demonstrate his hegemonic masculinity often elicits enthusiasm and pride, other and arguably subordinated guards are unable to challenge these practices for fear of reprisal.

> Dwaine: They just call security … you never know … the patient … can be refusing to do something that's completely within his rights to refuse. And just because the nurse doesn't like it, you know, tie him to a bed … And you wouldn't want to uh … go against the nurse's order and then … have that patient actually harm somebody. You definitely … you're at fault pretty much. Sometimes … it's better to take that path than the alternative.

Like Joey, a sense that patient restraint is the lesser of two evils allows Dwaine to escape blame for his role in administering pain to patients (Federman 2012). Despite the knowledge that their actions violate the patient's right to undergo a fair medical assessment by an attending physician before being restrained (Ontario Mental Health Act, section 15.1), the alpha guard implies that preventing the always/already unstable or incorrigible patient (Mason-Whitehead and Mason 2012: 229) from inflicting harm on herself or on a nurse is a necessary, albeit vindictive, victory the security team must preserve. Any guard who refuses to participate in a violent patient confrontation risks being met with contempt, belittlement, and emasculation from the nurse, who consequently dismisses him as weak, insubordinate, and ineffective in his work (Connell 1987). Since many patients will only encounter security staff in a stressful scenario where they are frightened, hurt, and humiliated, it is all the more important that physical intervention and chemical restraint only take place after concerted efforts have been made to communicate with and calm the patient verbally (Moylan 2009). Yet pressures from nursing staff to restrain a patient for chemical sedation who, in the guard's eyes, has not behaved unreasonably, reinforces his hegemonic masculine status within the hospital and destroys his chances of being perceived by the patient as empathetic and friendly.

Alternatively, not all guards link their resentment of nursing staff to the suffering that is done unto patients, but rather to the subjugated role they are seen as adopting when they take orders from a woman. Obeying the demands of a woman, that is, a person with a subordinated gender status, brings out a sexist anger in some guards – one of the only emotions hegemonic masculinity permits (Connell 1987, 2009). For example, Joey is able to reassert his hyper-masculine status by dismissing the discourse of a female nurse he characterizes as authoritative and thus "unfeminine" (Connell et al. 1987, Dell, Fillmore, and Kilty 2009). Confident that any outbursts from female nurses are a reflection of their physical and gendered insecurities, he suggests that orders that come from a woman's mouth may be taken with a grain of salt.

> Joey: Sometimes … like the nursing staff or whatever are oversensitive, and they're like "He just told me I was a fat bitch. Get him out of here". And if you go and talk to the patient yeah … they called her a fat bitch, but I mean like … they're gonna be calm, they're frustrated, you hear the story, you get them calmed down, you get them to agree not to open their mouths to the nurse again. And you don't hear from them again. Meanwhile if I took the nurse's advice … how many patients would I throw on [a local street] a day? Just because someone said something the wrong way or called some nurse a fat piggy. And she is fat. And she is fat. Would I bang her? Yeah. (laughs)

Here, the alpha guard is dismissive of the effects these kinds of sexist statements may have on a woman's ontological security in a culture that coincidentally demands she present herself in a gentle, nurturing, sympathetic way (Korobov 2011). And while Joey is completely insensitive on this front, he then also sexualizes the same nurse he constructs as unattractive in order to reassert his heterosexual prowess, and thus hegemonic masculine security performative (Connell 1987: 186).

One last point of tension in nurse-guard-patient relations that affects the production of hegemonic masculinity is the use of chemical injections, a common feature of hospital culture and forensic settings. The guards that participated in this study described their efforts to recognize the pain patients experience by encouraging the use of physical force and restraint in lieu of the injection of chemical tranquilizers. In spite of any emotional (read feminine) outbursts the guard may hear during physical confrontations with patients, Ed suggests that physical restraint practices avoid the potential for overdose, and eventually work to relax the patient (Delaney 2006, Doeselaar, Sleegers, and Hutschemaekers 2008) without the need to invoke chemical injections against the will of the patient.

> Ed: And my main concern … is over potential for over-medication … usually what I find works is if you just simply strap 'em down, eventually they'll calm down. They'll probably scream for an hour or two. But … usually once they're in restraints … after an hour, two, three hours, they'll calm themselves down. Uh I, I don't think it's necessary to keep giving them more and more and more Haldol®.[11]
>
> Matthew: Is there an incident where you … where you had a concern about it?
>
> Ed: Um … who was it? (…) He liked to walk around a lot and it seems like they gave him a ton of medication. It wasn't quite enough to knock him out. But he was groggy as all hell and unstable on his feet. And they wanted to give him even more to see if they could knock him out and I'm thinking to myself, well … just restrain him … it was ridiculous … we never did knock the guy out in the end. We ended up … restraining him and he stayed awake the whole time. Like the guy's resiliency was off the charts.

Illogically, the guard's solution to what he characterizes as an unnecessary measure to subdue a patient, is to implement what he thinks is a "softer" (Evans and Wallace 2008), but which remains, a brutal display of physical subordination. As such, Ed's passage stresses how hegemonic masculinity leaves the guard no alternative but to confine, humiliate, and dehumanize patients until they are silent and compliant. It also illustrates the gendered differences between predominantly female nurses and predominantly male guards in terms of their preferred methods of securing control of resistant, rowdy, or "unruly" (Monaghan 2002) patients. Dangerous enough to be described as what Connell (2009) calls "the most striking case" (p. 143), hegemonic or "alpha guard" masculinity is closely linked to the preservation and enforcement of violent punishments, hierarchy, and the carceral-like institution's heavily surveilling codes of conduct. Put simply, the end

11 Haloperidol (Haldol) is an antipsychotic medication used not only for punitive purposes (as described above), but also for the treatment of schizophrenia and acute phases of delirium or mania.

(neutralizing the patient) justifies the means (use of force, restraints, and chemical injections), irrespective of how traumatic and lasting these encounters may be for the patient (Hem, Steen, and Opjordsmoen 2001, Holmes and Federman 2003, Mason-Whitehead and Mason 2012: 224).

Conclusion

This research is a testament to how the struggle for gendered power and hegemonic masculine status entangles the relations, discourses, and associated practices of hospital nurses, patients, and guards. In this particular setting, security guards reproduce hegemonic masculinity either through physical/chemical force, punishment, intimidation (verbally or symbolically through their uniformed presence), and through perpetual expressions of ambivalence towards feminized displays of compassion, sympathy, and concern for the safety, respect, and care of patients. As Federman (2012) contends, there is no scientifically accepted definition of "dangerousness", and without empirically supported evidence gleaned through rigorous standards of speculation and deductive analysis (Guba and Lincoln 2005), it is thus fair to caution forensic healthcare workers, policy makers, psychiatrists, and hospital staff alike of the physical and emotional harms that are associated with physical/chemical incarceration and labelling patients dangerous. We suggest that one of the greatest harms is the discursive and practical transformation of hospital and forensic settings into prison or carceral-like environments (Donald 2001, Jain and Murphy 2006, Wright 1997). For example, as one participant stated:

> Joey: You can't go anywhere like usually you can't leave the floor. Because they expect that maybe you'll take off. You may have somebody watching you 24–7. Um … if you're somewhat immobile you'll have someone help you to the washroom; some of the most personal things you do at home that you think nothing of … you go take a piss in the toilet. What if someone had to hold your dick for ya?
>
> Matthew: Right. Sounds like a prison.
>
> Joey: Yeah … not even. Prisoners I'm pretty sure can go on their own.

This passage from Joey illustrates the degree of surveillance to which involuntarily committed hospital patients are subject. We encourage forensic healthcare researchers and facilities administrators to critically examine the value and necessity of physical and chemical restraint practices, which notably do not have any international standard for safe definition and form (Steinert et al. 2010). This is not to say that these mechanisms do not have a place in health care management, but rather, we suggest that they should be used as last resorts (Ashcraft and Anthony 2008, Barton, Johnson, and Price 2009, Cleary, Hunt, and Walter 2010).

The absence of women's voices in this study prevents us from accessing the lived experiences of female security guards. Since no women agreed to participate in the study, a comprehensive portrait of women's experiences as hospital private security officers cannot be fully illustrated. Instead, participants mirror the ways in which dominant outsiders understand and interact with subordinate groups. With trepidation, we speculate on the lived "reality" of the female guard, that is, the ways in which she accomplishes, or fails to accomplish, gender in a hyper-masculine culture. The male guards in this study provided us with only preliminary insight into how women negotiate and resist the gendered pains of their subordinated status in relation to their male, alpha peers. Of course, the plethora of references and allusions to widespread practices of sexual harassment and discrimination warrant scholars to critically explore how other gendered voices (i.e. women, gay men) are uniquely marginalized in this hyper-masculine culture.

To depart on an encouraging note, one of the participants informed the first author that the institution studied in this research implemented a policy following his resignation that restricts male-bodied security staff from restraining or interacting on their own with women. Hopefully, this policy will help to ensure that vulnerable women are protected from the less subtle, more visible forms of masculine assault. That said, this measure will not safeguard the female-bodied patient from enduring the lived experience of feeling that she is being sexually assaulted as she is pinned down by the thick hands of security men, who hold the autonomy to gaze at the exposed bare flesh on her buttocks while she is injected against her will with a chemical restraint, a scenario described in the opening of this chapter. Nor will this measure prevent women from experiencing an unjust violation of their human rights to privacy, security of the person, and bodily integrity as guards surveil her room while she undresses and changes into her hospital "uniform". As it is our hope that every hospital can greatly limit the practice of coercive interventions, this research indicates that we can do better to make the hospital mission of compassion, dignity, and respect a reality.

References

Acker, J. 1990. Hierarchies, jobs, bodies: A theory of gendered organizations. *Gender & Society*, *4*, 139–158.

Acker, J. 1992. Gender institutions: From sex roles to gendered institutions. *Contemporary Sociology*, *21*(5), 565–568.

Albuquerque, C.L. and Paes-Machado, E. 2004. The hazing machine: The shaping of Brazilian military police recruits. *Policing & Society*, *14*(2), 175–192.

Allen, D., Lowe, K., Brophy, S., and Moore, K. 2009. Predictors of restrictive reactive strategy use in people with challenging behaviour. *Journal of Applied Research in Intellectual Disabilities*, *22*, 159–168.

Ashcraft, L. and Anthony, W. 2008. Eliminating seclusion and restraint in recovery oriented crisis services. *Psychiatric Services*, *59*(10), 1198–1202.

Bandyopadhyay, M. 2006. Competing masculinities in a prison. *Men and Masculinities*, *9*(2), 186–203.

Barton, S., Johnson, R., and Price, L. 2009. Achieving restraint-free on an inpatient behavioural health unit. *Journal of Psychosocial Nursing*, *47*(1), 34–40.

Bosworth, M. and Carrabine, E. 2001. Reassessing resistance: Race, gender and sexuality in prison. *Punishment & Society*, *3*(4), 501–515.

Carlson, J.R., Anson, R.H. and Thomas, G. 2003. Correctional officer burnout and stress: Does gender matter? *The Prison Journal*, *83*(3), 277–288.

Carlson, M. 2009. *Man up or punk out: The role of masculinity in prison rape* (Doctoral dissertation). Retrieved from ProQuest Dissertations and Theses database. (Umi No. 3383649)

Carrigan, T., Connell, R.W., and Lee, J. 1985.Towards a new sociology of masculinity. *Theory and Society*, *14*(5), 551–604.

Cleary, M., Hunt, G., and Walter, G. 2010. Seclusion and its context in acute inpatient Psychiatric care. *J Med Ethics*, *36*, 459–462.

Cohn, C. 2000. "How can she claim equal rights when she doesn't have to do as many push-ups as I do?": The framing of men's opposition to women's equality in the military. *Men and Masculinities*, *3*(2), 131–151.

Connell, R.W. 1985. Theorising gender. *Sociology*, *19*(2), 260–272.

Connell, R.W. 1987. *Gender and Power: Society, the Person, and Sexual Politics*. Oxford, England: Polity Press.

Connell, R.W. 2009. *Gender*. Cambridge: Polity Press.

Connell, R.W and Messerschmidt, J.W. 2005. Hegemonic masculinity: Rethinking the concept. *Gender & Society*, *19*(6), 829–859.

Crocker, J.W., Stargatt, R., and Denton, C. 2010. Prediction of aggression and restraint in child inpatient units. *Australian and New Zealand Journal of Psychiatry*, *44*, 443–449.

Crouch, B. 1985. Pandora's box: Women guards in men's prisons. *Journal of Criminal Justice*, *13*(6), 535–548.

Delaney, K. 2006. Evidence base for practice: Reduction of restraint and seclusion use during child and adolescent psychiatric inpatient treatment. *Worldviews on Evidence-Based Nursing*, *3*, 19–30.

Dell, C.A., Fillmore, C.J. and Kilty, J.M. 2009. Looking back 10 years after the arbour inquiry: Ideology, policy, practice, and the federal female prisoner. *The Prison Journal*, *89*(3), 286–308.

Dickson-Swift, V., James, E.L., Kippen, S., and Liamputtong, P. 2009. Researching sensitive topics: Qualitative research as emotion work. *Qualitative Research*, *9*(1), 61–79.

Doeselaar, M., Sleegers, P., and Hutschemaekers, G. 2008. Professionals' attitudes toward reducing restraint: The case of seclusion in the Netherlands. *Psychiatr Q*, *78*, 97–109.

Donald, A. 2001. The wal-marting of American psychiatry: An ethnography of psychiatric practice in the late 20th century. *Culture, Medicine and Psychiatry*, *25*, 427–439.

Donaldson, S.D. 2001. A million jockers, punks, and queens. In D.F. Salo, T.A. Kupers, and W.K. London (Eds). *Prison Masculinities*. Philadelphia, PA: Temple University Press, 118–126.

Donat, D.C. 2003. An analysis of successful efforts to reduce the use of seclusion and restraint at a public psychiatric hospital. *Psychiatric Serv*, *54*, 1119–1123.

Duncanson, C. 2009. Forces for good? Narratives of military masculinity in peacekeeping operations. *International Feminist Journal of Politics*, *11*(1), 63–80.

Eigenberg, H. 2000. Correctional officer and their perceptions of homosexuality, rape, and prostitution in male prisoners. *Prison Journal*, *80*, 415–433.

Evans, T. and Wallace, P. 2008. A prison within a prison? The masculinity narratives of male prisoners. *Men and Masculinities*, *10*(4), 484–507.

Fairman, J. and Happ, M.B. 1998. For their own good?: A historical examination of restraint use. *H E C Forum*, *10*, (3–4), 290–299.

Federman, C. 2012. The mentally ill and civil commitment: Assessing dangerousness in law and psychiatry. In D. Holmes et al. (Eds). *(Re)thinking violence in health care settings: A critical approach*. Surrey: Ashgate, 297–314.

Fenstermaker, S. and West, C. 2002. Doing Gender, Doing Difference: Inequality, Power, and Institutional Change. London, UK: Routledge.

Fletcher, C. 1996. "The 250lb man in an alley": Police storytelling. *Journal of Organizational Change*, *9*(5), 36–42.

Foucault, M. 1977. *Discipline and Punish*. New York: Pantheon.

Foucault, M. 2003. *Society Must be Defended: Lectures at the Collège de France, 1975–1976*. New York: Picador.

Gillespie, G.L., Gates, D.M., Miller, M., and Howard, P.K. 2010. Workplace violence in healthcare settings: Risk factors and protective strategies. *Rehabilitation Nursing*, *35*(5), 177–184.

Gramsci, A. 1971. *Selections from the Prison Notebooks*. London: Lawrence and Wishart.

Guba, E.G. and Lincoln, Y.S. 2005. Paradigmatic controversies, contradictions, and emerging confluences. In N. Denzin, and Y.S. Lincoln (Eds). *The Sage Handbook of Qualitative Research – Second ed.* Thousand Oaks: Sage Publications, 253–291.

Hem, E., Steen, O., and Opjordsmoen, S. 2001. Thrombosis associated with physical restraints. *Acta Psychiatr Scand*, *103*, 73–75.

Hearn, J. 2004. From hegemonic masculinity to the hegemony of men. *Feminist Theory*, *5*(1), 49–72.

Herbert, S. 2001. "Hard charger" or "station queen"? Policing and the masculinist state. *Criminology*, *36*(2), 343–369.

Holmes, D. and Federman, C. 2003. Constructing monsters: Correctional discourse and nursing practice. *International Journal of Psychiatric Nursing Research*, *8*(3), 942–962.

Holmes, D. and Federman, C. 2006. Organizations as evil structures. In T. Mason (Ed.). *Forensic Psychiatry: Influences of Evil*. New Jersey: Humana Press, 15–30.

Holmes, D. and Murray, J. 2011. Civilizing the 'barbarian': A critical analysis of behaviour modification programs in forensic psychiatry settings. *Journal of Nursing Management*, *19*, 293–301.

Holmes, D. and Murray, J. 2012. A critical reflection on the use of behaviour modification programs in forensic psychiatry settings. In D. Holmes et al. (Eds). *(Re)thinking Violence in Health Care Settings: A Critical Approach*. Surrey: Ashgate, 21–30.

Holmes, D., Rudge, T., Perron, A., and St-Pierre. 2012. Introduction. In D. Holmes et al. (Eds). *Re-thinking Violence in Health Care Settings: A Critical Approach*. Surrey: Ashgate.

Huey, L.J., Ericson, R.V., and Haggerty, K.D. 2005. Policing Fantasy City. In D. Cooley (Ed.). *Re-Imagining Policing in Canada*. Toronto: University of Toronto Press, 140–208.

Jain, S. and Murthy, P. 2006. Madmen and specialists: The clientele and the staff of the lunatic asylum, Bangalore. *International Review of Psychiatry*, *18*(4), 345–354.

Jewkes, Y. 2005. Men behind bars: "Doing" masculinity as an adaptation to prison. *Men and Masculinities*, *8*(1), 44–63.

Johnson, B. 2010. A few good boys: Masculinity at a military-style charter school. *Men and Masculinities*, *12*(5), 575–596.

Jones, K. 1984. Robert Gardiner and the non-restraint movement. *Can J Psychiatry*, *29*, 121–124.

Kilty, J.M. 2012. It's like they don't want you to get better: Psy control of women in the carceral context. *Feminism & Psychology*, *22*(2), 162–182.

Korobov, N. 2011. Young men's vulnerability in relation to women's resistance to emphasized femininity. *Men and Masculinities*, *14*(1), 51–75.

Lakeridge Health 2011. *Mission & Values*. Retrieved March 26, 2012, from http://www.lakeridgehealth.on.ca/article.php?id=9TB-69U&navID=listMenuRootH

Leifer, R. 1990. Introduction: The medical model as the ideology of the therapeutic state. *The Journal of Mind and Behaviour*, *11*(3 and 4), 247–258.

Liberman, R.P. 2006. Elimination of seclusion and restraint: A reasonable goal? *Psychiatric Services*, *57*, 576.

Mason, T. 2006. *Forensic Psychiatry: Influences of Evil*. Totowa, New Jersey: Humana Press.

Mason-Whitehead, E. and Mason, T. 2012. Assessment of risk and special observations in mental health practice: A comparison of forensic and non-forensic settings. In D. Holmes, T. Rudge, and A. Perron (Eds). (Re)Thinking Violence in Health Care Settings. Surrey: Ashgate.

McLean Hospital Harvard. 2012. *McLean Hospital Values*. [Online]. Available at: http://www.mclean.harvard.edu/about/values/ [accessed: Sept 09, 2012].

McGill University Health Centre. 2012. *Our Vision, Mission and Values.* [Online]. Available at: http://muhc.ca/homepage/page/our-vision-mission-and-values [accessed : Sept 09, 2012].

Micucci, A. 1998. A typology of private policing operational styles. *Journal of Criminal Justice*, *26*(1), 41–51.

Miller, S.L., Forest, K.B., and Jurik, N.C. 2003. Diversity in blue: Lesbian and gay police officers in a masculine occupation. *Men and Masculinities*, *5*(4), 355–385.

Monaghan, L. 2002. Regulating "unruly" bodies: Work tasks, conflict and violence in Britain's night-time economy. *British Journal of Sociology*, *53*(3), 403–429.

Moylan, L.B. 2009. Physical restraint in acute care psychiatry: A humanistic and realistic nursing approach. *Journal of Psychosocial Nursing*, *47*(3), 41–47.

National Health Centre UK. 2012. *Mission Statement.* [Online]. Available at: http://www.stockporthealth.nwest.nhs.uk/about-us/mission-statement/ [accessed: Sept 09, 2012].

Ontario Mental Health Act. 1990. R.S.O. 1990, Chapter M.7. [Online]. Available at:http://www.search.e-laws.gov.on.ca/en/isysquery/89dfb48a-0d96-492a-90ea 28d7e7433cd7z/12/doc/?search=browseStatutes&context=#hit1 [accessed: November 06, 2010].

Prokos, A. and Padavic, I. 2002. "There oughtta be a law against bitches": Masculinity lesson in police academy training. *Gender, Work & Organization*, *9*(4), 439–459.

Rabe-Hemp, C.E. 2007. Survival in an "all boys club": Policewomen and their fight for acceptance. *Policing: An International Journal of Police Strategies & Management*, *31*(2), 251–270.

Rabe-Hemp, C. 2009. POLICEwomen or PoliceWOMEN? Doing gender and police work. *Feminist Criminology*, *4*(2), 114–129.

Remmington, P. 1983. Women in police: Integration or separation? *Qualitative Sociology*, *6*(2), 118–135.

Rigakos, G.S. 2002. *The New Parapolice: Risk Markets and Commodified Social Control.* Toronto: University of Toronto Press

The Scarborough Hospital. 2012. *Mission, Vision & Values.* [Online]. Available at: http://www.tsh.to/pages/Mission-Vision--Values [accessed: March 26, 2012].

Shefer, T. and Mankayi, N. 2007. The (hetero)sexualization of the military and the militarization of (hetero)sex: Discourses on male (hetero)sexual practices among a group of young men in the South African military. *Sexualities*, *10*(2), 189–207.

Simpson, R. 2004. Masculinity at work: The experiences of men in female dominated occupations. *Work, Employment & Society*, *18*(2), 349–368.

Steinert, T., Lepping, P., Bernhardsgrutter, et al. 2010. Incidence of seclusion and restraint in psychiatric hospitals: A literature review and survey of international trends. *Soc Psychiat Epidemiol*, *45*, 889–897.

St. Paul's Hospital Saskatoon. 2012. *St. Paul's Hospital Mission, Vision and Values.* [Online]. Available at: http://www.saskatoonhealthregion.ca/your_health/ch_sph_home.htm [accessed: Sept 09, 2012].

University Health Network. 2008. *A Message from our CEO.* [Online]. Available at: http://www.uhn.ca/About_UHN/ceo/index.asp [accessed: March 26, 2012].

Victoria General Hospital. 2003. *Mission Statement.* [Online]. Available at: http://www.vgh.mb.ca/hospital/main.asp?contentID=51 [accessed: Sept 09, 2012].

Walby, K. 2009. "He asked me if I was looking for fags … " Ottawa's national capital commission conservation officers and the policing of public park sex. *Surveillance & Society*, *6*(4), 367–379.

The Wesley Hospital Australia. 2012. *Wesley Mission & Values.* [Online]. Available at: http://wesley.uchealth.com.au/2012–01–30–06–02–46 [accessed: Sept 09, 2012].

West, C. and Zimmerman, D.H. 1987. "Doing gender". *Gender & Society*, *1*, 125–151.

Wickramasinghe, M. 2006. An epistemology of gender: An aspect of being as a way of knowing. *Women's Studies International Forum*, *29*, 606–611.

Wright, D. 1997. Getting out of the asylum: Understanding the confinement of the insane in the nineteenth century. *Social History of Medicine*, *10*(1), 137–155.

Young, J. 2011. The bogus of positivism. In J. Young (Chapter 4) *The Criminological Imagination*. Cambridge: Polity Press.

Chapter 5
Containment Practices in Psychiatric Care

Eimear Muir-Cochrane and Adam Gerace

> Many people have told us that high use of seclusion and restraint in mental health facilities are often an early sign of a system under pressure. They can deny people their rights. There is little evidence to support seclusion as an effective and positive clinical intervention to people when they are at their most vulnerable. (Mental Health Commission Report Card 2012)

Introduction

This chapter explores containment practices in psychiatric settings, specifically focusing on research into these practices and the implications for care of patients in a range of inpatient settings. Acute inpatient units, aged-care psychiatry wards, and emergency departments are the main settings discussed in this chapter. Restraint here refers to any form of confinement of inpatients and includes physical, chemical, and environmental restraint, including locked ward doors and seclusion. Such restrictive measures remain controversial, albeit commonplace, and in contradiction to global policies about the need for humane and least restrictive care for people with a mental illness (United Nations 1991). These practices produce an uneasy dyad in which restraint is deemed an acceptable strategy to control patient behaviour, generally as a last resort, but as such lies in direct opposition to United Nations' principles on the protection of the mentally ill (United Nations 1991). The authors will discuss the prevalence of these intrusive and controlling practices, and the physical, social, and psychological consequences for patients subjected to them. In addition, we will explore the possibilities for care that improves patients' experiences of hospitalization and potential recovery from their illness.

The Practice of Restraint

Restraint has been used in a range of healthcare settings and has had a long and notorious history in psychiatry (Szasz 2007). It has been used to manage patients deemed aggressive or violent (Van Der Zwan et al. 2011, Hodge and Marshall 2007, Rintoul, Wynaden, and McGowan 2008), or as "an emergency measure to prevent imminent harm to the patient or other persons when other means of control are not effective or appropriate" (Metzner et al. 2007: 417). Restraint is defined as "restricting a patient's movement and actions by the use of mechanical devices or physical means" (De Bellis et al. 2013: 94). There are various techniques for restraining patients, which may include different methods according to specific settings. Restraint can be enacted through physical holding, or the use of leather or fibre belts, straps for hands and feet, handcuffs, shackles, cotton or leather ties, and other devices (Bak et al. 2012). Seclusion (where patients are confined to a barely furnished room and are unable to leave), other environmental restraints such as locking day-room doors or ward front doors, and chemical restraint (using medication to heavily sedate) are other forms of restraint (Van Der Zwan et al. 2011). Restraint has been used in a variety of healthcare settings, including emergency departments, acute care institutions, psychiatric settings, aged-care residential homes, intensive care units, surgical or medical wards, as well as in paediatric wards or facilities housing people with an intellectual disability.

Reducing and eliminating these practices is a priority for psychiatric care worldwide, and attempts at reduction are underpinned by relevant initiatives at state, national, and international levels (National Association of State Mental Health Program Directors 2007, Department of Health 2008, Te Pou 2008). In her discussion of restraint use on older patients with dementia, Cotter suggests that "[t]he legal standard has moved from liability associated with the failure to restrain to one that presumes appropriate care relies on interventions other than restraints" (2005: 81). However, there is "considerable variation in the clinical standards governing the use of restraint and seclusion in mental health services and guiding the appropriate use of the interventions or the use of alternative strategies" (National Mental Health Working Group 2005: 17).

In Australia, the reduction and potential elimination of restraint and seclusion practices have been identified as one of four key national priority areas for increasing safety and reducing harm in mental health care (National Mental Health Working Group 2005). This is in line with the United Nations' (1991) *Principles on the Protection of People with Mental Illness*, which specifies that physical restraint and seclusion can be used only in cases "when it is the only means available to prevent immediate or imminent harm to the patient or others" (11.11); when it follows policy and procedure and is in place for the shortest time possible; and when its use is accompanied by constant patient supervision. Thus, when a patient's behaviour poses a risk either to themselves, other patients, or to staff, restraint and seclusion may be used to maintain ward safety (Bowers et al. 2004) despite opposition from governments and consumer organizations. These practices are contrary to international recommendations and government reports from prominent individuals, mental health service policies, and other scholarly literature which advocate that restraint and seclusion should be used as little as possible or eliminated when dealing with people with disturbed behaviour.

Legal and Ethical Issues

The use of restraint can pose a number of ethical and legal issues for mental health professionals, who have regarded the issue of restraint as an embarrassing reality (Soloff 1979) and a breach of human rights (Holmes 1998). Many jurisdictions deem restraint lawful under strict policy and practice guidelines when it is necessary to protect people from imminent risk to their health or safety (Muir-Cochrane and Holmes 2001) but it is this assessment that is problematic in terms of whether or not the use of restraint is warranted. From an ethical perspective coercive interventions can only be justified when the imminent risk or danger to the patient or others is deemed paramount over the autonomy of individuals and the removal of their liberty. Yet the overuse of seclusion in some population groups, for example psychiatric in-patient units indicates that there is potential for misuse of restraint in certain circumstances (Fernando 1991). Autonomy is closely associated with assessment of competency (Kendrick 1991). Restraining an individual implies that he or she is incompetent and it is often justified based on paternalistic principles of care. However, the proactive restraining of a patient based on a risk assessment may not be legally justified because such predictions of aggression and violence are notably unreliable (Muir-Cochrane and Holmes 2001). Given the legal and ethical implications for the restraint of patients, it is useful to consider both the perspective of people with a mental illness and the relatively recent emergence of the recovery approach, as the next section describes.

Recovery

The recovery approach emerged in the 1990s as a person-centred, pragmatic method underpinned by tenets of social justice, autonomy, and equity (Barker and Buchanan-Barker 2010). It is a philosophy, a framework, and a model with many different sub-genres, but is essentially on the person's potential, on symptom management, and the avoidance of labelling. While the recovery approach emerged alongside mental health reforms in the western world, it continues to sit in uncomfortable juxtaposition to traditional mainstream biomedical psychiatry. Nonetheless, recovery-oriented mental health service approaches exist in many parts of the world; New Zealand, for example, has recovery competencies for mental health workers (Mental Health Commission of New Zealand 2001). Principles of the recovery approach include protecting patients' rights, understanding discrimination and social exclusion and the impact these have on people with a mental illness, and supporting patients' personal resourcefulness. How the recovery approach sits alongside restraint practices in psychiatric units has received little attention in the research literature to date and is an area that requires further investigation. Despite the calls for the elimination of seclusion and restraint, restraint remains commonplace, acceptable, if not vital, to many health professionals, who believe that they cannot provide a safe environment without such strategies. The next section explores how the concept of risk and zero tolerance has affected practices in psychiatric settings and how these concepts have reinforced the removal of autonomy from psychiatric patients.

Risk in Psychiatric Practice

Exploring the influence that conceptualizations of risk have on the continued and widespread use of restraint in health care settings is useful. Risk assessment in the field of health care is acknowledged as existing within a contemporary framework of "a risk aversive culture" (Cleary et al. 2009: 644). MacNeela et al. (2010) suggest that such an orientation toward risk assessment in inpatient settings is a function of the types of patients admitted, while authors such as Crowe and Carlye (2003) have pointed to an increase in a focus on risk across a range of social settings, tying its predominance in mental health care to key historical, cultural, political, and economic processes.

Prior to the late 1990s, the concept of risk was not widely used in relation to a patient's condition. As Lupton (1999) outlined, the idea of risk entered mainstream health and social policies without critical analysis. A risk-aversive culture emerged in school playgrounds in the United Kingdom when children were prevented from climbing trees to collect conkers (horse chestnuts) (Drennan and McConnell 2007). It has also emerged in other aspects of society, including psychiatric wards where it was used to reduce the possibility of harm to patients (Brooke 2006).

Today, risk assessment has been identified as a significant part of everyday clinical psychiatric practice (Godin 2004, Muir-Cochrane and Wand 2005). Since its introduction, the term "needs assessment", which included a professional assessment of a person's abilities and disabilities (symptoms) and helped to create individualized care plans, has all but vanished, with risk assessment now the core mandatory assessment task of mental health professionals for patients admitted to a hospital ward or acute care unit.

Risk in psychiatric practice primarily refers to negative outcomes – a range of potentially adverse events that need to be avoided at all costs (Kettles et al. 2004, Muir-Cochrane and Wand 2005). The UK Department of Health defines risk as "[t]he nature, severity, imminence, frequency/duration and likelihood of harm to self or others" and as a "hazard that is to be identified, measured and ultimately, prevented" (2007: 57). Specifically, these risks include violence, aggression, absconding (leaving without permission), and substance abuse (Muir-Cochrane and Mosel 2009). Focusing solely on risk assessment creates an immediate deficit in approaches to care, in that a person's level of psychosis, aggression, capacity for self-harm and/or suicidal behaviour becomes a problem to be thwarted or forestalled and not a "need" to be attended to. Under the umbrella of safety, risks have to be managed, reduced and eliminated despite this being an impossible task that results in increased control and surveillance of psychiatric patients.

The most basic example of coercive care to eliminate risk can be seen under official Mental Health Acts, where individuals can be subjected to confinement in a psychiatric facility against their own volition. For example, the *Mental Health Act 2009* (SA), s.2 (21;1) states that a person can be held involuntarily if a) it is decided that he or she has a mental illness; (b) that because of the mental illness, the person requires treatment for his or her own protection from harm (including harm involved in the continuation or deterioration of the person's condition) or for the protection of others from harm; and (c) that there is no less restrictive means than detention to ensure appropriate treatment of the person's illness.

Risk assessment requires a careful consideration of the consequences of the risk behaviour (the hazard) –an understanding of the harmful behaviour, the likelihood of it occurring and its severity (Vinestock 1996). Cutcliffe and Stevenson (2008), in their discussion of suicide prevention initiatives, believe that definitions of mental illness and policy focus on control and management, and result in a situation where "the 'problem of suicide' is seen to reside in individuals who thus need to be controlled, contained, and/or managed, and this inevitably means controlling, and/or containing, and/or managing the risk" (345). Indeed, risk assessment and management in mental health care occurs within wider discourses regarding methods and approaches to assessing risk, how the process is undertaken by mental health professionals, and the nature of this assessment and management (Godin 2004, Littlechild and Hawley 2010).

While a risk assessment is meant to protect the individual, family and community, it can also be seen as a safety measure for the health care providers as well as a way to minimize litigation for the institution involved (Raven and Rix 1999). While there is evidence that aggression and violence towards health professionals is increasing, the imposition of zero tolerance policies to manage verbal and physical aggression in psychiatric units denies a place for normal expression of heightened emotions for patients who are severely unwell or under duress. This is not to say that aggression is acceptable but allowing patients to verbally let off steam may be more appropriate and helpful than forcibly restraining them and placing them in seclusion because they lost their temper. In such circumstances it is not difficult to understand how patients might interpret these practices as punishment rather than therapeutic measures for their behaviour. Further, despite risk assessments being mandatory on psychiatric inpatients, relatively little literature examines "how" health professionals empirically assess risk (Littlechild and Hawley 2010), or how effective zero tolerance is in psychiatric practice in general (Skiba 2000). Holmes (2006) argued that zero tolerance is indeed an ineffective response to the management of violence and that its adoption in Australian mental health services should be reversed. Associated research also suggests that the problem of violence may be misunderstood – that organizations that focus on training as the first approach fail to recognize that the violence is primarily a function of interpersonal conflict (Paterson, Leadbetter, and Miller 2005).

Perhaps as a consequence of zero tolerance and risk management policies, there appears to be a re-stigmatization of patients with a mental illness in mainstream health care. In Australia, for example, the Royal Flying Doctor Service will not transfer any patients with a mental illness unless they are first sedated intravenously.

This restraint approach has crept into ambulance services in at least two Australian states and ambulances now carry "netting" that physically restrains psychiatric patients in the vehicle as a safety management tool.

This shift away from care to control has been debated in the mental health nursing literature. Much attention has been focused on the increased emphasis on risk management and "defensive and coercive practices such as locked voluntary units, increased rates of involuntary detention, restraint, sedation and seclusion, formal observation levels, zero tolerance policies and a preoccupation with the assessment of risk" (Wand and White 2007: 785). These strategies and practices have occurred without a reflection on an evidence-based practice that questions the accuracy and efficacy of risk assessment approaches in health care (McNiel and Binder 1995, Kapur et al. 2005). The next section discusses the current research on conflict and containment in psychiatric units.

Contemporary Research into Restraint and Seclusion

Factors influencing Restraint and Seclusion

Research has identified a number of factors which influence the use of coercive measures. These include patient demographics and clinical presentation (Gerace et al. 2013, Keski-Valkama et al. 2010); ward culture, such as when restraint is considered appropriate and for which types of behaviour (Fisher 1994); staff characteristics such as gender mix and experience (Bowers et al. 2013); administrative and staff changes (Fisher 1994, O'Connor et al. 2004); physical ward environment (Borckardt et al. 2011); level of training provided to staff in handling risk situations (Fisher 2003); and individual attitudes toward restraint and seclusion and beliefs about alternatives to restraint (Happell and Koehn 2011, Strumpf and Evans 1988). Factors such as these are also likely to be interactive. For example, an individual's diagnosis (e.g., dementia or psychosis) and the prevalent diagnoses in a ward (e.g., number of patients with such a diagnosis) are likely to influence the ward environment, resources required of nursing staff, and the nature of care needed. Indeed, factors which have been identified by Fisher (2003) as reducing restraint, including high level administrative endorsement, recipient participation, culture change, training, data analysis, and individualized treatment, likely have a role to play in restraint and seclusion differences within and between services.

Outcomes for Patients

Restraint and seclusion have received research and clinical attention as a result of the potential "serious deleterious physical and (more often) psychological effects on patients" (Fisher 1994: 1588). A series of reports in the U.S. newspaper, the *Hartford Courant*, in 1998 (Weiss et al. 1998) brought national community attention to the dangers of containment measures and called for legislative change. Based on a 50-state survey, the articles documented 142 deaths over a decade during or following the use of restraint and seclusion in psychiatric and intellectual disability facilities and group homes in the U.S. A later systematic review by Evans, Wood and Lambert (2003) reported sudden deaths following mechanical restraint, and that patients can die through vest strangulation or being caught in bedrails. The literature has also documented outcomes including infection, falls and fall-related injury, declines in cognitive functioning, declines in activities of daily living, and subsequent mortality (Engberg, Castle, and McCaffrey 2008, Evans, Wood, and Lambert 2003)

Patients view restraint and seclusion as highly coercive interventions. One study found that of 11 interventions used in inpatient settings, net beds, mechanical restraint, intramuscular medication, locked-door seclusion, and physical restraint had the lowest approval ratings among service users (Whittington et al. 2009). Meehan, Vermeer and Windsor (2000) found that patients perceived the practices associated with seclusion (e.g., removal of clothing, force) as consistent with punishment. Participants felt that they had not been given information about either ward rules that might lead to seclusion or about seclusion itself (e.g., how long it would last), but "were also acutely aware of what they considered were the unspoken 'rules' of seclusion" (374). They also found that patients were dissatisfied with the interaction with staff during and after the seclusion (e.g., lack of debriefing).

A range of negative emotions have been documented from those who have undergone restraint and seclusion, including anger, fear, humiliation, resistance, powerlessness, and resignation (Mayers et al. 2010, Meehan, Vermmer, and Windsor 2000, Strumpf and Evans 1988), as well as exacerbation of previous trauma (Brockardt et al. 2011, Cusack et al. 2003, Sambrano and Cox 2013). Patients may view basic needs, such as toileting, eating, and drinking, as not being adequately met (Kontio et al. 2012). Patients have reported that they did not think seclusion and restraint were necessary interventions during their treatment (Soininen et al. 2013). While some patients report positive aspects to these coercive measures (e.g., seclusion allowing them to feel safe and regain control), this often relates to factors such as the nature of the seclusion room and staff observation and interaction during the episode (Van Der Merwe et al. 2013). In addition, although research has found that health professionals are aware of the negative experiences of patients who are secluded, they nonetheless believe that seclusion is a therapeutic and necessary intervention (Van Der Merwe et al. 2013).

We now turn to selected contemporary research conducted in different care settings that use containment measures.

Acute Adult Care

Patients admitted to psychiatric facilities in an acute phase of psychiatric illness are of particular risk to themselves or others and are often hospitalized involuntarily (Bowers et al. 2008, Mosel, Gerace and Muir-Cochrane 2010). Aggression and violence toward staff and other patients are frequent behaviours in these acute-care psychiatric settings (Daffern and Howells 2002, Frueh et al. 2005, Gudjonsson, Rabe-Hesketh, and Szmukler 2004). Not surprisingly, issues of conflict and containment come into play here as staff attempt to provide a safe *and* therapeutic environment. This is particularly important for, as Knutzen et al. (2011: 492) contend, "[f]or some patients, the inpatient admission is their first experience of mental health services". A substantial number of hospitalized psychiatric patients have experienced seclusion and/or restraint (Cusack et al. 2003), and perceive it to be extremely distressing (Frueh et al. 2005). The use of restraint and seclusion can adversely affect patient attitudes toward subsequent treatment and engagement with services (Grunbaugh et al. 2007).

Rates of restraint and seclusion vary due to factors such as methods of calculation, data available, and particular ward structure and procedures (Bowers 2000). However, recent studies shed light on the continued use of the procedures. Studies in Canada, the United States, and Australia have reported rates of seclusion and restraint of between 15–31% of admitted patients over a one- or two-year period (Dumais et al. 2011, Hendryx et al. 2010, Tunde-Ayinmode and Little 2004). On five English acute psychiatric wards seclusion was used in 35.9% (aggression toward staff) and 25% (aggression toward another patient) of aggressive incidents, and restraint used in 12.4% (staff) and 6.3% (patients) of incidents (Foster, Bowers and Nijman 2007). Studies conducted over lengthier periods of time have suggested little change or some increase in the use of restraint and seclusion (Keski-Valkama et al. 2010, Luckhoff et al. 2013).

In terms of patient and admission characteristics associated with the use of restraint and seclusion in this setting (see Dumais et al. 2011, Keski-Valkama et al. 2010, Knutzen et al. 2011, Tunde-Ayinmode and Little 2004), having a diagnosis of a schizophrenic disorder or psychosis, substance use-related disorder, bipolar disorder, or personality disorder have emerged as being associated with the use of restraint or seclusion. Restraint and seclusion often occur early in admission, with patients who have a longer hospitalization and those under an involuntary hospitalization order. Gender and age have been more inconsistent in their relationship with seclusion and restraint. In a study by Gudjonsson et al. (2004) of violent incidents in 14 general adult wards, consistent predictors of emergency medication, seclusion or physical restraint included a nurse being the target of the incident, patient agitation, and attempting to abscond.

Of concern are the hours some patients spend in restraint or seclusion (e.g., median seclusion room stay of 12.5 hours in a study by Dumais et al. 2011), the repeated use of the methods with patients (Hendryx et al. 2010), and how an intervention prior to the use of restrictive measures is often not documented (Tunde-Ayinmode and Little 2004). This makes particularly pertinent the conclusions of Knutzen et al. (2011: 496) that "use of restraint must be regarded as an indication of mutual distrust", suggesting that individual, collaborative, and trauma-informed care from an early stage of the admission is needed to reduce coercive measures.

Emergency Care

There has been surprisingly little research into restraint and seclusion use in emergency departments and services (D'Orio et al. 2004). Work, however, is needed as emergency department health professionals encounter psychiatric presentations in increasing numbers due to changes to inpatient and outpatient services, and the consequent increasing role of emergency departments in both emergency and routine treatment (Allen and Currier 2004, Dolan and Fein 2011). The potential relationship of the nature of emergency departments and restraint and seclusion is also compelling. The nature of emergency departments being "a high-stimulation environment" (Dolan and Fein 2011: e1357) could be particularly problematic for those presenting with psychiatric issues, and encounters between patients and staff are of a time-limited nature or may not be specialized (Woo et al. 2007). Knox and Holloman (2012) conceptualized the emergency department similarly to that of Knutzen et al. (2011) in their discussion of acute care (see above), and contend that "the goal [is] of getting that patient into ongoing psychiatric treatment to minimize the likelihood of another decompensation and emergency department encounter" (39).

One study of US hospitals with an emergency department reported that 27.8% used seclusion, with most seclusion rooms located in the department (Zun and Downey 2005). Recent research has indicated that rates of restraint and seclusion and their duration vary across emergency departments. Psychosis and substance use-related presentations, as well as younger age, are associated with the use of the measures, and these methods are often accompanied by other methods such as chemical restraint or involuntary medication (Allen and Currier 2004, Currier, Walsh and Lawrence 2011, Pamungkas 2012, Zun 2003, Zun and Downey 2005).

The relationship between restraint and seclusion and subsequent outcomes are complex. Patients have been found to have a lower probability of subsequent psychiatric inpatient hospitalization (Unick et al. 2011), but also a lower probability of attending their first outpatient psychiatry appointment (Currier, Walsh and Lawrence 2011) when restrained in an emergency service. Indeed, while some researchers have considered seclusion a lesser restrictive measure than restraints (Huf, Coutinho, and Adams 2012), these same researchers have documented low levels of satisfaction as well as adverse effects associated with either method. This would suggest the need for prevention of seclusion or restraint use. Indeed, there is some evidence that procedures for early assessment and management of problematic behaviours, including verbal de-escalation, time out, medication for symptoms, and increased monitoring of patients are associated with statistically significant reductions in restraint and seclusion in a psychiatric emergency service (D'Orio et al. 2004).

Older Persons' Care

The containment of older persons is a particularly unique consideration when discussing its use in psychiatric settings. One reason is because of the potential outcomes to physical and mental capacity (e.g., cognitive functioning, activities of daily living, walking dependence) subsequent to restraint (Engberg, Castle, and McCaffrey 2008). Health professionals treating older persons must also address issues of patient autonomy and understanding (Strumpf and Evans 1988), and how promotion of physical wellbeing can exist alongside consideration of overall wellbeing (Gastmans and Milisen 2006). Minnick et al. (2007) suggest that it was concerns regarding the use of restraint with older persons that drove initial attempts to reduce use of the practice.

Restraint use with older persons has been associated with dementia and cognitive impairment, patient mobility and need for assistance in walking, functioning in activities of daily living, impaired speech, and behaviours such as shouting, aggression, and restlessness (DeSantis, Engberg, and Rogers 1997, Karlsson et al. 1996). Rates of restraint and seclusion in older persons' psychiatric settings have been reported to be quite high (27.1% of patients in DeSantis et al., and 45% in Karlsson et al.) and, like other care settings, to vary widely (O'Connor et al. 2004). In our own work investigating the use of restraint in acute and extended psychiatric services for older persons in one psychiatric hospital (Gerace et al. 2013), there was considerable variation in the use of physical and mechanical restraint between five wards. Restraint was associated with a diagnosis of an organic, including symptomatic mental disorder (dementia being the main diagnosis), and was predominantly used to manage aggression and falls. Restraint occurred quite early in admission (50% of patients in the ward with the most restraint were restrained 17.50 hours into their admission). Other wards exhibited considerably lesser restraint, with factors such as differences in acuity and patient diagnoses emerging as potential explanations. Indeed, on the basis of two of their studied wards not having seclusion rooms, O'Connor et al. (2004: 799) questioned whether this method has "a valid place in modern aged psychiatric practice".

In our research and that of others, the importance of increased attention to the purposes of aggressive, self-harming, or wandering behaviours in older persons has been advocated (Gerace et al. 2013). Frameworks for understanding these behaviours include the need-driven, dementia-compromised behaviour model (Algase et al. 1996) and the Progressively Lowered Stress Threshold model (Hall and Buckwalter 1987, Smith et al. 2004). The continued use of restraint to prevent falls is also concerning, as evidence for restraint being a method of fall and injury prevention is lacking (Oliver et al. 2007).

Chemical Restraint

In comparison to other forms of restraint and containment, chemical restraint has received much less attention in the literature (Bilanakis, Papamichael, and Peritogiannis 2011). Chemical restraint is defined as the use of pharmaceuticals to sedate patients deemed "out of control" and includes the administration of medication intramuscularly or by rapid intravenous injection. Many professional associations, including the American Medical Association, American Psychiatric

Association, and British Psychiatric Association, emphasize the use of the least restrictive measures being implemented prior to the use of any form of restraint. However, the concept of chemical restraint involves a discussion as to whether the medication is given as part of a treatment regimen or to control a patient's behaviour (Currier and Allen 2000), or, indeed, both. Further, the use of chemical restraint is often used in combination with other forms of restraint so determination of the effectiveness of individual forms of restraint is not easily possible.

In one study there was no difference in the number of males or females being chemically restrained, nor whether they were homeless or under the influence of drugs on admission. Having a diagnosis of schizophrenia was, however, significant (Husum et al. 2010). As discussed in relation to other forms of restraint in the adult inpatient population, having a diagnosis of schizophrenia and being psychotic is a risk factor for experiencing chemical restraint. In a study by Grenyer et al. (2013) of patients classified as repeatedly aggressive, 41.9% of aggressive incidents were handled with intramuscular injection, with fewer incidents handled with oral medication (12.9%) and intravenous injection (3.2%). Dack, Ross and Bowers (2012) found that higher use of intramuscular medication on an acute ward (regardless of whether a patient reported being subject to it) was associated with lesser approval from patients of other types of coercive measure.

Locked Doors

Locking doors to control entry to or exit from acute care wards has undergone change, particularly since the middle of the twentieth century when there was an increased move to providing care in open wards (Ashmore 2008). Increases in locking of acute, non-forensic wards have been documented, with some wards permanently locked or locked for substantial periods of time (Van Der Merwe et al. 2009).

A review of locked doors literature found that "[b]oth staff and patients recognized the need for staff to be in control, but they felt that this control came at the expense of the patients' freedom" (Van Der Merwe et al. 2009: 297). Patients have reported feeling safe when the ward doors are locked, such as through the ability to control entry by unwanted visitors (Adams 2000, Haglund and Von Essen 2005). At the same time, they report feelings of depression and sadness when a ward door is locked; a sense of constraint and frustration; and perception of the ward space as one of incarceration and control by staff, rather than one of therapeutic interaction between staff and patients (Muir-Cochrane et al. 2012).

The implications of locking doors are both physical and psychological. Voluntary patients need to ask a nurse to open the door to allow them to leave the space, which leads to questions regarding their rights as non-compulsory held patients. Patients have reported that "the locked door symbolized their outcast status, and an open door inclusion in the normal everyday world" (Muir-Cochrane et al. 2012: 45). Indeed, Bowers et al. (1999) found that patients who had absconded reported that they had felt isolated from family and friends, as well as unable to meet everyday responsibilities pertaining to their own roles as carers or maintenance of their homes. They could also feel "trapped and claustrophobic" (202). This is in contradiction to research suggesting that staff lock doors to prevent absconding (Van Der Merwe et al. 2009). Nurses acknowledge that patients are often not given information or communication about changes in a door's status or the reasons for it (Ashmore 2008).

Adams (2000) described a locked-door policy on four acute psychiatric wards, resulting from risk management requirements and increases in close observation (with consequent lesser time for nurse therapeutic activity), sentinel events, unwanted visitors, and substance use. Adams commented that "[n]owadays most people keep their house door locked during the day as well as at night. There is a parallel with the requirements of safety for in-patients" (327). While the duty of care of health care staff to maintain patient and ward safety is indeed paramount, restriction of patient movement via locked doors is a somewhat different case to a homeowner making a decision to lock the doors on their personal property.

Indeed, while a locked door policy may have a number of potential desirable elements, patients and staff can feel uneasy during the process. Ashmore (2008) found that nursing staff were often unaware of policy around locking doors, and patients often not informed or informed with little information on reasons. In addition, the use of locking doors and other exit security measures to reduce the use of alcohol and other substances has been questioned in recent research (Simpson et al. 2011). An ethnographic study by Johansson, Skarsater, and Danielson (2006) conceptualized the environment on a locked psychiatric ward as involving staff exerting control through legal rules and procedures, with patients (and sometimes staff) often lacking control and trying to be heard.

Absconding

Absconding from inpatient psychiatric care, while not a coercive intervention, is an important issue for the present discussion. This is because of its relationship with locking wards doors, and the use of restraint and seclusion to prevent its occurrence (Bowers et al. 2010, Bowers et al. 2011). Absconding affects the patients, staff, and families. Since absconding is often defined and recorded as an involuntary patient who is held under mental health legislation leaving the ward/hospital (Muir-Cochrane and Mosel 2008), there are legal implications of absconding. These include the need to notify authorities, and to report and search for the patient (Meehan, Morrison and McDougall 1999). Patients leaving hospital without permission can come to harm or pose a risk to others, with Dickens and Campbell (2001) reporting 16.2% of absconding episodes they studied resulted in "serious adverse outcomes" (self-harm, violence, committing offences, and sexual exploitation) (548). Missed treatment and medication are also of concern.

In our own research in Australia we found that over a one-year period, approximately 12% of detained patients on acute and extended care psychiatric wards absconded (Muir-Cochrane et al. 2011). These patients were younger than patients who did not abscond, and nearly 80% of them had a schizophrenic disorder. Patients often abscond early in their admission, and a significant minority do so repeatedly (Meehan, Morrison, and McDougall 1999, Mosel, Gerace, and Muir-Cochrane 2010). In spite of being used as a strategy to prevent absconding (Muir-Cochrane et al. 2012), whether a ward was predominantly "open" or "locked" was not found to be a significant predictor of preventing absconding (Muir-Cochrane et al. 2011, see also Dickens and Campbell 2001).

Identified reasons for absconding in studies which have interviewed patients shortly after returning to the ward have found that fear, boredom, dislike of activities and rules, stress of the ward, believing they did not need to be there, and leaving to attend to issues at home were raised (Meehan, Morrison and McDougall 1999). Utilizing Moore's conceptualization of "opportunity-takers" and "opportunity-makers" in absconding events, Dickens and Campbell (2001: 550) stress "the need to address issues both of physical security and skilful mental health care in managing absconding risk". Indeed, as Bowers et al. (1999: 204) outlined, "[m]ental disorder clearly plays some role in absconding, but not by itself. To write everything off as irrational behaviour means that listening to the patients will cease and understanding disappear".

In a recent study (Muir-Cochrane et al. 2013) we drew on work on therapeutic landscapes to examine how person and place interact in the psychiatric ward, and can be used to understand absconding. The overarching finding was that the ward could be perceived as a "safe" or "unsafe" place by patients. This perception was influenced by individual illness factors; positive or negative interactions and relationships with caregivers, including feeling listened to, staff being available, and being respected; fear of other consumers; and the physical space. The space could also represent unfamiliarity and fear, lack of autonomy, and "being jailed" in a prison-like environment. Participants differed on how they perceived these aspects as either safe or unsafe, stressing the importance of individualized treatment and communication. This highlights the importance of environment and other ward factors in attempting to manage conflict on the ward and the use of containment measures (Dickens and Campbell 2001, Papadopoulos et al. 2012).

Discussion

As Szasz (1997) identified, the use of coercive measures in psychiatry is culturally engrained and accepted as a practice of "care". The risk aversive and zero tolerant landscape in health care generally and in psychiatry specifically, facilitates continuing acceptance of containment measures that would not be deemed reasonable or appropriate in any other setting. When such containment measures are implemented as punishment (which patients believe they often are), this constitutes a humiliating breach of human rights, violating principles within the Universal Declaration of Human Rights (Morrall and Muir-Cochrane 2002).

The research evidence discussed in this chapter provides a comprehensive analysis of issues associated with the use of containment measures in psychiatric care. There are many factors affecting the decision to use restrictive measures, including environmental, social, physical, and economic, which influence staff decision-making and serve to perpetuate their use.

The safety and dignity of patients within psychiatric settings is being given increasing attention in the literature (Robins et al. 2005). Patients have reported negative experiences of aspects of hospitalization that include insensitive, neglectful, inappropriate care that has been named "sanctuary harm" (Robins et al. 2005). Such treatment appears to be provided in environments which have a philosophy of physical separation with an emphasis on physical boundaries and exclusion (Bowers et al. 2010). These environments also operate using situation and environmental variables aimed at complete control of the ward. Such a conformist and controlling discourse reinforces the acceptability of de-humanizing practices and the misuse of restraint and seclusion, and the need for staff to remain in complete control at all times (Paterson et al. 2013).

In the past decades authors have posited that high levels of control in psychiatric institutions enabled staff to maintain high levels of efficiency, in a conformist environment designed to maintain the *status quo* of the ward routine and reduce anxiety associated with the working environment (Menzies 1970, Brown 1973, Beardshaw 1981). As this chapter has described, it seems little has changed other than the justification of containment measures within an alternative ideology, that of risk assessment and zero tolerance. The need in health care to mitigate risk requires a trade-off (Smithson 2010); and that is patient freedom. Although "violence by people with mental illness commonly evokes moral outrage" (Szmukler and Rose 2013: 126), serious violence and homicide by people with a mental illness is not a common event, although media reports suggest otherwise.

There are many sequelae for the provision of care when risk assessment is the dominant discourse in psychiatric wards. Risk assessment and management are time consuming and take time away from other more therapeutic engagement activities with patients. Further, risk assessment can be seen to reduce the potential for trust between staff and patients and reinforce stigma and discrimination against people with a mental illness. At the same time, the current focus in mental health care on a recovery framework (Anthony 1993, Deegan 1988) has important implications for risk assessment and management. Theories and models have been developed such as the Tidal Model of Mental Health Recovery (Barker and Buchanan-Barker 2005), which focuses on consumers' individual goals, voice, and resources, the potential for change and growth, and a transparent and collaborative relationship between the consumer and the professional. However, a "philosophical tension between the *person*-focus of recovery and the *patient* (or illness) focus of psychiatric medicine" (Buchanan-Barker and Barker 2008: 94) can exist, and consumer perspectives on recovery often differ from more traditional notions of mental illness. Within Australia, policy and service reform to implement the main principles has been identified as important to maintaining a recovery focus (Ramon, Healy, and Renouf 2007, Rickwood 2005), and inherent in such principles is, indeed, the notion of risk:

> [recovery] is a complex and multifaceted concept, both a process and an outcome, the features of which include strength, self-agency and hope, interdependency and giving, and systematic effort, which entails risk-taking (Ramon, Healy, and Renouf 2007: 119).

The challenge exists, therefore, in the practical implementation of a balance between a focus on the risk a consumer is seen to pose, particularly in areas where risk to others and self is involved, and the development of "a respectful and considered therapeutic relationship [which] assists the patient to achieve a sense of ownership and responsibility for their mental illness, treatment and risk management" (Kelly, Simmons, and Gregory 2002: 208).

If we consider restraint and seclusion as treatment failure (Paterson et al. 2013) then we can address the problem of coercion by exploring ways to improve the practices of health professionals and use restraint strategies as a last resort only. Nevertheless it is important to remember the impact of the media on the attitude of the public to people with a mental illness and the pressure that health professionals are under to prevent harm to patients at any cost. The fear of litigation for health professionals is another motivating factor to use controlling mechanisms to attempt to guarantee patient safety. It is a paradox that in doing so, patients are subjected to psychological ill effects in staff's attempts to reduce physical harm. At a fundamental level, relationships between patients and staff need to be a priority of effective care. Trust, mutual respect, and shared care planning can reduce the likelihood of conflict between patients and staff. If positive and respectful communication between staff and patients can become a basic expectation of care in acute psychiatric units, the reduction and potential elimination of restrictive practices can be a realistic, achievable goal. One such contemporary approach is sensory modulation, detailed below.

Possibilities for Care

Sensory modulation is a relatively new approach, which emerged from Occupational Therapy (Champagne 2003) to assist patients regain a sense of calm. In acute psychiatric units, dedicated sensory modulation rooms with sensory equipment (sensory rooms/chill rooms) can be used when patients are distressed (Te Pou 2010). Sensory tools can include weighted blankets, aromatherapy, lava lamps, music, fish tanks, and squeeze balls. Although there is limited evidence of the efficacy of this approach (Champagne and Sayer 2003), the literature suggests that sensory modulation is better than no treatment and as effective as traditional methods. Certainly this approach is humane, person-centred, and fits well within a recovery framework, as it empowers patients to establish self-soothing strategies that can be used to assist them to remain in control when they are agitated when acutely unwell, as well as in everyday life when having left hospital. For the implementation of this approach to occur there needs to be the political will within institutions as well as financial support to make required environmental changes. Further training and education of health professionals is required to ensure effective and sustainable culture change. This is certainly possible as has been demonstrated in New Zealand where widespread adoption of sensory modulation has seen the reduction of the use of restraint and seclusion and improved patient experience of hospitalization.

Conclusion

Containment practices, including restraint of various kinds, seclusion, locked doors, and conflict behaviours such as absconding are negative experiences for both patients and staff and occur in a climate in psychiatric settings of control versus care. The dominant discourse of a risk-averse and zero-tolerant environment has facilitated such an environment, one which is antithetical to a recovery-based, patient-centred approach. There are many possibilities to move the function of psychiatric settings from coercion to care as have also been described in this chapter. The importance of evidenced based interventions and a collaborative partnership between health professionals and patients cannot be overstated.

References

Adams, B. 2000. Locked doors or sentinel nurses? *Psychiatric Bulletin, 24*, 327–328.

Algase, D.L., Beck, C.B., Kolanowski, A., Whall, A., Berent, S., Richards, K., and Beattie, E. 1996. Need-driven dementia-compromised behavior: An alternative view of disruptive behavior. *American Journal of Alzheimer's Disease, 11*(6), 10–19.

Allen, M.H. and Currier, G.W. 2004. Use of restraints and pharmacotherapy in academic psychiatric emergency services. *General Hospital Psychiatry, 26*, 42–49.

Anthony, W. 1993. Recovery from mental illness: The guiding vision of the mental health service system in the 1990s. *Psychosocial Rehabilitation Journal, 16*, 11–23.

Ashmore, R. 2008. Nurses' accounts of locked ward doors: Ghosts of the asylum or acute care in the 21st century. *Journal of Psychiatric and Mental Health Nursing, 15*, 175–185.

Bak, J., Brandt-Christensen, M., Sestoft, D., and Zoffmann, V. 2012. Mechanical restraint – which interventions prevent episodes of mechanical restraint – a systematic review. *Perspectives in Psychiatric Care, 48*, 83–94.

Barker, P. and Buchanan-Barker, P. 2005. *The Tidal Model: A Guide for Mental Health Professionals*. London: Brunner-Routledge.

Barker, P. and Buchanan-Barker, P. 2010. The Tidal Model of Mental Health Recovery and Reclamation: Application in acute care settings. *Issues in Mental Health Nursing, 31*, 171–180.

Beardshaw, V. 1981. *Conscientious Objectors at Work, Mental Hospital Nurses: A Case Study*. London: Social Audit.

Bilanakis, N., Papamichael, G., and Peritogiannis, V. 2011. Chemical restraint in routine clinical practice: A report from a general hospital psychiatric ward in greece. *Annals of General Psychiatry, 10*, 4.

Bowers, L. 2000. The expression and comparison of ward incident rates. *Issues in Mental Health Nursing, 21*, 365–374.

Bowers, L., Flood, C., Brennan, G., and Allan, T. 2008. A replication study of the City nurse intervention: Reducing conflict and containment on three acute psychiatric wards. *Journal of Psychiatric and Mental Health Nursing, 15*, 737–742.

Bowers, L., Jarrett, M., Clark, N., Kiyimba, F., and Mcfarlane, L. 1999. Absconding: Why patients leave. *Journal of Psychiatric and Mental Health Nursing, 6*, 199–205.

Bowers, L., Simpson, A., Alexander, J., Ryan, C., and Carr-Walker, P. 2004. Cultures of psychiatry and the professional socialization process: The case of containment methods for disturbed patients. *Nurse Education Today, 24*, 435–442.

Bowers, L., Stewart, D., Papadopoulos, C., and Iennaco, J.D. 2013. Correlation between levels of conflict and containment on acute psychiatric wards: the City-128 study. *Psychiatric Services, 64*, 423-430.

Bowers, L., Van Der Merwe, M., Nijman, H., Hamilton, B., Noorthoorn, E., Stewart, D., and Muir-Cochrane, E. 2010. The practice of seclusion and time-out on english acute psychiatric wards: The city-128 study. *Archives of Psychiatric Nursing, 24*, 275–286.

Brockardt, J.J., Madan, A., Grunbaugh, A.L., Danielson, C.K., Pelic, C.G., and Hardesty, S.J. 2011. Systematic investigation of initiatives to reduce seclusion and restraint in a state psychiatric hospital. *Psychiatric Services, 62*, 477–483.

Brooke, C. 2006. Killjoy officials accused of 'nanny state' madness as they take children's conkers. *Mail Online* [Online, 9 October] Available at: http://www.dailymail.co.uk/news/article-409507/Killjoy-officials-accused-nanny-state-madness-childrens-conkers.html [accessed: 18 March 2013].

Brown, G. 1973. The mental hospital as an institution. *Journal of Social Science and Medicine, 7*, 407–424.

Buchanan-Barker, P. and Barker, P. 2008. The tidal commitments: Extending the value base of mental health recovery. *Journal of Psychiatric and Mental Health Nursing, 15*, 93–100.

Champagne, T. 2003. *Sensory Modulation and Environment: Elements of Occupation*. Southampton, MA: Champagne Conferences.

Champagne, T. and Sayer, E. 2003. *The Effects of the Use of the Sensory Room in Psychiatry* [Online] Available at: http://www.ot-innovations.com/pdf_files/QI_STUDY_Sensory_Room.pdf [accessed 27 March 2013].

Cleary, M., Hunt, G.E., Walter, G., and Robertson, M. 2009. Locked inpatient units in modern mental health care: values and practice issues. *Journal of Medical Ethics, 35*, 644–646.

Cotter, V. 2005. Restraint free care in older adults with dementia. *The Keio Journal of Medicine, 54*, 80–84.

Crowe, M. and Carlyle, D. 2003. Deconstructing risk assessment and management in mental health nursing. *Journal of Advanced Nursing, 43*, 19–27.

Currier, G.W. and Allen, M.H. 2000. Physical and chemical restraint in the psychiatric emergency service. *Psychiatric Services, 51*, 717–719.

Currier, G.W., Walsh, P., and Lawrence, D. 2011. Physical restraints in the emergency department and attendance at subsequent outpatient psychiatric treatment. *Journal of Psychiatric Practice, 17*, 387–393.

Cusack, K.J., Frueh, B.C., Hiers, T.G., Suffoletta-Maierle, S., and Bennett, S. 2003. Trauma within the psychiatric setting: A preliminary empirical report. *Administration and Policy in Mental Health, 30*, 453–460.

Cutcliffe, J. and Stevenson, C. 2008. Never the twain? Reconciling national suicide prevention strategies with the practice, educational and policy needs of mental health nurses. *International Journal of Mental Health Nursing, 17*, 341–350.

Dack, C., Ross, J., and Bowers, L. 2012. The relationship between attitudes towards different containment measures and their usage in a nationl sample of psychiatric inpatients. *Journal of Psychiatric and Mental Health Nursing, 19*, 577–586.

Daffern, M. and Howells, K. 2002. Psychiatric inpatient aggression: A review of structural and functional assessment approaches. *Aggression and Violent Behavior, 7*, 477–497.

De Bellis, A., Mosel, K., Curren, D., Prendergast, J., Harrington, A., and Muir-Cochrane, E. 2013. Education on physical restraint reduction in dementia care: A review of the literature. *Dementia, 12*, 93–110.

Deegan, P. 1988. Recovery: The lived experience of rehabilitlation. *Psychosocial Rehabilitation Journal, 11*, 11–19.

D'Orio, B.M., Purselle, D., Stevens, D., and Garlow, S.J. 2004. Reduction of episodes of seclusion and restraint in a psychiatric emergency service. *Psychiatric Services, 55*, 581–583.

Department of Health. 2007. *Best Practice in Managing Risk: Principles and Evidence for Best Practice in the Assessment and Management of Risk to Self and Others in Mental Health Services*. United Kingdom: Department of Health.

Department of Health. 2008. *Code of Practice: Mental Health Act 1983*. London: TSO.

DeSantis, J., Engberg, S., and Rogers, J. 1997. Geropsychiatric restraint use. *Journal of the American Geriatrics Society, 45*, 1515–1518.

Dickens, G.L. and Campbell, J. 2001. Absconding of patients from an independent UK psychiatric hospital: a 3-year retrospective analysis of events and characteristics of absconders. *Journal of Psychiatric and Mental Health Nursing, 8*, 543–550.

Dolan, M.A. and Fein, J.A. 2011. Technical report – Pediatric and adolescent mental health emergencies in the emergency medical services system [Online]. Available at: http://pediatrics.aappublications.org/content/early/2011/04/25/peds.2011-0522.abstract [accessed 29 February 2012].

Drennan, L. and McConnell, A. 2007. *Risk and Crisis Management in the Public Sector*. Australia: Routledge.

Dumais, A., Larue, C., Drapeau, A., Menard, G., and Giguere Allard, M. 2011. Prevalence and correlates of seclusion with or without restraint in a canadian psychiatric hospital: A 2-year retrospective audit. *Journal of Psychiatric and Mental Health Nursing, 18*, 394–402.

Engberg, J., Castle, N., and McCaffrey, D. 2008. Physical restraint initiation in nursing homes and subsequent resident health. *The Gerontologist, 48*, 442–452.

Evans, D., Wood, J., and Lambert, L. 2003. Patient injury and physical restraint devices: A systematic review. *Journal of Advanced Nursing, 41*, 274–282.

Fernando, S. 1991. *Mental health, race and culture*. London: Macmillan.

Fisher, W.A. 1994. Restraint and seclusion: a review of the literature. *American Journal of Psychiatry, 151*, 1584–1591.

Fisher, W.A. 2003. Elements of successful restraint and seclusion reduction programs and their application in a large, urban, state psychiatric hospital. *Journal of Psychiatric Practice, 9*, 7–15.

Foster, C., Bowers, L., and Nijman, H. 2007. Aggressive behaviour on acute psychiatric wards: Prevalence, severity and management. *Journal of Advanced Nursing, 58*(2), 140–149.

Frueh, B.C., Knapp, R.G., Cusack, K.J., Grubaugh, A.L., Sauvageot, J.A., Cousins, V.C., Yim, E., Robins, C.S., Monnier, J., and Hiers, T.G. 2005. Patients' reports of traumatic or harmful experiences within the psychiatric setting. *Psychiatric Services, 56*,1123–1133.

Gastmans, C. and Milisen, K. 2006. Use of physical restraint in nursing homes: Clinical-ethical considerations. *Journal of Medical Ethics, 32*, 148–152.

Gerace, A., Mosel, K., Oster, C., and Muir-Cochrane, E. 2013. Restraint use in acute and extended mental health services for older persons. *International Journal of Mental Health Nursing, 22,* 545-557.

Godin, P.M. 2004. 'You don't tick boxes on a form': A study of how community mental health nurses assess and manage risk. *Health, Risk and Society, 6*, 347–360.

Grenyer, B.F.S., Lewis, K.L., Ilkiw-Lavalle, O., Deane, R., Milicevic, D., and Pai, N. 2013. The developmental and social history of repetitively aggressive mental health patients. *Australian and New Zealand Journal of Psychiatry* [Online], Online Early View. Available at: http://anp.sagepub.com/content/early/2013/01/21/0004867412474106.long [accessed 20 March 2013].

Gudjonsson, G.H., Rabe-Hesketh, S., and Szmukler, G. 2004. Management of psychiatric in-patient violence: Patient ethnicity and use of medication, restraint and seclusion. *British Journal of Psychiatry*, *184*, 258–262.

Haglund, K. and von Essen, L. 2005. Locked entrance doors at psychiatric wards: Advantages and disadvantages according to voluntary admitted patients. *Nordic Journal of Psychiatry*, *59*(6), 511–515.

Hall, G.R. and Buckwalter, K.C. 1987. Progressively lowered stress threshold: A conceptual model for care of adults with Alzheimer's disease. *Archives of Psychiatric Nursing*, *1*, 399–406.

Happell, B. and Koehn, S. 2011. Seclusion as a necessary intervention: the relationship between burnout, job satisfaction and therapeutic optimism and justification for the use of seclusion. *Journal of Advanced Nursing*, *67*, 1222–1231.

Hendryx, M., Trusevich, Y., Coyle, F., Short, R., and Roll, J. 2010. The distribution and frequency of seclusion and/or restraint among psychiatric inpatients. *The Journal of Behavioral Health Services and Research*, *37*(2), 272–281.

Hodge, A.N. and Marshall, A.P. 2007. Violence and aggression in the emergency department: A critical care perspective. *Australian Critical Care*, *20*, 61–67.

Holmes, C.A. 1998. *The Policies and Practices of Seclusion: An Advisory Report for the Western Sydney Area Mental Health Service*. Parramatta, NSW: Western Sydney Area Mental Health Service.

Holmes, C.A. 2006. Violence, zero tolerance and the subversion of professional practice. *Contemporary Nurse*, *21*, 212–227.

Huf, G., Coutinho, E.S.F., and Adams, C.E. 2012. Physical restraints versus seclusion room for management of people with acute aggression or agitation due to psychotic illness (TREC-SAVE): a randomized trial. *Psychological Medicine*, *42*, 2265–2273.

Husum, T.L., Bjorngaard, J.H., Finset, A., and Ruud, T. 2010. A cross-sectional prospective study of seclusion, restraint and involuntary medication in acute psychiatric wards: Patient, staff and ward characteristics. *BMC Health Services Research*, *10*, 89.

Johansson, I.M., Skarsater, I., and Danielson, E. 2006. The health-care environment on a locked psychiatric ward: an ethnographic study. *International Journal of Mental Health Nursing*, *15*, 242–250.

Karlsson, S., Bucht, G., Eriksson, S., and Sandman, P.O. 1996. Physical restraints in geriatric care in Sweden: prevalence and patient characteristics. *Journal of the American Geriatrics Society*, *44*, 1348–1354.

Kapur, N., Cooper, J., Rodway, C., Kelly, J., Guthrie, E., and Mackway-Jones, K. 2005. Predicting the risk of repetition after self harm: cohort study. *British Medical Journal*, *330*, 394–395.

Kelly, T., Simmons, W., and Gregory, E. 2002. Risk assessment and management: A community forensic mental health practice model. *International Journal of Mental Health Nursing*, *11*, 206–213.

Kendrick, K. 1991. A baseline for practice. *Nursing*, 4, 34.

Keski-Valkama, A., Sailas, E., Eronen, M., Koivisto, A-M., Lonnqvist, J., and Kaltiala-Heino, R. 2010. Who are the restrained and secluded patients: A 15-year nationwide study. *Social Psychiatry and Psychiatric Epidemiology*, *45*, 1087–1093.

Kettles, A.M., Moir, E., Woods, P., Porter, S., and Sutherland, E. 2004. Is there a relationship between risk assessment and observation level? *Journal of Psychiatric and Mental Health Nursing*, *11*, 156–164.

Knox, D.K. and Holloman, G.H. 2012. Use and avoidance of seclusion and restraint: consensus statement of the American Association for Emergency Psychiatry Project BETA Seclusion and Restraint Workgroup. *Western Journal of Emergency Medicine*, *13*, 35–40.

Knutzen, M., Mjosund, N.H., Eidhammer, G., Lorentzen, S., Opjordsmoen, S., Sandvik, L., and Friis, S. 2011. Characteristics of psychiatric inpatients who experienced restraint and those who did not: A case-control study. *Psychiatric Services*, *62*, 492–497.

Kontio, R., Joffe, G., Putkonen, H., Kuosmanen, L., Hane, K., Holi, M., and Valimaki, M. 2012. Seclusion and restraint in psychiatry: patients' experiences and practical suggestions on how to improve practices and use alternatives. *Perspectives in Psychiatric Care*, *48*, 16–24.

Littlechild, B. and Hawley, C. 2010. Risk assessment for mental health service users: Ethical, valid and reliable? *Journal of Social Work*, *10*, 211–229.

Luckhoff, M., Jordaan, E., Swart, Y., Cloete, K.J., Koen, L., and Niehaus, J.H. 2013. Retrospective review of trends in assaults and seclusion at an acute psychiatric ward over a 5-year period. *Journal of Psychiatric and Mental Health Nursing*, *20*, 687–695.

Lupton, D. 1999. *Risk*. London: Routledge.

MacNeela, P., Scott, A., Treacy, P., and Hyde, A. 2010. In the know: Cognitive and social factors in mental health nursing assessment. *Journal of Clinical Nursing*, *19*, 1298–1306.

Mayers, P., Keet, N., Winkler, G., and Flisher, A.J. 2010. Mental health service users' perceptions and experiences of sedation, seclusion and restraint. *International Journal of Social Psychiatry*, *56*, 60–73.

McNiel, D.E. and Binder, R.L. 1995. Correlates of accuracy in the assessment of psychiatric inpatients' risk of violence. *The American Journal of Psychiatry*, *152*, 901–906.

Meehan, T., Morrison, P., and McDougall, S. 1999. Absconding behaviour: an exploratory investigation in an acute inpatient unit. *Australian and New Zealand Journal of Psychiatry*, *33*, 533–537.

Meehan, T., Vermeer, C., and Windsor, C. 2000. Patients' perceptions of seclusion: a qualitative investigation. *Journal of Advanced Nursing*, *31*, 370–377.

Mental Health Commission. 2001. *Recovery Competencies for New Zealand Mental Health Workers*. Wellington: Mental Health Commission.

Menzies, I.E.P. 1970. *The Function of Social Systems as a Defence Against Anxiety – A Report of a Study on the Nursing Service of a General Hospital.* London: Tavistock Institute.

Metzner, J.L., Tardiff, K., Lion, J., Reid, W.H., Recupero, P.R., Schetky, D.H., Edenfield, B.M., Mattson, M., and Janofsky, J.S. 2007. Resource document on the use of restraint and seclusion in correctional mental health care. *Journal of the American Academy of Psychiatry and the Law, 35*, 417–425.

Minnick, A.F., Mion, L.C., Johnson, M.E., Catrambone, C., and Leipzig, R. 2007. Prevalence and variation of physical restraint use in acute care settings in the US. *Journal of Nursing Scholarship, 39*, 30–37.

Morral, P. and Muir-Cochrane, E. 2002. Naked social control: Seclusion and psychiatric nursing in post-liberal society. *Australian e-Journal for the Advancement of Mental Health, 1*, 1–12.

Mosel, K., Gerace, A., and Muir-Cochrane, E. 2010. Retrospective analysis of absconding behaviour by acute care consumers in one psychiatric hospital campus in Australia. *International Journal of Mental Health Nursing*, 19, 177–185.

Muir-Cochrane, E. and Holmes, C.A. 2001. Legal and ethical aspects of seclusion: An Australian perspective. *Journal of Psychiatric and Mental Health Nursing, 8*, 501–506.

Muir-Cochrane, E. and Mosel, K. 2009. A retrospective analysis of absconding behaviours by psychiatric inpatients in one psychiatric hospital campus in Australia. *Journal of Psychiatric and Mental Health Nursing, 16*, 211–213.

Muir-Cochrane, E., Mosel, K., Gerace, A., Esterman, A., and Bowers, L. 2011. The profile of absconding psychiatric inpatients in Australia. *Journal of Clinical Nursing, 20*, 706–713.

Muir-Cochrane, E., Oster, C., Grotto, J., Gerace, A., and Jones, J. 2013. The inpatient psychiatric unit as both a safe and unsafe place: implications for absconding. *International Journal of Mental Health Nursing, 22,* 304-312. Muir-Cochrane, E., Van Der Merwe, M., Nijman, H., Haglund, K., Simpson, A., and Bowers, L. 2012. Investigation into the acceptability of door locking to staff, patients, and visitors on acute psychiatric wards. *International Journal of Mental Health Nursing, 21*, 41–49.

Muir-Cochrane, E. and Wand, T. 2005. *Contemporary Issues in Risk Assessment and Management in Mental Health.* South Australia: Australian and New Zealand College of Mental Health Nurses.

National Association of State Mental Health Program Directors. 2007. NASMHPD's position statement on seclusion and restraint. Virginia, USA: NASMHPD. Available at: http://www.nasmhpd.org/Policy/position_statement-posses1.aspx.

National Mental Health Working Group. 2005. *National Safety Priorities in Mental Health: A National Plan for Reducing Harm.* Canberra: Health Priorities and Suicide Prevention Branch, Department of Health and Ageing, Commonwealth of Australia.

O'Connor, D., Horgan, L., Cheung, A., Fisher, D., George, K., and Stafrace, S. 2004. An audit of physical restraint and seclusion in five psychogeriatric admission wards in Victoria, Australia. *International Journal of Geriatric Psychiatry*, *19*, 797–799.

Oliver, D., Connelly, J.B., Victor, C.R., Shaw, F.E., Whitehead, A., Genc., Vanoli, A., Martin, F.C., and Gosney, M.A. 2007. Strategies to prevent falls and fractures in hospitals and care homes and effect of cognitive impairment: Systematic review and metaanalyses. *BMJ (Clinical Research Ed.)*, *334* (7584), 82–85.

Pamungkas, D.R. 2012. *The Use of Physical Restraint with Adults Psychiatric Patients in Emergency Departments* (Unpublished masters thesis). Adelaide, Australia: School of Nursing & Midwifery, Flinders University.

Papadopoulos, C., Bowers, L., Quirk, A., and H. Khanom. 2012. Events preceding changes in conflict and containment rates on acute psychiatric wards. *Psychiatric Services*, *63*, 40–47.

Paterson, B., Leadbetter, D., and Miller, G. 2005. Beyond zero tolerance: A varied approach to workplace violence. *British Journal of Nursing*, *14*, 810–815.

Paterson, B., McIntosh, I., Wilkinson, D., McComish, S., and Smith, I. 2013. Corrupted cultures in mental health inpatient settings. Is restraint reduction the answer? *Journal of Psychiatric and Mental Health Nursing*, *20*, 228–235.

Ramon, S., Healy, B., and Renouf, N. 2007. Recovery from mental illness as an emergent concept and practice in Australia and the UK. *International Journal of Social Psychiatry*, *53*, 108–122.

Raven, J. and Rix, P. 1999. Managing the unmanageable: risk assessment and risk management in contemporary professional practice. *Journal of Nursing Management*, *7*, 201–206.

Rickwood, D. 2005. *Pathways of Recovery: 4as Framework for Preventing Further Episodes of Mental Illness*. Canberra, Australian Capital Territory: Commonwealth of Australia.

Rintoul, Y., D. Wynaden and S. McGowan. 2009. Managing aggression in the emergency department: Promoting an interdisciplinary approach. *International Emergency Nursing*, *17*, 122–127.

Robins, C.S., Sauvageot, JA., Cusack, KJ., Suffoletta-Maierle, S., and Frueh, BC. 2005. Consumer's perceptions of negative experiences and 'sanctuary harm' in psychiatric settings. *Psychiatric Services*, *56*, 1134–1138.

Sambrano, R. and Cox, L. 2013. 'I sang *Amazing Grace* for about 3 hours that day': Understanding Indigenous Australians' experience of seclusion. *International Journal of Mental Health Nursing, 22,* 522–531.

Simpson, A., Bowers, L., Haglund, K., Muir-Cochrane, E., Nijman, H., and van der Merwe, M. 2011. The relationship between substance use and exit security on psychiatric wards. *Journal of Advanced Nursing*, *67*, 519–530.

Skiba, R.J. 2000. *Zero Tolerance, Zero Evidence: An Analysis of School Disciplinary Practice*. In Policy Research Report #SRS2. Indiana, U.S.A: Indiana Education Policy Center. Available at: http://www.indiana.edu/~safeschl/ztze.pdf.

Smith, M., Gerdner, LA., Hall, GR., and Buckwalter, KC. 2004. History, development, and future of the progressively lowered stress threshold: a conceptual model for dementia care. *Journal of the American Geriatrics Society*, *52*, 1755–1760.

Smithson, M. 2010. Understanding uncertainty, in *Dealing with Uncertainties in Policing Serious Crime*, edited by G. Bammer. Canberra, Australia: ANU E Press, 27–48.

Soininen, P., Valimaki, M., Noda, T., Puuka, P., Korkeila, J., Joffe, G., and Putkonen, H. 2013. Secluded and restrained patients' perceptions of their treatment. *International Journal of Mental Health Nursing*, *22*, 47–55.

Soloff, P.H. 1979. Physical restraint and the nonpsychotic patient: Clinical and legal perspectives. *Journal of Clinical Psychiatry*, *40*, 302–305.

Strumpf, N.E. and Evans, L.K. 1988. Physical restraint of the hospitalized elderly: perceptions of patients and nurses. *Nursing Research*, *37*, 132–137.

Szasz, T. 1997. *Insanity: The Idea and Its Consequences*. New York: Syracuse University Press.

Szasz, T. 2007. *The Medicalisation of Everyday Life – Selected Essays*. New York: Syracuse University Press.

Szmukler, G. and Rose, N. 2013. Risk assessment in mental health care: Values and costs. *Behavioral Sciences and the Law*, *31*, 125–140.

Te Pou. 2008. *Developing Alternatives to the Use of Seclusion and Restraint in New Zealand Mental Health Inpatient Setting*. Auckland, New Zealand: Te Pou, the National Centre of Mental Health Research, Information and Workforce Development.

Te Pou. 2010. *Impact of Sensory Modulation in Mental Health Acute Wards on Reducing the Use of Seclusion*. Auckland, New Zealand: Te Pou, the National Centre of Mental Health Research, Information and Workforce Development.

Tunde-Ayinmode, M. and Little, J. 2004. Use of seclusion in a psychiatric acute inpatient unit. *Australasian Psychiatry*, *12*(4), 347–351.

Unick, G.J., Kessell, E., Woodward, E.K., Leary, M., Dilley, J.W., and Shumway, M. 2011. Factors affecting psychiatric inpatient hospitalization from a psychiatric emergency service. *General Hospital Psychiatry*, *33*, 618–625.

United Nations. 1991. *The Protection of Persons with Mental Illness and the Improvement of Mental Health Care*. New York: United Nations.

Van der Merwe, M., Bowers, L., Jones, J., Simpson, A., and Haglund, K. 2009. Locked doors in acute inpatient psychiatry: A literature review. *Journal of Psychiatric and Mental Health Nursing*, *16*, 293–299.

Van Der Merwe, M., Muir-Cochrane, E., Jones, J., Tziggili, M., and Bowers, L. 2013. Improving seclusion practice: Implications of a review of staff and patient views. *Journal of Psychiatric and Mental Health Nursing*, *20*, 203–215.

Van der Zwan, R., Davies, L., Andrews, D., and Brooks, A. 2011. Aggression and violence in the ED: Issues associated with the implementation of restraint and seclusion. *Health Promotion Journal of Australia*, *22*, 124–127.

Vinestock, M. 1996. Risk asssessment: 'A word to the wise'? *Advances in Psychiatric Treatment*, *2*, 3–10.

Wand, T. and White, K. 2007. Examining models of mental health service delivery in the emergency department. *Australian and New Zealand Journal of Psychiatry*, *41*, 784–791.

Weiss, E.M., Altimari, D., Blint, D.F., and Megan, K. 1998. Deadly restraint: A *Hartford Courant* investigative report. *Hartford Courant*, 11–15 October.

Whittington, R., Bowers, L., Nolan, P., Simpson, A., and Neil, L. 2009. Approval ratings of inpatient coercive interventions in a national sample of mental health service users and staff in England. *Psychiatric Services*, *60*, 792–798.

Woo, B., Chan, V.T., Ghobrial, N., and Sevilla, C.C. 2007. Comparison of two models for delivery of services in psychiatric emergencies. *General Hospital Psychiatry*, *29*, 489–491.

Zun, L.S. 2003. A prospective study of the complication rate of use of patient restraint in the emergency department. *The Journal of Emergency Medicine*, *24*, 119–124.

Zun, L.S. and Downey, L. 2005. The use of seclusion in emergency medicine. *General Hospital Psychiatry*, *27*, 365–371.

Chapter 6
Pediatric Bipolar Disorder: An Object of Study in the Creation of an Illness[1]

David Healy and Joanna Le Noury

Introduction

The diagnosis of bipolar disorder is rapidly increasing in frequency in North America. It seems commonly assumed that pharmaceutical companies must have engineered this.[2] However, no company has a license for treating bipolar disorder in children and hence no company can advertise their drug for use in children in either academic or lay outlets. As such this disease cannot be mongered as readily as social anxiety disorder, panic disorder or other such entities.

This paper seeks to explore the capacities of companies to create a culture that legitimizes practices that would otherwise appear extra-ordinary. The article aims at offering a historically accurate narrative that shares many background themes in common with developments in other medical disorders, but which has in its foreground a comparatively small number of actors whose roles may merit further research. The narrative illustrates how company strategies in one domain can resonate in another, in this case the pediatric domain. To bring this point out, we first describe the marketing of adult bipolar disorder.

The Marketing of Adult Bipolar Disorder

Just as other corporations do, pharmaceutical companies attempt to establish what marketing departments refer to as the unmet needs of their market (Applebaum 2004). One mechanism is to use focus groups; in the case of psychotropic drugs, focus groups consist of academic psychiatrists, also termed opinion leaders. In this process, academics have three roles. As repositories of psychiatric knowledge they help companies understand what the average clinician

1 From Healy, D. and Le Noury, J. (2007). Pediatric bipolar disorder: An object of study in the creation of an illness. *International Journal of Risk & Safety in Medicine*, *19*, 209–221. Copyright 2007, with permission from ISO Press.

2 It seems to the authors that this assumption is common and it seems unlikely that this increase in diagnosis would be happening in the absence of possible treatments clinicians could give.

might perceive as a development. As opinion leaders they help deliver the company message to non-academic clinicians. As academics, they lend their names to the authorship lines of journal articles and presentations at professional meetings reporting the results of company studies or discussing clinical topics of strategic interest to marketing departments (Healy 2004).

From work like this with opinion leaders in the early 1990s, a series of unmet mental health needs clustering around the concept of bipolar disorder were identified. The field was prepared to believe that bipolar disorder could affect up to 5% of the population; that it was an unacknowledged and under researched disorder; that antidepressants might not be good for this disorder; that treatment might be better focused on the use of a "mood stabilizer"; and that everybody stood to gain by encouraging patients to self monitor.

Early market research was linked to the introduction of Depakote. In the form of sodium valproate, this anticonvulsant had been available and shown to be helpful in manic-depressive illness from the mid- 1960s. Abbott Laboratories reformulated it as semi-sodium valproate,[3] which it was claimed formed a more stable solution than sodium valproate. This trivial distinction was sufficient to enable the company to gain a patent on the new compound, which as Depakote was introduced in 1995 for the treatment of mania. Depakote was approved by the Food and Drugs Administration on the basis of trials that showed this very sedative agent could produce beneficial effects in acute manic states (Psychopharmacologic Drugs Advisory Committee 1995). Any sedative agent can produce clinical trial benefits in acute manic states but no company had chosen to do this up till then, as manic states were comparatively rare and were adequately controlled by available treatments.

Depakote was advertised as a "mood stabilizer." Had it been advertised as prophylactic for manic-depressive disorder, FDA would have had to rule the advertisement illegal, as a prophylactic effect for valproate had not been demonstrated to the standards required for licensing. The term mood stabilizer in contrast was a term that had no precise clinical or neuroscientific meaning (Ghaemi 2001). As such it was not open to legal sanction. It was a new brand.[4]

Depakote was referred to exclusively as a mood stabilizer rather than an anticonvulsant, even though there still have not been any studies that prove it to be prophylactic for manic-depressive illness. This branding played a major role in leading to increased sales of the compound compared for instance to sodium valproate, which had better evidence for efficacy but was never referred to as a mood stabilizer. Although the term still has no precise clinical or neuroscientific

3 United States Patent 4,988,731. Date of Patent Jan. 29th 1991; United States Patent 5,212,326. Date of Patent May 18th 1993.

4 While the term mood-stabilizer is not a trade-marked term, this use of the word brand here is deliberate. While the drugs are products, the identification of these previously existing products under one advertising rubric such as mood-stabilizer or SSRI appears to conform to the notion of a brand.

meaning, mood stabilizers have become the rage, with a range of other agents passing themselves off as mood stabilizers. Before 1995 there were almost no articles in the medical literature on mood-stabilizers but now there are over one hundred a year (Healy 2006). Both clinicians and patients seem happy to endorse this rebranding of sedatives despite a continuing lack of evidence that these drugs will achieve their stated aim.

But in addition to branding a new class of psychotropic drugs, the 1990s saw the rebranding of an old illness. Manic-depressive illness became bipolar disorder. While the term bipolar disorder had been introduced in DSM-III in 1980, as late as 1990 the leading book on this disease was called Manic-Depressive Disease (Goodwin and Jamison 1990). It is rare to hear the term manic-depressive illness now. This combination of a brand new disease and brand new drug class is historically unprecedented within psychiatry.

Lilly, Janssen and Astra-Zeneca, the makers of the antipsychotic drugs, olanzapine (Zyprexa), risperidone (Risperdal) and quetiapine (Seroquel), respectively sought indications in this area and the steps they have taken to market their compounds as mood stabilizers illustrate how companies go about making markets. We will outline six such steps.

First, each company has produced patient literature and website material aimed at telling people more about bipolar disorder, often without mentioning medication; this is a feature of what has been termed disease mongering (Moynihan and Cassels 2005). In the case of Zyprexa, patient leaflets and booklets—routed in Britain through a patient group, the Manic-Depressive Fellowship—aim at telling patients what they need to do to stay well. Among the claims are "that bipolar disorder is a life long illness needing lifelong treatment; that symptoms come and go but the illness stays; that people feel better because the medication is working; that almost everyone who stops taking the medication will get ill again and that the more episodes you have the more difficult they are to treat."[5]

A similar message is found in a self-help guide for people with bipolar disorder sponsored by Janssen Pharmaceuticals which under a heading 'the right medicine at the right time' states: "Medicines are crucially important in the treatment of bipolar disorders. Studies over the past 20 years have shown without a shadow of doubt that people who have received the appropriate drugs are better off in the long term than those who receive no medicine" (De Hert et al. 2005).

If studies had shown this, there would be a number of drugs licensed for the prophylaxis of bipolar disorder when in fact until recently lithium was the only drug that had demonstrable evidence for prophylactic efficacy but even this had not received a license from the FDA. More to the point all studies of life expectancy on antipsychotics show a doubling of mortality rates on treatment compared to the non-treated state and this doubling increases again for every extra antipsychotic

5 Staying Well ... with bipolar disorder. Relapse Prevention Booklet. Produced in Association with the Manic-Depressive Fellowship of Great Britain, Sponsored by Eli Lilly and Company (2004), page 17.

drug that the patient takes (Joukamaa et al. 2006). Patients taking these drugs show a reduction of life expectancy of up to 20 years compared to population norms (Colton and Manderscheid 2006).

Furthermore, to date when all placebo-controlled studies of Depakote, Zyprexa and Risperdal in the prophylaxis of bipolar disorder are combined they show a doubling of the risk of suicidal acts on active treatment compared to placebo (Healy 2006, Storosum et al. 2005). In addition, valproate and other anticonvulsants are among the most teratogenic in medicine (Ernst and Goldberg 2002).

These claims about the benefits of treatment therefore appear misleading. No company could make such public statements without the regulators intervening. But by using patient groups or academics, companies can palm off the legal liability for such claims (Healy 2004).

A second aspect of the marketing of the drugs uses celebrities such as writers, poets, playwrights, artists and composers who have supposedly been bipolar. Lists circulate featuring most of the major artists of the nineteenth and twentieth centuries intimating they have been bipolar, when in fact very few if any had a diagnosis of manic-depressive illness.

A third aspect of the marketing has involved the use of mood diaries. These break up the day into hourly segments and ask people to rate their moods on a scale that might go from +5 to −5. For example, on the Lilly sponsored mood diary,[6] one would rate a +2 if one was very productive, doing things to excess such as phone calls, writing, having tea, smoking, being charming and talkative. For a score of +1 your self-esteem would be good, you are optimistic, sociable and articulate, make good decisions and get work done. Minus 1 involves slight withdrawal from social situations, less concentration than usual and perhaps slight agitation. Minus 2 involves feelings of panic and anxiety with poor concentration and memory and some comfort in routine activities. Most normal people during the course of the week will probably cycle between at least +2 and −2, which is almost precisely the point behind this mood-watching. Most normal people will show a variation in their moods that might be construed as an incipient bipolar disorder.

On IsItReallyDepression.com,[7] Astra-Zeneca, the makers of Seroquel (quetiapine), provide a mood questionnaire which asks whether there has been a period when you were more irritable than usual, more self-confident than usual, got less sleep than usual and found you didn't really miss it, were more talkative than usual, had thoughts race through your mind, had more energy than usual, were more active than usual, were more social or outgoing than usual, or had more libido than usual.

These are all functions that show some variation in everyone. Answering Yes to 7 of these, leads to two further questions one of which is whether you have ever

6 Mood diary produced in consultation with the Manic-Depressive Fellowship of Great Britain, Sponsored by Eli Lilly & Company (2004). Other companies have similarly sponsored mood diaries.

7 Accessed April 27th 2006.

had more than one of these at any one time and the second of which is whether you have ended up in any trouble as a result of this. If you answer yes to these two questions you may meet criteria for bipolar disorder and are advised to seek a review by a mental health professional. Whether or not you meet criteria, if concerned, it is suggested you might want to seek a mental health review.

This measurement induced mood watching has an historical parallel in the behavior of weight watching that came with the introduction of weighing scales (Healy 2002). This new behavior coincided with the emergence of eating disorders in the 1870s. There was subsequently an increase in frequency in eating disorders in the 1920s that paralleled a much wider availability of weighing scales and the emergence of norms for weight that had a rather immediate impact on our ideas of what is beautiful and healthy. In the 1960s there was a further increase in the frequency of eating disorders and again this paralleled the development of smaller bathroom scales and their migration into the home. While there are undoubtedly other social factors involved in eating disorders, it is a moot point as to whether eating disorders could have become epidemic without the development of this measurement technology.

There is an informational reductionism with mood diaries that is perhaps even more potent that the biological reductionism to which critics of psychiatry often point. Measuring is not inherently a problem and figures may provide potent reinforcement to behaviors, but the abstraction that is measurement can lead to an oversight for context and other dimensions of an individual's functioning or situation that are not open to measurement or that are simply not being measured. If these oversights involve significant domains of personal functioning, we are arguably being pseudoscientific rather than modestly scientific in measuring what we can.

A fourth aspect of the current marketing of all medical disorders involves the marketing of risk. This is true for the marketing of depression and bipolar disorder as well disorders like osteoporosis, hypertension and others. In the case of osteoporosis, companies will typically present pictures of a top model looking her best in her mid-20s and juxtapose that image with a computer generated image of how the same person might look during her 60s or 70s with osteoporosis. On the one hand a beautiful woman, on the other a shrunken crone. The message is "one can never be too safe." If one wants to retain beauty and vitality it is best to monitor for osteoporosis from an early age and even treat prophylactically. In the case of bipolar disorder the risks of suicide, alcoholism, divorce, and career failure are marketed.

All of the above come together in a fifth strategy in North America—direct to consumer advertising. A now famous advertisement produced by Lilly, the makers of Zyprexa (olanzapine) begins with a vibrant woman dancing late into the night. A background voice says, "Your doctor never sees you like this." The advert cuts to a shrunken and glum figure, and the voiceover now says, "This is who your doctor sees." Cutting again to the woman, in active shopping mode, clutching bags with the latest brand names, we hear: "That is why so many people being treated for bipolar disorder are being treated for depression and aren't getting any better—because depression is only half the story." We see the woman depressed, looking at bills that have arrived in the post before switching to seeing her again energetically painting her apartment. "That fast talking, energetic, quick tempered, up-all-night you," says the voiceover, "probably never shows up in the doctor's office."

Viewers are encouraged to log onto bipolarawareness.com, which takes them to a "Bipolar Help Center," sponsored by Lilly Pharmaceuticals. This contains a "mood disorder questionnaire."[8] In the television advert, we see our heroine logging onto bipolarawareness.com and finding this questionnaire. The voice encourages the viewer to follow her example: "Take the test you can take to your doctor, it can change your life. Getting a correct diagnosis is the first step in helping your doctor to help you."

No drugs are mentioned. The advert markets bipolar disorder. Whether this is a genuine attempt to alert people who may be suffering from a debilitating disease, or an example of disease mongering, it will reach beyond those suffering from a clearcut mood disorder to others who as a consequence will be more likely to see aspects of their personal experiences in a way that will lead to medical consultations and will shape the outcome of those consultations. "Mood-watching" like this risks transforming variations from an emotional even keel into indicators of latent or actual bipolar disorder. This advert appeared in 2002 shortly after Zyprexa had received a license for treating mania, when the company was running trials to establish olanzapine as a "mood stabilizer."

The sixth strategy involves the co-option of academia and is of particular relevance to the pediatric bipolar domain. The American Psychiatric Association meeting in San Francisco in 2003 offers a good symbol of what happened. Satellite symposia linked to the main APA meeting, as of 2000, could cost a company up to $250,000. The price of entry is too high for treatment modalities like psychotherapy. There can be up to 40 such satellites per meeting. Companies usually bring hundreds of delegates to their satellite. The satellites are ordinarily distributed across topics like depression, schizophrenia, OCD, social phobia, anxiety, dementia and ADHD. At the 2003 meeting, an unprecedented 35% of the satellites were for just one disorder—bipolar disorder.[9] These symposia have to have lecturers and a Chair,[10] and 57 senior figures in American psychiatry were involved in presenting material on bipolar disorder at these satellites, not counting other speakers on the main meeting program. One of these satellite symposia, a first ever at a major meeting, was on juvenile bipolar disorder.

The upshot of this marketing has been to alter dramatically the landscape of mental disorders. Until recently manic depressive illness was a rare disorder in the United States and Canada involving 10 per million new cases per year or 3300 new cases per year. This was a disorder that was 8 times less common than schizophrenia. In contrast bipolar disorder is now marketed as affecting 5% of the United States

8 http://www.bipolarhelpcenter.com/resources/mdq.jsp.

9 American Psychiatric Association (2003). Meeting Program.

10 All of which comes with a fee, unlike symposia on the main program.

and Canada—that is 16.5 million North Americans, which would make it is as common as depression and 10 times more common than schizophrenia. Clinicians are being encouraged to detect and treat it. They are educated to suspect that many cases of depression, anxiety or schizophrenia may be bipolar disorder and that treatment should be adjusted accordingly (Hebert 2005). And, where recently no clinicians would have accepted this disorder began before adolescence, many it seems are now prepared to accept that it can be detected in preschoolers.

Bipolar Disorder in Children

The emergence of bipolar disorder in children needs to be reviewed against the background outlined above. Until very recently manic-depressive illness was not thought to start before the teenage years and even an adolescent onset was atypically early. The clearest indicator of change came with the publication of *The Bipolar Child* by Papolos and Papolos (2000). This sold 70,000 hardback copies in half a year. Published in January 2000, by May it was in a 10th printing. Other books followed, claiming that we were facing an epidemic of bipolar disorders in children (Isaac 2001) and that children needed to be treated aggressively with drugs from a young age if they were to have any hope of a normal life (Findling, Kowatch and Post 2003). Newspapers throughout the United States reported increasingly on cases of bipolar children, as outlined below.

A series of books aimed at children with pastel colored scenes in fairy tale style also appeared. In *My Bipolar Roller Coaster Feelings Book* (Hebert 2005), a young boy called Robert tells us he has bipolar disorder. As Robert defines it doctors say you are bipolar if your feelings go to the top and bottom of the world, in roller coaster fashion. When Robert is happy he apparently hugs everybody, he starts giggling and feels like doing backflips. His parents call it bouncing off the walls. His doctor, Doctor Janet, calls it silly, giddy and goofy.

Aside from giddiness, Robert has three other features that seem to make the diagnosis of pediatric bipolar disorder. One is temper tantrums. He is shown going into the grocery store with his Mum and asking for candy. When she refuses, he gets mad and throws the bag of candy at her. His mum calls this rage and he is described as feeling bad afterwards.

Second, when he goes to bed at night Robert has nightmares. His brain goes like a movie in fast forward and he seemingly can't stop it. And third, he can be cranky. Everything irritates him—from the seams in his socks, to his sister's voice, and the smell of food cooking. This can go on to depression when he is sad and lonely, and he just wants to curl up in his bed and pull the blanket over his head. He feels as though it's the end of the world and no one cares about him. His doctor has told him that at times like this he needs to tell his parents or his doctor and he needs to get help.

Dr. Janet gives Robert medication. His view on this is that while he doesn't like having bipolar disorder, he can't change that. He also doesn't like having to take all those pills but, the bad nightmares have gone away and they help him have more good days. His father says a lot of kids have something wrong with their bodies, like asthma and diabetes and they have to take medicine and be careful, and so from this point of view he's just like many other children.

His parents have told him that his bipolar disorder is just a part of who he is, not all of who he is. That they love him and always will. Finally his doctor indicates that it's only been a little while since doctors knew that children could have bipolar disorder, and that they are working hard to help these children feel better.

In another book, *Brandon and the Bipolar Bear*, we are introduced to Brandon, who has features in common with Robert that the unwary might fail to realize indicate bipolar disorder (Anglada 2004). When we are introduced to Brandon, he has just woken up from a nightmare. Second, when requested to do things that he doesn't want to do he flies into a rage. And third, he can be silly and giddy.

His mother takes both Brandon and his bear to Dr. Samuel for help, where Brandon is told that he has bipolar disorder. Dr. Samuel explains that the way we feel is controlled by chemicals in our brain. In people with bipolar disorder these chemicals can't do their job right so their feelings get jumbled inside. You might feel wonderfully happy, horribly angry, very excited, terribly sad or extremely irritated, all in the same day. This can be scary and confusing—so confusing that it can make living seem too hard.

When Brandon responds that he thinks he got bipolar disorder because he is bad, Dr. Samuel responds that many children have bipolar disorder, and they come to the doctor for help. Neither they nor Brandon are bad—it's a case of having an illness that makes you feel bad.

Brandon moves on to asking how he got bipolar disorder if he didn't get it from being bad, to which Dr. Samuel responds by asking him how he got his green eyes and brown hair. Brandon and his mother respond that these came from his parents. And Dr. Samuel tells them it's the same with bipolar disorder. That it can be inherited. That someone else in the family may have it also.

The final exchange involves Brandon asking whether he will ever feel better. Dr. Samuel response is upbeat—there are now good medicines to help people with bipolar disorder, and that Brandon can start by taking one right away. Brandon is asked to promise that he will take his medicine when told by his mother.

Brandon and the Bipolar Bear comes with an associated coloring book, in which Brandon's Dad makes it clear that a lot of kids have things wrong with their bodies, like asthma and diabetes, and they have to take medicine and be careful too.

Janice Papolos, co-author of *The Bipolar Child*, in a review on the back cover of Brandon and the Bipolar Bear says:

> children will follow (and relate to) Brandon's experience with rapid mood swings, irritability, his sense of always being uncomfortable and his sadness that he can't control himself and no one can fix him. The comforting explanation that Dr. Samuel gives him makes Brandon feel not alone, not bad, but hopeful that the medicine will make him feel better. We were so moved by the power of

> this little book and we feel better that we can now highly recommend a book for children aged 4 through 11.

The book *The Bipolar Child* arrived at Sheri Lee Norris' home in Hurst, Texas, in February 2000. When it did Karen Brooks, a reporter in the Dallas Star-Telegram describes Norris as tearing open the package with a familiar mix of emotions: hope, skepticism, fear, guilt, shame, love. But as she reads in the book about violent rages, animal abuse, inability to feel pain, self-abuse and erratic sleeping patterns, Norris is reported as feeling relief for the first time in over a year. Now she finally knew what was wrong with her daughter ... Within days, Heather Norris, then 2, became the youngest child in Tarrant County with a diagnosis of bipolar disorder (Brooks 2000).

Brooks goes on to note that families with mentally ill children are plagued with insurance woes, a lack of treatment options and weak support systems but that parents of the very young face additional challenges. It is particularly hard to get the proper diagnosis and treatment because there has been scant research into childhood mental illness and drug treatments to combat them. Routine childcare is difficult to find, because day-care centers, worried about the effect on other children, won't accept mentally ill children or will remove them when they are aggressive. Few baby sitters have the expertise or the desire to handle difficult children, leaving parents with little choice but to quit work or work from home.

Having outlined these difficulties, Brooks also notes that the lack of public awareness of childhood mental illness means that parents are judged when their children behave badly. They are accused of being poor parents, of failing to discipline their children properly, or even of sexual or physical abuse or neglect. The sense of hopelessness is aggravated when they hear about mentally ill adults; this leaves them wondering whether the battles they and their children are fighting will go on forever.

In a few short paragraphs here Brooks outlines the once and future dynamics of disease from ancient to modern times—the reflection on parents or family, the concerns for the future, the hope for an intervention. But she also covers a set of modern and specifically American dynamics. Heather Norris's problems began with temper tantrums at 18 months old. Sheri-Lee Norris had a visit from the Child Protective Services. Someone had turned her in because Heather behaved abnormally. Sheri-Lee was furious and felt betrayed. She brought Heather to pediatricians, play therapists and psychiatrists, where

Heather was diagnosed with ADHD and given Ritalin. This made everything worse. Faced with all this, a psychiatrist did not make the diagnosis of bipolar disorder because the family had no history of it. But Sheri-Lee began asking relatives and discovered that mental illness was, indeed, in her family's history. She presented that information along with a copy of *The Bipolar Child* to her psychiatrist, and Heather got a diagnosis of bipolar disorder immediately.

Heather Norris' story is not unusual. The mania for diagnosing bipolar disorders in children hit the front cover of *Time* in August 2002, which featured 9-year-old Ian Palmer and a cover title Young and Bipolar (Kluger and Song 2002), with a strapline, why are so many kids being diagnosed with the disorder, once known as manic-depression? The Time article and other articles report surveys that show 20% of adolescents nationwide have some form of diagnosable mental disorder. Ian Palmer, we are told, just like Heather Norris, had begun treatment early—at the age of 3—but failed to respond to either Prozac or stimulants, and was now on anticonvulsants.

While Heather Norris was in 2000 the youngest child in Tarrant County to be diagnosed as bipolar, Papolos and Papolos in *The Bipolar Child* indicate that many of the mothers they interviewed for their book remembered their baby's excessive activity *in utero*, and the authors seem happy to draw continuities between this and later bipolar disorder. The excessive activity amounts to hard kicking, rolling and tumbling and then later keeping the ward awake with screaming when born. Or in some instances being told by the sonographer and obstetrician that it was difficult to get a picture of the baby's face or to sample the amniotic fluid because of constant, unpredictable activity (Papolos and Papolos 2000). It is not unusual to meet clinicians who take such reports seriously.

Anyone searching the Internet for information on bipolar disorder in children are now likely to land at BPChildren.com, run by Tracy Anglada and other co-authors of the books mentioned above. Or at the Juvenile Bipolar Research Foundation (JBRF), linked to the Papoloses and *The Bipolar Child.* Or at a third site, bpkids.org, linked to a Child and Adolescent Bipolar Foundation, which is supported by unrestricted educational grants from major pharmaceutical companies.

In common with the mood-watching questionnaires in the adult field, all three sites offer mood watching questionnaires for children. The Juvenile Bipolar Research Foundation has a 65-item Child Bipolar Questionnaire, which also featured in the *Time* magazine piece above; on this scale most normal children would score at least modestly.[11]

The growing newsworthiness of childhood bipolar disorder also hit the editorial columns of the American Journal of Psychiatry in 2002 (Volkmar 2002). But where one might have expected academia to act as a brake on this new enthusiasm, its role has been in fact quite the opposite.

The Academic Voice

As outlined above until very recently manic-depressive illness was not thought to start before the teenage years. The standard view stemmed from Theodore Ziehen, who in the early years of the twentieth century established, against opposition, that it was possible for the illness to start in adolescence (Baethge, Glovinsky, and Baldessarini 2004). This was the received wisdom for 100 years.

---

11 www.jbrf.org/cbq/cbq_survey.cfm. Accessed December 1st 2005.

As of 2006, European articles on the issue of pre-pubertal bipolar disorder continued to express agnosticism as to whether there was such an entity (Kyte, Carlsson, and Goodyer 2006) . The view was that patterns of overactivity could be seen in patients with learning disabilities/mental retardation, or for example in Asberger's syndrome, but it was not clear that these should be regarded as indicative of manic-depressive disease.

Geller and colleagues in St. Louis framed the first set of criteria for possible bipolar disorder in children in 1996 as part of an NIMH funded study (Geller, Williams, Zimmerman, and Frazier 1996). Using these criteria the first studies reporting in 2002 suggested that essentially very little was known about the condition. There were children who might meet the criteria, but these had a very severe condition that in other circumstances have been likely to be diagnosed as childhood schizophrenia or else they displayed patterns of overactivity against a background of mental retardation (Geller 2003).

The course of this study and the entire debate had however been derailed by the time the Geller study reported. In 1996, a paper from an influential group, based at Massachusetts' General Hospital, working primarily on ADHD, suggested there were patients who might appear to have ADHD who in fact had mania or bipolar disorder (Biederman et al. 1996, Faraone et al. 1997). This study had used lay raters, did not interview the children about themselves, did not use prepubertal age specific mania items, and used an instrument designed for studying the epidemiology of ADHD. Nevertheless the message stuck. Cases of bipolar disorder were being misdiagnosed as ADHD. Given the many children diagnosed with ADHD who do not respond to stimulants, and who are already in the treatment system, this was a potent message for clinicians casting round for some other option.

A further study by Lewinsohn and colleagues in 2000 added fuel to the fire (Lewinson, Klein and Seeley 2000). Even though this study primarily involved adolescents and pointed toward ill-defined overactivity rather than proper bipolar disorder, the message that came out was that there was a greater frequency of bipolar disorder in minors that had been previously suspected.

These developments led in 2001 to an NIMH roundtable meeting on prepubertal bipolar disorder (National Institute of Mental Health Research Roundtable on Prepubertal Bipolar Disorder 2001) to discuss the issues further. But by then any meeting or publication, even one skeptical in tone, was likely to add fuel to the fire. Simply talking about pediatric bipolar disorder endorsed it. The Juvenile Bipolar Research Foundation website around this time noted that bipolar disorder in children simply does not look like bipolar disorder in adults, in that children's moods swing several times a day—they do not show the several weeks or months of elevated mood found in adults. They baldly state that "The DSM needs to be updated to reflect what the illness looks like in childhood."[12]

The Child and Adolescent Bipolar Foundation convened a meeting and treatment guideline process in July 2003 that was supported by unrestricted

12 www.jbrf.org/juv_bipolar/faq.html. Accessed December 1st 2005.

educational grants from Abbott Astra-Zeneca, Eli Lilly, Forrest, Janssen, Novartis, and Pfizer. This assumed the widespread existence of pediatric bipolar disorder and the need to map out treatment algorithms involving cocktails of multiple drugs (Kowatch 2005).

There are many ambiguities here. First is the willingness it seems of all parties to set aside all evidence from adult manic-depressive illness which involves mood states that persist for weeks or months and argue that children's moods may oscillate rapidly, up to several times per day, while still holding the position that this disorder is in some way continuous with the adult illness and therefore by extrapolation should be treated with the drugs used for adults.

Another ambiguity that the framers of the American position fail to advert to is a problem with DSM-IV. Advocates of pediatric bipolar disorder repeatedly point to problems with DSM-IV that hold them back from making diagnoses. But in fact, DSM-IV is more permissive than the rest of world in requiring a diagnosis of bipolar disorder following a manic episode—in practice any sustained episode of overactivity. The International Classification of Disease in contrast allows several manic episodes to be diagnosed without a commitment to the diagnosis of bipolar disorder. The rest of the world believes it simply does not know enough even about the relatively well understood adult illness to achieve diagnostic consistency worldwide. DSM-IV in fact therefore makes it easier to diagnose bipolar disorder than any other classification system, but therapeutic enthusiasts want an even further loosening of these already lax criteria.

Finally, we appear to have entered a world of operational criteria by proxy. Clinicians making these diagnoses are not making diagnoses based on publicly visible signs in the patients in front of them, or publicly demonstrable on diagnostic tests, as is traditional in medicine. Nor are they making the diagnoses based on what their patients say, as has been standard in adult psychiatry, but rather these are diagnoses made on the basis of what third parties, such as parents or teachers, say without apparently any method to assess the range of influences that might trigger parents or teachers to say such things—the range of influences brought out vividly by Karen Brooks in her Star-Telegram articles.

When clinicians raise just this point (Harris 2005), the response has been aggressive.

> Mood need not be elevated, irritable etc. for a week to fulfill criteria ... A period of 4 days suffices for hypomania. This is ... itself an arbitrary figure under scrutiny ... Dr. Harris is incorrect ... that the prevalence of adult bipolar disorder is only 1–2%. When all variants are considered the disease is likely to be present in more than 6% of the adult pop. There are still those who will not accept that children commonly suffer from bipolar illness regardless of how weighty the evidence. One cannot help but wonder whether there are not political and economic reasons for this stubborn refusal to allow the outmoded way of thought articulated by Dr. Harris to die a peaceful death. It is a disservice to our patients to do otherwise. (Dilsaver 2005)

Where one might have thought some of the more distinguished institutions would bring a skeptical note to bear on this, they appear instead to be fueling the fire. Massachusetts's General Hospital (MGH) have run trials of the antipsychotics risperidone and olanzapine on children with a mean age of 4 years old (Mick et al. 2004). A mean age of 4 all but guarantees three and possibly two year olds have been recruited to these studies.

MGH in fact recruited juvenile subjects for these trials by running its own DTC adverts featuring clinicians and parents alerting parents to the fact that difficult and aggressive behavior in children aged 4 and up might stem from bipolar disorder. Given that it is all but impossible for a short term trial of sedative agents in pediatric states characterized by overactivity not to show some rating scale changes that can be regarded as beneficial, the research can only cement the apparent reality of juvenile bipolar disorder into place.

As a result where it is still rare for clinicians elsewhere in the world to make the diagnosis of manic-depressive illness before patients reach their mid to late teens, drugs like olanzapine and risperidone are now in extensive and increasing use for children including preschoolers in America with relatively little questioning of this development (Cooper 2006).

Studies run by academics that apparently display some benefits for a compound have possibly become even more attractive to pharmaceutical companies than submitting the data to the FDA in order to seek a license for the treatment of children. Companies can rely on clinicians to follow a lead given by academics speaking on meeting platforms or in published articles. The first satellite symposium on juvenile bipolar disorder at a major mainstream meeting, the American Psychiatric Association meeting in 2003 featured the distinguished clinical faculty of MGH. The symposium was supported by an unrestricted educational grant. None of the speakers will have been asked to say anything other than what they would have said in any event. The power of companies does not lie in dictating what a speaker will say but in providing platforms for particular views. If significant numbers of clinicians in the audience are persuaded by what distinguished experts say, companies may not need to submit data to FDA and risk having lawyers or others pry through their archives to see what the actual results of studies look like. As an additional benefit, academics come a lot cheaper than putting a sales force in the field.

It would seem only a matter of time before this American trend spreads to the rest of the world. In a set of guidelines on bipolar disorder issued in 2006, Britain's National Institute of Health and Clinical Excellence (NICE), which is widely regarded as being completely independent of the pharmaceutical industry, has a section on children and adolescents (National Institute for Health & Clinical Excellence 2006). The guideline contains this section because if there are treatment studies on a topic, NICE has to perforce consider them; it cannot make the point that hitherto unanimous clinical opinion has held that bipolar disorders do not start in childhood. But simply by considering the treatment for bipolar disorders in childhood, NICE effectively brings it into existence, illustrating in the process the ability of companies to capture guidelines (Healy, submitted). And again, the need for a company to seek an indication for treatment in children recedes if influential guidelines tacitly endorse such treatment.

Munchausen's Syndrome New Variant?

As outlined above, a number of forces appear to have swept aside traditional academic skepticism with the result that an increasing number of children and infants are being put on cocktails of potent drugs without any evidence of benefit.

One of the features of the story is how a comparatively few players have been able to effect an extraordinary change. There the academics noted above and a handful of others. One was Robert Post who was among the first to propose that anticonvulsants might be useful for adult manic-depressive disease, who when the frequency of the disorder began to increase rather than decrease as usually happens when treatments work, promoted the idea that the reason we were failing was because we had failed to catch affected individuals early enough. No age was too early.

> One would encourage major efforts at earlier recognition and treatment of this potentially incapacitating and lethal recurrent central nervous system disorder. It would be hoped that instituting such early, effective, and sustained prophylactic intervention would not only lessen illness-related morbidity over this interval, but also change the course of illness toward a better trajectory and more favorable prognosis. (Post 2002)

Another group consists of evangelical parents and clinicians, who bring to the process of proselytizing about bipolar disorder a real fervor. Some of these parents and clinicians readily contemplate the possibility of making a diagnosis *in utero*. When those challenging such viewpoints are subject to opprobrium, one has to ask what has happened to the academic voices that should be questioning what is happening here.

Finally there is the role of companies who make available the psychoactive drugs without which the diagnoses would not be made, unrestricted educational grants, and access to academic platforms. This has clearly facilitated the process outlined above. While companies cannot market directly to children, it is now clear that documents from 1997 show that at least one company was aware of the commercial opportunities offered by juvenile bipolar disorder (Tollefson 1997).

If the process outlined here was one that could reasonably be expected to lead to benefits it could regarded as therapeutic. But given that there is no evidence for benefit and abundant prima facie evidence that giving the drugs in question to vulnerable subjects in such quantities cannot but produce consequent difficulties for many of these minors, one has to wonder whether we are not witnessing instead a variation on Munchausen's syndrome, where some significant other wants the individual to be ill and these significant others derive some gain from these proxy illnesses.

The contrast between the developing situation and the historical record is striking. The records of all admissions to the asylum in North Wales from North West Wales for the years from 1875 to 1924 show that close to 3,500 individuals were admitted, from a population base of slightly more than a quarter of a million per annum (12,500,000 person years). Of these, only 123 individuals were admitted for manic-depressive disease. The youngest admission for manic-depression was aged 17. The youngest age of onset may have been EJ, who was first admitted in 1921 at the age of 26, but whose admission record notes that she "has had several slight attacks in the last 12 years, since 13 years of age." All told there were 12 individuals in 50 years with a clear onset of illness under the age of 20 (Harris, Chandran, Chakroborty and Healy 2005). But it would seem almost inevitable that there will be a greater frequency of hospital admissions for juveniles in future diagnosed with bipolar disorder. This is not what ordinarily happens when medical treatments work.

References

Anglada, T. 2004. *Brandon and the Bipolar Bear*. Victoria, BC: Trafford Publishing.

Applbaum, K. 2004. *The Marketing Era*. New York: Routledge.

Baethge, C., Glovinsky, R., and Baldessarini, R.J. 2004. Manic-depressive illness in children: An early twentieth century view by Theodore Ziehen (1862–1950). *Hist. Psychiatr*, *15*, 201–226.

Biederman, J., Faraone, S., Mick, E., Wozniak, J., Chen, L., Ouellette, C., Marrs, A., Moore, P., Garcia, J., Mennin, D., and Lelon, E. 1996. Attention-deficit hyperactivity disorder and juvenile mania: An overlooked co-morbidity? *J. Am. Acad. Child Adolesc. Psychiatr*, *35*, 997–1008.

Brooks, K. 2000. No Small Burden, Families with mentally ill children confront health care shortcomings, undeserved stigma of "bad parenting." *Dallas Star Telegram* [Online]. Available at: DOI: 1%3A00MENTALHEALTH170719100.html. [accessed: July 19th, 2000].

Colton, C.W. and Manderscheid, R.W. 2006. Congruencies in increased mortality rates, years of potential life lost, and causes of death among public mental health clients in eight states. *Prev. Chronic Dis.* [Online]. Available at: http://www.cdc.gov/pcd/issues/2006/apr/05_0180.htm [accessed: 2006].

Cooper, W., Arbogast, P.G., Ding, H., Hickson, G.B., Fuchs, C., and Ray, W.A. 2006. Trends in prescribing of antipsychotic medications for US children. *Ambul. Pediatr. 6*, 79–83.

De Hert, M., Thys, E., Magiels, G. and Wyckaert, S. 2005. *Anything or Nothing. Self-Guide for People with Bipolar Disorder*. Antwerp: Uitgeverij Houtekiet.

Dilsaver, S. 2005. Review of J. Harris. *J. Bipolar Disorders*, *4*, 8–9.

Ernst, C.L. and Goldberg, J.F. 2002. The reproductive safety profile of mood-stabilizers, atypical antipsychotics and broad- spectrum psychotropics. *J. Clin. Psychiatr*, *63*(Suppl. 4), 42–55.

Faraone, S.V., Biederman, J., Mennin, D., Wozniak, J., and Spencer, T. 1997. Attention-deficit hyperactivity disorder with bipolar disorder: A familial subtype?. *J. Am. Acad. Child. Adolesc. Psychiatr*, *36*, 1378–1387.

Findling, R.L., Kowatch, R.A., and Post, R.M. 2003. *Pediatric Bipolar Disorder. A Handbook for Clinicians*. London: Martin Dunitz.

Geller, B., Williams, M., Zimmerman, B., and Frazier, J. 1996. *Washington University in St. Louis Kiddie Schedule for Affective Disorders and Schizophrenia (Wash-U-KSADS)*. St. Louis: Washington University.

Geller, B., Craney, J., Bolhoffer, K., DelBello, M.P., Axelson, D., Luby, J., Williams, M., Zimerman, B., Nickelsburg, M.J., Frazier, J., and Beringer, L. 2003. Phenomenology and longitudinal course of children with a prepubertal and early adolescent bipolar disorder phenotype. In B. Geller and M.P. DelBello (Eds). *Bipolar Disorder in Childhood and Early Adolescence*. New York: The Guilford Press, 25–50.

Ghaemi, S.N. 2001. On defining 'mood stabilizer.' *Bipolar Disorder*, *3*, 154–158.

Goodwin, F.K. and Jamison, K.R. 1990. *Manic Depressive Illness*. New York: Oxford University Press.

Harris, J. 2005. The increased diagnosis of juvenile "bipolar disorder," what are we treating?. *Psychiatr. Serv.*, *56*, 529–531.

Harris, M., Chandran, S., Chakroborty, N., and Healy, D. 2005. Service utilization in bipolar disorders, 1890 and 1990 compared. *Hist. Psychiatr.*, *16*, 423–434.

Healy, D. 2002. *The Creation of Psychopharmacology*. Cambridge, MA: Harvard University Press.

Healy, D. 2004. *Let Them Eat Prozac*. New York: New York University Press.

Healy, D. 2006. The Latest Mania. Selling Bipolar Disorder. *PloS Medicine*. [Online]. Available at: http://dx.doi.org/10.1371/journal.pmed.0030185 [accessed: 2006].

Healy, D. 2008. *Mania*. Baltimore, MD: Johns Hopkins University Press.

Hebert, B. 2005. *My Bipolar Roller Coaster Feeling Book*. Victoria, BC: Trafford Publishing.

Isaac, G. 2001. *Bipolar not ADHD. Unrecognized Epidemic of Manic-Depressive Illness in Children*. Lincoln, NE: Writers' Club Press.

Joukamaa, M., Heliovaara, M., Knekt, P., Aromaa, A., Partosalo, R., and Lehtinen, R. 2006. Schizophrenia, neuroleptic medication and mortality. *Br. J. Psychiatr.*, *188*, 122–127.

Kluger, J. and Song, S. 2002. Young and Bipolar. Once called Manic Depression, the disorder afflicted adults. Now it's striking kids. Why? *TIME Magazine*, *160*, 30–41.

Kowatch, R.A., Fristad, M., Birmaher, B., Wagner, K.D., Findling, R.L., Hellander, M., and The Child Psychiatric Workgroup on Bipolar Disorder. 2005. Treatment guidelines for children and adolescents with bipolar disorder. *J. Am. Acad. Child Adolesc. Psychiatr.*, *44*, 213–235.

Kyte, Z.A., Carlsson, G.A., and Goodyer, I.M. 2006. Clinical and neuropsychological characteristics of child and adolescent bipolar disorder. *Psychol. Med*, *36*, 1197–1211.

Lewinsohn, P., Klein, D. and Seeley, J. 2000. Bipolar disorder during adolescence and young adulthood in a community sample. *Bipolar Disorder*, *2*(2000), 281–293.

Mick, E., Biederman, J., Dougherty, M., and Aleardi, M. 2004. Comparative efficacy of atypical antipsychotics for pediatric bipolar disorder [abstract]. *Acta Psychiatr. Scand.*, *110*, P50, 29.

Mick, E., Biederman, J., Dougherty, M., and Aleardi, M. 2004. Open trial of atypical antipsychotics in pre-schoolers with bipolar disorder [abstract]. *Acta Psychiatr. Scand.*, *110*, P51, 29.

Moynihan, R. and Cassels, A. 2005. *Selling Sickness*. New York: Nation Books.

National Institute for Health & Clinical Excellence (NICE). 2006. *Bipolar disorder, Clinical Guideline* 38. [Online]. Available at www.nice.org.uk [accessed: 2006].

National Institute of Mental Health Research Roundtable on Prepubertal Bipolar Disorder. 2001. *J. Am. Acad. Child Adolesc. Psychiat.*, *40*, 871–878.

Papolos D. and Papolos, J. 2000. *The Bipolar Child*. New York: Random House.

Post, R.M. 2002. Treatment resistance in bipolar disorder, in *Royal College of Psychiatrists Meeting*, Newcastle, England, October 17th, 2002.

Psychopharmacologic Drugs Advisory Committee, in: *Forty-Fourth Meeting*, NDA 20–320: Depakote, Transcript of Proceedings, Department of Health and Human Services, Washington, DC, February 6th, 1995.

Storosum, J.G., Wohlfarth, T., Gispen-de Wied, C.C., Linszen, D.H., Gersons, B.P., van Zwieten, B., and van den Brink, W. 2005. Suicide-risk in placebo controlled trials of treatment for acute manic episode and prevention of manic-depressive episode. *Am. J. Psychiatr.*, *162*, 799–802.

Tollefson, G.D. 1997. Zyprexa Product Team: 4 Column Summary. Zyprexa MultiDistrict Litigation 1596, Document ZY200270343.

Volkmar, F.R. 2002. Changing perspectives on mood disorders in children. *Am. J. Psychiatr.*, *159*(2002), 893–894.

Chapter 7
Delinquent Life: Forensic Psychiatry and Neoliberal Biopolitics

Stuart J. Murray and Sarah Burgess

Introduction

In *Discipline and Punish*, Michel Foucault claims that a "curious substitution" takes place within the "penitentiary apparatus": the convicted *offender* is substituted by the *delinquent*. While the "offender" was a product of a legal judgment corresponding to that individual's criminal act(s), for the "delinquent" it is "not so much his act as his life that is relevant in characterizing him" (Foucault 1977: 251). Delinquency is in large part a product of a moral judgment that bears upon the person's life or *bios*, less a matter of what one *does* and more a psychiatric question of who one *is*, "a whole bundle of complex threads (instincts, drives, tendencies, character)" (1977: 253). In treating the delinquent, correctional and psychiatric techniques represent a moral orthopedics that constellates around a vital norm, fixing on the precise manner in which that norm has been transgressed, and implementing new technologies of rectification. In this respect, as Foucault describes it, the prison becomes "a sort of artificial and coercive theatre in which his life will be examined from top to bottom" (1977: 251–252). At once—and often indistinguishably—both correctional and psychiatric, the prison is a theatre for the coercive production of a relatively new and emergent form of subjectivity—one produced through the regulation of an individual's "disposition."

This chapter examines the role of forensic psychiatry in the production and treatment of what we are calling *delinquent life*. We argue that forensic psychiatry has, wittingly or not, led the way toward a new form of power, evident in the place of expert psychiatric testimony in the legal arena and in the design and execution of treatment plans in prisons. Specifically, we develop the following claim from *Abnormal*, Foucault's 1974–1975 lectures at the Collège de France: "a certain type of power—distinct from both medical and judicial power—has in fact colonized and forced back both medical knowledge and judicial power throughout modern society" (Foucault 2003b: 26). The "distinct" power that has "colonized" and "forced back" both medicine and law is the power of normalization—a normalization which we interpret specifically as the combined effect of biopolitics and neoliberalism, as discussed throughout Foucault's 1978–1979 lectures at the Collège de France, *The Birth of Biopolitics* (2008). Forensic psychiatry is perhaps uniquely susceptible to such "colonization," since it is situated at the nexus of the assiduous bureaucracy of the biomedical and prison-industrial complexes, which produce regimes of truth and truth-effects in their own right. Forensic psychiatry is thus caught between conflicting and intersecting roles: an ethico-medical duty to care, a moral obligation to pass paralegal judgments in the form of expert testimony, and a professional responsibility to design and administer treatment plans in a correctional milieu—a total institution devised to carry out the punishment and legal judgment that his or her "expert opinion" may well have helped to determine in the first place.

Biopower and the Management of Life

Given what are arguably its incompatible allegiances, forensic psychiatry is a particularly rich site at which to investigate the ongoing historical shift taking place, from disciplinary forms of medical power-knowledge to biopolitical ones. These forms of biopower often intersect and overlap, although they are not mutually exclusive. Foucault writes: "Medicine is a power-knowledge that can be applied to both the body and the population, both the organism and biological processes, and it will therefore have both disciplinary effects and regulatory effects" (Foucault 2003: 252). In the first form of biopower, the body is subject to a *disciplinary* power that takes the individual organism as its object of treatment. In the second, that body is understood primarily as a member of a population subject to *biopolitical* regulation and normalization. Effectively, the body is doubled along this axis, both a disciplinary body and a biopolitical body. This doubling is all the more salient when the body in question belongs to someone who has been diagnosed with a mental illness, and more complex still when that body belongs to an inmate in a correctional facility. As the convicted offender is gradually substituted by the delinquent, we see a shift from disciplinary power to the colonizing force of a specific form of biopolitics supported by and constituted in neoliberalism—a shift that marks not simply a distinction between corrections and psychiatry, but, increasingly, their indistinguishability, their colonization, and coerced collusion.

In Foucault's terms, disciplinary and biopolitical biopower have specific objects and objectives: where discipline "individualizes," biopolitics "massifies," the latter treating "populations" by regulating and regularizing them *en masse*. To be sure, both law and medicine will disavow their "massifying" role; if pressed, they would prefer to align themselves with disciplinary biopower in order to preserve and privilege the *individual* who is said to be free, rational, and autonomous—i.e., the foundation of personal rights, responsibility, consent, and dignity within the tradition of liberalism (and without which modern law and medicine become unrecognizable, inoperable). But consider Foucault's description of biopolitics and we see how traditional liberalism is increasingly untenable, and how law and medicine have been colonized, perverted:

> The mechanisms introduced by biopolitics include forecasts, statistical estimates, and overall measures. And their purpose is not to modify any

> given phenomenon as such, or to modify a given individual insofar as he is an individual, but, essentially, to intervene at the level at which these general phenomena are determined … . [R]egulatory mechanisms must be established to establish an equilibrium, maintain an average, establish a sort of homeostasis, and compensate for variations within this general population and its aleatory field. In a word, security mechanisms have to be installed around the random element inherent in a population of living beings so as to optimize a state of life. (2003a: 246)

Management on this scale demands a vast network of experts, much in the ways that public health and epidemiology are mobilized as a form of population-based power-knowledge. We have left the "individual" of traditional liberalism far behind. While neoliberalism promotes hyper-individualism—one who is responsibilized to manage and assume various personal risks—this individuality is a ruse because individual "choices" have come increasingly to rely on a cadre of "experts," whose expertise is managed and delivered through corporate structures which are increasingly privatized, deregulated, commodified. Expertise is purchased on the open market; the citizen is transformed into a consumer whose "freedom" is tied to his or her socioeconomic class, race, sexual orientation, etc.

There can be no doubt that medical knowledge and judicial power increasingly rely on statistical estimates and measures—to better understand risk, to regulate and mitigate it amongst "at-risk" populations. Indeed, we expect medicine and law to make use of advances in science and technology to "optimize" the lives of the living. At the same time, however, they have little choice: biopolitical "massification" is driven by the inexorable demand for economies of scale, the maximization of efficiencies, the minimization of costs, and the eradication of randomness. Under neoliberalism, market forces drive computerization and e-health, dictate permissible cost-benefit analyses, promote "affordable" and "reasonable" treatment plans (typically in line with multinational pharmaceutical and insurance industry profits and quarterly stock reports), and constellate around the statistically "average" patient of evidence-based medicine and its randomized controlled trials. Not just today, but in the future: hence, the rise of predictive rationalities, quantitative forecasts, epidemiological pattern recognition, vectors of infection, the analysis of past behaviors and trends, extrapolating them, in order to regulate and regularize, and to act pre-emptively, to thwart, to prevent, and when this is not possible, to prohibit and proscribe.

The result has less to do with treating illness or managing epidemics and more to do with the biopolitical regulation of living populations in their generality—their health, hygiene, productivity, and vitality. Epidemics have been substituted by "endemics":

> illnesses that were difficult to eradicate and that were not regarded as epidemics that caused more frequent deaths, but as permanent factors which … sapped the population's strength, shortened the working week, wasted energy, and cost

> money, both because they led to a fall in production and because treating them was expensive. (Foucault 2003a: 244)

In brief, neoliberal biopolitics has as its object and its objective the (re)production and circulation of human capital. According to Henry A. Giroux, neoliberalism is "a form of terrorism because it abstracts economics from ethics and social costs, makes a mockery of democracy, works to dismantle the welfare state, thrives on militarization, undermines any public sphere not governed by market values, and transforms people into commodities" (Giroux and Letizia 2012). Thus, neoliberal biopolitics consists in this voracious, violent, near-totalizing economic ideology, together with the increasingly abstract "populations" it both constitutes and serves, in tandem with and further driven by the burgeoning technological capacities of the biomedical and military-industrial complexes.

Under the aegis of neoliberal biopolitics, Foucault's claim in *Abnormal* (2003b) takes on added significance. When read alongside *The Birth of Biopolitics* (2008), we get a better understanding of the "certain type of power—distinct from both medical and judicial power" that has "colonized and forced back both medical knowledge and judicial power" (2003b: 26). Somewhat paradoxically, medical knowledge and judicial power are "forced back" through what might be called the "advances" of science and technology, driven by the joint efficiencies of neoliberal economics and biopolitics. They must constitute as normative a juridico-biological field in which the (re)production and circulation of human capital will flourish; and as with any colonizing discourse, this "ground" is hegemonic, operating as originary and natural, fuelling false-consciousness. In *Abnormal*, Foucault traces a genealogy of the abnormal individual, a historical trajectory of three colonizing (his word again) "elements" or "figures" or "circles in which the problem of abnormality is gradually posed" (2003b: 55). The first in this trajectory is the "human monster," followed by the "individual to be corrected," and then the "masturbator" (particularly the child). The genealogy proceeds through increasingly circumscribed fields of application; while the frame of reference for the "human monster" was nature and society, for the "individual to be corrected" it is "the family and its entourage," while for the "masturbator" it is "a much narrower space … the bedroom, the bed, the body; it is the parents, immediate supervisors, brothers and sisters; it is the doctor: it is a kind of microcell around the individual and his body" (2003b: 59). In some respects, the trajectory traces for us the rise of disciplinary biopower, which "individualizes" in and through a meticulous technical infrastructure, a politico-medical micromanagement. But this history is incomplete.

Resurrection of Human Monstrosity

If, more recently, there has been a "colonization" and a "forcing back," we are suggesting here that there has been a resurrection of human monstrosity—but a monstrosity that incorporates, that has itself been colonized by neoliberal economies and biopolitical forces. Recall that the "human monster" is "not only a violation of the laws of society but also a violation of the laws of nature … . The field in which the monster appears can thus be called a 'juridico-biological' domain" (2003b: 55–56). Today, this juridico-biological field is occupied, we contend, by forensic (bio)psychiatry. And so we have passed from the "individual to be corrected," which was the object of nineteenth-century penality and psychiatry, to what we are calling *delinquent life*, which is at once monstrous in the classical sense, but whose monstrosity now secretes the hidden truth of the dangerous—or potentially dangerous—population it characterizes.

The high-profile American forensic psychiatrist Michael Welner prefers the term "depravity," a term that captures very well our understanding of the role of forensic psychiatry in the production of delinquent life. Welner is a media darling, appearing on talk shows following particularly horrific violent crimes, such as the Sandy Hook school massacre, after which he propounded on the mental condition of the gunman, Adam Lanza, and others like him:

> It starts with someone who is fundamentally resentful and alienated, and blames others. Alright? Then it progresses from there to someone who identifies with the idea of destruction as a matter of stature. And then, the person becomes increasingly withdrawn and they get a little older and they have social or sexual frustration and incompetence. (*Forensic Psychiatrist Dr. Michael Welner on the Newtown Shooting, Part 1,* 2012)

Of course, Welner cannot discuss the Lanza case with any authority, but he does not hesitate to provide a profile, a "type," right down to the character's sexual dysfunctions. He is resentful, he feels alienated, and so forth—hardly profound insights, but these alone are not crimes and the causal link to the criminal acts are tenuous at best. These dispositions are irregularities in his psychology, his relationships, his moral or spiritual life—irregularities characteristic of the profile but attached to Lanza seamlessly. In Foucault's words: "Expert psychiatric opinion makes it possible to transfer the point of application of punishment from the offense defined by the law to criminality evaluated from a psychologico-moral point of view" (Foucault 2003b: 18). Welner's status as forensic expert, his authority to pronounce a moral judgment on an individual he has never met, precedes him, part of the "CSI Effect" (Podlas 2005, Schweitzer and Saks 2007) in which the public exhibit an unrealistic faith in the capabilities and reliability of forensics, thanks to popular television shows like *CSI: Crime Scene Investigation.*

With the label "forensic," it hardly matters that psychiatry cannot be considered analogous to blood spatter analysis and ballistic fingerprinting. Welner capitalizes on the perceived authority of forensics, offering us "The Depravity Scale," which is proclaimed to be the latest in "evidence-based forensics." The Depravity Scale is meant to *objectively* define evil in everyday human interactions, criminal or otherwise. The Depravity Scale boasts a website, http://depravityscale.org/, which also includes a depravity survey for those who are interested (and whose participation, apparently, will contribute to this research). In response to the question, "What is the Standard helping to judge? The act, or the person?" the website tells us:

> The Depravity Standard will measure the crime itself, and not the perpetrator—that is, it will judge the "what" of a crime, as opposed to the "who." This instrument will provide an objective, evidence-based standard by which to assess the intents, actions, and attitudes associated with a given crime that distinguish it as worse than other crimes. (https://depravityscale.org/depscale/faq.php#q6)

"Depravity" and "evil" are patently subjective categories, and not absolute at that; a person's intents, actions, and attitudes cannot be abstracted from "who" he or she is. Some scholars are critical about whether categories such as these ought to be used as testimony (e.g., Simon 2003), noting that since the Supreme Court case of *Daubert v. Merrell Dow Pharmaceuticals, Inc.* (1993), courts must consider the admissibility of scientific evidence—whether it is testable, supported by peer review, and so forth. Certainly, "depravity" and "evil" can only fail the test of scientific objectivity. As Simon observes, "Some perpetrators of the worst atrocities do not have a diagnosable psychiatric disorder" (Simon 2003: 415). But this is all the more reason, Welner retorts, that his Standard is necessary: "Evil behavior bedevils the law and the behavioral sciences, and it will not go away. Defining evil is only the latest frontier where psychiatry, confronting the challenge of ambiguity, will bring light out of darkness" (Welner 2003: 421). In his view, psychiatry has an obligation to challenge "ambiguity," to expand its diagnostic arsenal to include tools that measure depravity and evil, and to operationalize this for judgment in a standardized fashion. According to Welner, the forensic psychiatrist is the person best equipped for this task:

> What gives forensic psychiatrists the expertise to make judgments about what is normal or not, with any greater expertise than lay people? What gives psychiatrists the qualification to brand someone "psychotic" or as sexually "deviant" in a world of millions of particularized internet erotica consumers? Is there not a philosophical or theological point to be considered about mental infirmity? Is mental sickness not influenced by cultural and political orientation? But of course. (2003: 418)

Remarkably, in Welner's terms the role of the forensic psychiatrist is to judge "what is normal or not"—to judge, to pathologize, and by implication, to criminalize *ab*normality according to particular philosophical or theological values, according to cultural and political orientations—the failure to embody arbitrary norms. Should there be a philosophy or a (political) theology of evil, Welner claims their definitions of good and evil, friend and enemy, for forensic psychiatry, installing (or securing) evidence-based psychiatry as both the organizing principle and natural *telos* of such musings on evil.

While Welner presents a limit case, he demonstrates clearly the ways that both law and psychiatry have been "pushed back" and "colonized" by neoliberal biopolitics: in the name of normalization and standardization, at the altar of efficiency and operationalizability, we produce populations who are divided according to perceptions of normality, abnormality, and tolerable risk. It is a vague "public" or "society" that is constituted as the population "at risk" of harm from an endemically "risky" or "dangerous" population. In the province of Ontario, Canada, the forensic mental health system is aligned with the Ministry of Community Safety and Correctional Services. The name itself is telling: one ministry is in charge of public security and corrections, as if these were synonymous. Here, the forensic mental health system operates to protect the "public," to help judge when the security of the public is deemed to be at risk, and to act so as to prevent risk. "The public" is constituted rhetorically as a population whose lives and livelihood are perpetually at risk, while the offender is judged according to the prevailing norms of an existing population of mentally ill offenders who are judged to be at risk of re-offending and threatening public security.

Forensic Psychiatry as Switchpoint

Biopolitically, forensic psychiatry is the switchpoint between public security and corrections; it functions within an aleatory field—a field saturated by risk and uncertainty, informed by mental health statistics, probabilities, rates of recidivism, and so on. It intervenes in the lives of populations or sub-populations conceived in statistical or average terms, and its intervention is a form of actuarialism. But it is unclear which population forensic psychiatrists truly represent, or whose "risk" is being assessed and managed—whether they are motivated more by the care of one population or the security of the other. Arguably, "risk" has very little to do with either population: if there is risk, it is the risk to normality as such, a risk to "normal" philosophical or theological values, "normal" cultural and political orientations, here exalted as a "way of life." In other words, abnormality threatens our normative symbolic system; it serves the reproduction of an ideological form. The discourse on risk, then, shores up normality by performatively producing perpetual risks and dangers. While there may in some instances be a credible threat, highly mediatized events depicting mass murders succeed in terrorizing the public, who in turn become all the more willing to enlist the support security "experts," to approve if not call for "pre-emptive strikes" and a sort of counter-insurgent psychiatry. The legal concept of the "dangerous offender" provides the juridical sanction for psychiatry to act pre-emptively. However, by allowing for the designation of "dangerous offender," the *Criminal Code* of Canada (15, Part XXIV) seems to contradict Canada's *Charter of Rights and Freedoms* (Kaiser 2009). The *Criminal Code* allows courts to assign harsher (or indeterminate) sentences for those deemed by forensic psychiatrists to be "dangerous." These measures are justified according to the logic of "preventive detentions" or "protective sentences," which are designed to protect the public from "likely harm" at some unspecified future moment. Responding to a challenge to such legislation, Canadian Supreme Court Justice La Forest clearly aligns risk and the need for security when discussing a criminal's disposition: "His being in the wrong by virtue of the risk he represents is what entitles us to consider imposing on him the risk of unnecessary measures to save the risk of harm to innocent victims" (*R. v. Lyons*). The proliferation of "risk" is dizzying: who is at risk, or at risk of risk? "Innocent victims" in this case means *potential* victims, those at risk of victimization, and thus not victims at all. And all this justifies what La Forest does not hesitate to name a judicial "entitlement" to heap risk upon risk. In this case, the "dangerous offender" is punished not merely for what he has done, but for who he is, what he might do, and for what he represents; it is an ontological claim, he *is* "in the wrong" by virtue of the risk he represents. And this depends on the testimony of forensic psychiatrists, who wear the mantle of the scientific expert.

But here the forensic psychiatrist must leave his/her professional and deontological obligations behind to adopt the legal reasoning of the *Criminal Code*. In Alan Stone's words, this amounts to a "legal assault on psychiatry" which has occurred over the last several decades (Stone 2008: 167). As forensic psychiatry has surrendered its "discretionary authority" to the courts, paradoxically, the courts have come to rely increasingly on expert testimony from forensic psychiatrists. Forensic psychiatry has been "juridicized," that is, taken over by juridical forms of discourse concerned primarily with criminal justice, rather than mental health. This raises a basic boundary question for the profession. Stone asks: "Does psychiatry have anything true to say that the courts should listen to?" (2008: 167). There is a question here of what constitutes truth and how—or whether—truth can be told in such a context (Gutheil, Hauser, White, Spruiell, and Strasburger 2003). What authority must psychiatrists possess or presume in order to wield scientific knowledge, as the psychiatrist moves from the clinic to the courtroom? After all, these two domains have largely incommensurable conventions governing evidence. Stone suggests that "forensic psychiatrists are without any clear guidelines as to what is proper and ethical" (2008: 167–168). The ethical—and irresolvable—dilemma that faces the psychiatrist becomes exacerbated in the courtroom. The Hippocratic tension between helping and, first of all, doing no harm, makes little sense in a juridical context; help and harm become supplanted by the logics of evidence, justice, and public security. The ethic of the physician and the ethic of the jurist should not coincide; they take a different object, they have a different purpose.

One way to close this gap involves reducing psychiatry, *grosso modo*, to jurisprudence. But what occurs when the language of law is imported into the psychiatric domain? Unsurprisingly, we find psychiatry adhering to increasingly rigid and refined diagnoses, adhering to the rhetoric of "evidence." Increasingly, forensic psychiatrists align themselves with the rather narrow field of evidence-based medicine (Cole 2007), with its emphasis on randomized controlled trials and treatment plans informed by best-practice guidelines. For the evidence-based practitioner, these guidelines function as quasi-legal precedents. But evidence-based medicine has many critics, within psychiatry and without, so it is troubling that this biomedical model has become the standard in courts of law. In the United States, evidence-based medicine has been endorsed by the Supreme Court in *Daubert* (1993), where the Court recognized trial judges as the gatekeepers of evidence, giving them the power to determine whether and which evidence is scientifically valid and relevant to the case at hand. In Canada, there are similar Supreme Court cases that treat the role of evidence and expert testimony, namely, *R. v. Mohan* (1994) and *R. v. J.-L.J.* (2000). Significantly, both involved cases of pedophilia, which provide additional leeway for expert testimony in light of judging the "disposition" of the accused: "the exception has been applied to abnormal behaviour usually connoting sexual deviance" (*R. v. Mohan* 1994). In *Mohan*, we read: "The trial judge should consider the opinion of the expert and whether the expert is merely expressing a personal opinion or whether the behavioral profile which the expert is putting forward is in common use as a reliable indicator of membership in a distinctive group" (*R. v. Mohan* 1994). Problematically, the decision to include expert testimony is made on the basis of the "common sense and experience" of the trial judge, but expert evidence is only deemed necessary to the trial if it is "outside the experience and knowledge of a judge or jury" (*R. v. Mohan* 1994), so psychiatric "expertise" and juridical "common sense" stand in some tension. Either way, the evidence does not speak to the crime, but seeks to establish "scientific" and "common sense" evidence for a "disposition," and whether or not by virtue of said disposition the accused can be reliably profiled as a member of an abnormal population or group. In Foucault's words, "penal sanction will not be brought to bear on a legal subject who is recognized as being responsible but on an element that is the correlate of a technique that consists in singling out dangerous individuals and of taking responsibility for those who are accessible to penal sanction in order to cure them or reform them" (Foucault 2003b: 25).

Conclusion

These "developments" in forensic psychiatry are perhaps merely symptomatic of a deeper illness afflicting the late modern psychiatric enterprise as a whole. If, as we have argued, forensic psychiatry is ripe for being "pushed back" and "colonized," this is because psychiatry has largely abandoned a psychodynamic-psychotherapeutic approach to mental health care and has turned to a biopsychiatric one that treats the brain pharmacologically. The talk of "dispositions," "attitudes," "character" or "intent" no longer makes sense; these are not attributes of brains, and it is highly reductive to speak of them as neurochemical. The accused is a person, a life lived in complex relation with others and with the world. The person is subject to criminal law, not the brain. So psychiatry has nothing worthwhile to say; it speaks in another idiom.

While we have focused on forensic psychiatrists acting as expert witnesses in the courtroom, the courtroom scene is instructive because it provides a dramatization of the dilemma that faces the psychiatrist working in a prison setting—where the patient/inmate may be confused about the roles that the psychiatric healthcare provider plays. Does s/he practice psychiatry, taking up the role of a healer, to relieve suffering but first of all to do no harm? Does s/he practice forensics, using science to establish the facts in a criminal case, and to understand his/her patient's mental health in relation to the administration of criminal justice? Is s/he an agent of care or an agent of the correctional apparatus? Are his/her treatment plans informed by neoliberal biopolitics, as they are with "incentivizing" behaviour modification plans based on token economies? It matters little whether the token economy adopts a "rewards" or "punishments" model: it is a process of socialization that capitulates to market values, "where individuals are seduced into seeing themselves as 'human capital' within a system that calculates, quantifies and otherwise measures all manner of human relationships according to the terminology of the 'free' market" (Holmes and Murray 2011: 299). The answer, then, is that s/he has a dual role, s/he is a "double agent" (Austin, Goble, and Kelecevic 2009, Robertson and Walter 2008). And s/he lacks a meta-ethics that might help him/her to navigate between his/her two obligations. What happens to his/her ethical duty to "help" a patient if this results in a miscarriage of "justice"? Or, will s/he be forced to do "harm" in the *name* of "justice"? And how, according to what—and whose—logic will s/he decide?

References

Austin, W., Goble, E., and Kelecevic, J. 2009. The ethics of forensic psychiatry: Moving beyond principles to a relational ethics approach. *Journal of Forensic Psychiatry & Psychology, 20*(6), 835–850.

Cole, S.A. 2007. Toward evidence-based evidence: Supporting forensic knowledge claims in the post-Daubert era. *Tulsa Law Review, 43*(2), 101–121.

Daubert v. Merrell Dow Pharmaceuticals, Inc., 509 U.S. 579 (1993). [Online]. Available at: http://caselaw.lp.findlaw.com/scripts/getcase.pl?court=us&vol.=509&invol=579.

Forensic Psychiatrist Dr. Michael Welner on the Newtown Shooting, Part 1. (2012). (The View) [ABC television broadcast, season 16, episode 2]. Available at: http://theview.abc.go.com/video/dr-michael-welner-forensic-psychiatrist-part-1.

Foucault, M. 1977. *Discipline and Punish.* New York: Vintage Books.

Foucault, M. 2003a. *"Society Must be Defended": Lectures at the Collège de France, 1975–1976.* New York: Picador.

Foucault, M. 2003b. *Abnormal: Lectures at the Collège de France, 1974–1975.* New York: Picador.

Foucault, M. 2008. *The Birth of Biopolitics: Lectures at the Collège de France, 1978–1979.* New York: Picador.

Giroux, H.A. and Letizia, A. 2012. Interview with Henry A. Giroux. *Figure/Ground Communication.* Available at: http://figureground.ca/interviews/henry-armand-giroux/.

Gutheil, T.G., Hauser, M., White, M.S., Spruiell, G., and Strasburger, L.H. 2003. "The whole truth" versus "the admissible truth": An ethics dilemma for expert witnesses. *Journal of the American Academy of Psychiatry and the Law Online*, *31*(4), 422–427.

Holmes, D. and Murray, S.J. 2011. Civilizing the "barbarian": A critical analysis of behaviour modification programmes in forensic psychiatry settings. *Journal of Nursing Management*, *19*(3), 293–301.

Kaiser, H.A. 2009. Canadian mental health law: The slow process of redirecting the ship of state. *Health Law Journal*, *17*, 139–194.

Podlas, K. 2005. "The CSI Effect": Exposing the media myth. *Fordham Intellectual Property, Media and Entertainment Law Journal*, *16*(2), 429–465.

R. v. J.-L.J. 2000. 2 S.C.R. 600. Available at: http://scc.lexum.org/decisia-scc-csc/scc-csc/scc-csc/en/item/1815/index.do.

R. v. Lyons. 1987. 2 S.C.R. 309. Available at: http://scc.lexum.org/decisia-scc-csc/scc-csc/scc-csc/en/item/248/index.do.

R. v. Mohan. 1994. 2 S.C.R. 9. Available at: http://scc.lexum.org/decisia-scc-csc/scc-csc/scc-csc/en/item/1131/index.do.

Robertson, M.D. and Walter, G. 2008. Many faces of the dual-role dilemma in psychiatric ethics. *Australian and New Zealand Journal of Psychiatry*, *42*(3), 228–235.

Schweitzer, N.J. and Saks, M.J. 2007. The CSI Effect: Popular fiction about forensic science affects the public's expectations about real forensic science. *Jurimetrics*, *47*, 357–364.

Simon, R.I. 2003. Should forensic psychiatrists testify about evil? *Journal of the American Academy of Psychiatry and the Law Online*, *31*(4), 413–416.

Stone, A.A. 2008. The ethical boundaries of forensic psychiatry: A view from the ivory tower. *Journal of the American Academy of Psychiatry and the Law Online*, *36*(2), 167–174.

Welner, M. 2003. Response to Simon: Legal relevance demands that evil be defined and standardized. *Journal of the American Academy of Psychiatry and the Law Online*, *31*(4), 417–421.

PART II
Transformation

Chapter 8

Structural Othering: Towards an Understanding of Place in the Construction of Disruptive Subjectivities

Jean Daniel Jacob, Amélie Perron, and Pascale Corneau

Introduction

In the inaugural edition of the nursing journal *Aporia*, Stuart Murray (2009) drew on the work of Susan Sontag (1990) and spoke of two kingdoms: the kingdom of the well and the kingdom of the sick—kingdoms to which we must identify as citizens at some point in our lives. In talking about health and illness as forms of citizenships, however, Murray (2009) problematized the system of binary identities through which we are expected to experience and make sense of our health—as if there were only two kingdoms, as if "[w]e are meant to 'inhabit' a space of sickness or health […] with no space in between" (p. x). In boundaries and boundary crossing, however, we are reminded of a power politics that separates the kingdom of the well and the kingdom of the sick, one that is often negotiated at the point of care. Here, we turn to the many ways in which conceptions and experiences of health and illness lead to a contested "power politics being mapped out in the landscape of place through symbols, language and materiality" (Wilbert and Kearns 1999: 2); a power politics that comes to define us and remind us of where we belong in the vast health care infrastructure. As members of a two-king society, we come to derive our identity, in part, from the prevailing and divisive definitions of health and illness. As with Murray (2009), we draw on the image of two kingdoms to problematize the experiences of health at the border of these kingdoms where some individuals are denied passage and "are unable to achieve entry into what is essentially the legitimate career of sickness" (Jeffery 1979: 90). If we speak of health and sickness as two kingdoms, what place is there for a subject position that does not fit in one kingdom or another?

As healthcare professionals, "we play our part in lending and legitimizing the meaningful terms by which health and sickness are negotiated" (Murray 2009: 10). Throughout this chapter, it is our intention to explore how nurses practicing in the emergency department (ED) patrol the borders of these kingdoms in ways that produce (and reproduce) conceptions of health and illness and, in the process, confer the terms by which those who are "legitimately" sick and those who are not find their place in the health care system. As such, we must conceptualize entry into the kingdom of the sick as a place of contestation that stops the safe transition of people from one kingdom to another, thus creating subject positions that do not belong to either kingdom. In the ED, those patients whom we come to define through various terms ("the overdose," "the homeless," "the violent," "the psychotic," "the borderline," etc.) and who continuously challenge the way we legitimize/value certain illnesses over others, are forced to navigate a complex system that positions them somewhere between health and illness—a subject position that we may define as *Other*.

In order to engage in such a discussion, this chapter draws on qualitative data from a research project that explored how both nurses and patients identify and manage violence in one psychiatric emergency department (PED). One element that is particularly important to highlight for this chapter is the context in which the PED under study operates. The PED was physically located in (and not separated from) the general ED of an urban Canadian general hospital. In this case, the PED did not have a formal space per se, other than a small section of the central nursing station and the immediate space in front of it (small hallway and access to a few individual rooms) where stretchers for psychiatric patients were located. In other words, the PED was considered to be an integral part of the ED, to the extent that very little formal divisions existed between the two—a reality that inevitably contributed to the discussion that follows. Guided by individual accounts from both providers of mental health services (nurses) and recipients of care (patients), the results of this research highlight the multiple contextual elements that inadvertently give therapeutic significance to controlling interventions and, more importantly, shape the way we come to define "Others"—those who do not fit in the mainstream (ex. people presenting with objective physical ailments). As an extreme site where bodies are scrutinized, analyzed, and controlled, the PED participates in the production of subjectivities rooted in location. Drawing on the works of Foucault, Goffman, and other critical scholars, our analysis highlights the tensions that exist between nursing care and the micro-politics involved in its place of practice, thus positioning the PED as an anomaly in an ED and a key factor in the way patients are conceptualized and subsequently treated.

Background

Over the past 60 years, the field of mental health has undergone significant changes. A particular landmark in Western history has been the movement of deinstitutionalization as a movement of both individual rights and neoliberal ideology. However, de-institutionalization combined with insufficient community resources, has led to various negative impacts such as homelessness, multiple hospital readmissions, increased criminalization, and notably, the increased solicitation of emergency departments to provide mental health services (Dorvil and Gutman 1999). As a result, it is now common to see psychiatric emergency services (albeit in various forms and levels of organization) in ED to address the growing demand for psychiatric care.

When looking at the literature on EDs, it is clear that these environments are not always conducive to psychiatric assessments, as patients often find themselves having to interact with health care professionals in crowded and/or noisy environments (Olsen and Sabin 2003). Too often are we confronted with statistics showing that emergency staff have over-relied on the use of coercive treatments in the form of restraints to deal with patients presenting with a psychiatric issue (CIHI 2011). Though they may be perceived to be highly effective (Downey, Zun, and Gonzales 2007), seclusion and restraints (including chemical restraints) remain highly contested practices in health care and need to be explored in relation to the factors that promote their application. If hospitals now address the increased demands for psychiatric care in the emergency department by developing psychiatric emergency services—services that are often called upon to deal with the bulk of behavioral disturbances (Vibha and Saddichha 2010)—we need to understand that ensuing practices are "influenced by a complex set of factors including the types of behaviors patients present with, staff attitudes and the organizational context within which decisions are made" (Lincoln et al. 2010: 2). That is, we need to acknowledge that emergency psychiatric practices cannot be understood outside of their context and necessitate that we speak of *place* in the delivery of care.

Understanding Place in the Construction of Subjectivities

In the context of health care, we must consider the fact that bodies are located in institutional places that are laden with significance. On the topic of place, socio-cultural geographer Robin Kearns (1993) writes: "what occurs in a place (in terms of the relations between people and elements of their environment) has a profound importance to health" (p. 141). Here, Kearns (1993) turns to the concept of place to highlight the contextual nature of health experiences as determined, in part, by the places (as opposed to spaces) in which care is provided.

The distinction between place and space is important to highlight for this paper. On the one hand, space may be conceived as an element of place and fairly neutral concept: a setting, a geometric variable or backdrop in which social relations are enacted (Poland 2005). It this sense, we may find this concept useful for its descriptive capability—helping us map out the physical (or virtual) world that makes up our environment. On the other hand, place may be thought of as "a particular or lived space" (Agnew 2001: 6), one that is considered to be an active player in the enactment of social relations. In looking at PEDs, the use of place (as opposed to space) forces us to shift our thinking and focus on the dialectical relationship between the elements that make up our environment (material, symbolic, human, etc.) and our subjective experiences (sense of place or feeling out of place) (Poland et al. 2005); how being in certain places effects how we come to understand ourselves and others. In this sense, place can be seen as emerging from a complex web of ongoing relations (material, social, and discursive), which in turn participate in the production of experiences and the composition of subjectivity (McGrath and Reavey 2013). The concept of place and its role in shaping individual subjectivities becomes meaningful to the extent that we take into account those interrelated elements that surround us (material, social, symbolic, discursive, etc.) and shape the way we come to see ourselves and others. It is precisely the contextual notion of place that directs our attention to the emergence of a "culture of place" (Poland et al. 2005: 172). Here, "culture" finds all of its significance in the way socially produced values and beliefs are enacted through interactions bounded in space (real and/or virtual). As part of a culture of place and our attempts to grasp the complexities of PEDs, it is imperative that we take into account how "place both represents and is represented within language, meaning, experience and subjectivity" (Poland et al. 2005: 172).

Place and Power

Inherent to our understanding of a culture of place is the concurrent understanding of how interactions within any given space (physical locale) are rife with power relations. In effect, any institutional space gives rise to discursive, material, and symbolic elements permeated by diffuse power relations. In this sense, place is as much about material divisions and the many ways in which they reflect and reinforce relations of power as it is about social dynamics, symbols, and discourses that are embedded in daily ways of thinking and doing. According to Foucault (1980), this system of relations between various elements may be defined as an apparatus which, in any given place, is designed to achieve a specific purpose. As Latour (2005) would argue, this complex network or set of relations between human and non-human elements enables these same elements to acquire certain attributes and meanings. As part of our understanding of place in the construction of subjectivities, the focus on relations between entities is of utmost importance. How we come to understand our place in the health care infrastructure results from various associations and dissociations between both human and non-human entities. If Foucault speaks of various forms of power in the government of self and others, then Latour further pushes our attention to the elements that enable this power to be produced and crystallized in ways of doing and thinking. Examining the intricacies of what we define as "emergency psychiatric services" within the ED is useful to understand how emergency psychiatric nursing care comes into being, is experienced within a situated set of relations, and becomes an active element in its own right in the production of practices and subjectivities.

In health care, and nursing more specifically, the way place and power intersect is perhaps most evident in the hierarchical structure of the hospital that dictates "who controls access, who sets the agenda, whose interests are served, and how those lower in the socio-institutional hierarchy are treated in ways that continually 'remind' them of—and keep them in—their 'place'" (Poland et al. 2005: 172). What is less evident, however, are the ways in which power is embedded, produced, and reproduced in practices of care (Holmes and Gastaldo 2002). Power is anything but irrelevant when we look at nursing interventions in the ED and the way they are associated with a set of complex contextual elements, whether they are human, material, legal, ideological, moral, etc. Using data obtained from our research, we wish to engage in a discussion that will highlight the *embeddedness* of practices and its effects in one psychiatric emergency department. Here, Foucault's (1995) work on places of discipline is seminal, as are the works of Goffman (2002) and Sibley (1995) on total institutions and geographies of exclusion, respectively. These theoretical works will be presented alongside empirical data in order to analyze practices in the PED and to generate new ways of thinking about them.

Places of Discipline

In *Discipline and Punish*, Foucault (1995) engages in a detailed history of confinement as well as the "microphysics" of power that seek to generate forces, make them grow, and order them (Rabinow 1984). Out of Foucault's account emerge places of discipline where power, discourses, practices, and space come to be aligned in the regulation of individual and group behavior. Foucault's work "focuses our attention on the interrelationship between spatial relation and spatial formation: he shows that particular discourses, networks of power, sets of material resources can all be stabilized in discrete spatial zones (the hospital, the prison, and so forth)" (Murdoch 2006: 53). Significant to the production/operation of disciplinary power and the ways in which it intersects with space and knowledge are the techniques (hierarchical observation, normalizing judgment, and examination) deployed in the control/production of docile bodies. A central concept related to the deployment of these techniques is that of panopticism—a metaphorical spatial organization that intensifies visibility and highlights power/knowledge dynamics "designed to observe, monitor, shape and control the behavior of individuals" (Gordon 1991: 3). As the participants in our study noted, the ED is designed in such a way to enable complete supervision of patients and immediate interventions.

> They tend to put you on a stretcher close to the nurses' station, where someone always can have an eye on you, […] if there is a problem they will intervene. (Patient)

While panopticism permits the emergence of new forms of knowledge though observation, "that knowledge is, in turn, employed to exercise more efficient and effective Panoptic power" (Roberts 2005: 35). As Foucault (1995) explains, the hospital, among other disciplinary places, tends to be "divided into as many sections as there are bodies […] in order to easily locate individuals, to set up useful communications, to interrupt others, to be able at each moment to supervise the conduct of each individual, to assess it, to judge it, to calculate its qualities or merits" (p. 143). The distribution of people in specific locations and the control of their activities ensure that everyone is assigned a place in the institution and can, therefore, be monitored, known, controlled, contained, and so forth. Clearly, ED patients are highly visible and subject to corrective interventions if they proved to be "disruptive" in this environment. However, it is the nurses' visibility and its disciplinary effects that were particularly striking in this research. That is, limiting the analysis of panopticism and disciplinary power to the distribution and discipline of patients in the hospital would not acknowledge the full complexity of this form of power and the ways in which psychiatric nurses are themselves disciplined in adopting new behaviors and practices in the ED. In effect, psychiatric nurses working in the emergency department are affected by disciplinary power, in that their practice proves to be governed, in part, by the gaze of other ED nurses and their expectations of control.

> [The psychiatric nurse] will be seen as being too permissive, as lacking ... experience, so [the ED nurse] will blame the [psychiatric] nurse as opposed to saying; "it is the patient who is responsible for his actions and it is him who decided to do this." […] in part, the medical side will make her accountable for the patient's behavior. (Nurse)

In effect, the concept of panopticism suggests that awareness of being under constant observation induces self-discipline (change in behavior) in those being observed. That is, nurses come to change their own practice knowing that their actions (or lack thereof) may be under the scrutiny of their colleagues—especially if observed behaviors may lead to sanctions such as blame for improper care. The difficulty in being permissive in the ED due to space constraints coupled with accountability of the patient's whereabouts/actions increases the need for control by psychiatric nurses.

> For example, if he starts wandering in the ED, […] I have the nurses from the medical side saying: "Ah! Look at what your patient is doing" […] It is the others who look at me and say: "Hey, look at your patient!" I know that my patient is OK. […] Even I can't stay on the bed for 6 hours doing nothing. I will wander. […] On the other hand, this is not a psychiatric ED, it is not closed. (Nurse)

Perceptions of being unpredictable coupled with the fact that patients are mobile becomes a key element in their subjectification as disruptive individuals in need of a separate, locked space.

> All patients in psychiatry, I think, have a potential to be aggressive—either because their mental state does not permit them to control themselves or … they are under the effects of drugs other than medications. (Nurse)

> If we could have a more structured environment, where we had more control, yes, there would be more flexibility. We could be more smooth with them. […] But in the ED we are scared that patients may leave; we are scared that they mix with other patients; we are scared that the ED staff come on our side […] (Nurse)

> A separated area for the psychiatric patients, a locked unit where I don't have to worry about them running away, and maybe an extra nurse … (Nurse)

In lieu of what the nurses consider an ideal workplace, the cohabitation of the PED and the ED produces complex dynamics in which controlling practices come to be seen as necessary to foster a "therapeutic environment." A common example given by participants is the unofficial request to medicate patients (often at bedtime) to limit any interventions during the night shift and avoid blame from other nurses if something were to happen. The notion of autonomy (or lack thereof) in decision making is particularly striking, as psychiatric nurses are compelled by other ED nurses to enforce control through PRN medication (medication given as needed)—a situation that creates its fair share of internal tension.

> Personally, I find it a little intrusive, a little bit controlling, that I give a PRN to someone who is OK for him to be more OK. But in the ED it is zero tolerance. They want nothing to do with psychiatry. (Nurse)

As the next excerpts demonstrate, some nurses address this internal tension by rationalizing the use of PRN medication within a therapeutic framework. Knowing that unmedicated patients run the risk of being restrained during the night given that there is no psychiatric staff and caring for such patients is often deemed to be a burden by other ED nurses, the use of PRN medication thus becomes a tool that protects patients from such invasive/coercive practices and safeguards nurses from future blame.

> We know that if the patient wanders in on the medical side, the medical team will call a code white, they will tie her up and they will inject her. It's about trying to contain the person in the most "least restrictive" way possible in the environment that we have in order to avoid less serious situations. (Nurse)

> There are no [psychiatric] nurses on nights. I have to give my patients to the nurses in the ED. It is something they don't really like. So, again, I have to use medication as a restraint for my patients and the benefits of everyone. I make my patients sleep. I give them medication so that they can sleep during the night and assure that they will not be a problem for the night nurses. (Nurse)

While Foucault explores how disciplinary power is closely linked to spatial configurations (architecture/division of space), knowledge and discipline (of the self and others), Goffman (2002) problematizes the existing tensions and contradictions between the therapeutic demands of care and the imperatives of social control in total institutions (including hospitals). As in the results of this research, we can appreciate how "health care places encompass normative considerations that reveal, materialize and extend significant aspects of professional cultures and dynamics" (Lehoux et al. 2007: 1537). In this sense, PEDs are inextricably linked to surveillance and control of the self and the other, relying on models of care that organize the work of nurses and the use of various technologies. In other words, current practices in the PED show the extent to which experiences of health are deeply structured by spatial regulations (Andrews 2002, Kearns 1993).

Places of Exclusion—Being Out of Place

In our conception of place, it is clear that every space has meaning. The way a space is divided and organized (both physically and discursively) suggests particular relationships between those who occupy (or not) that space: friendship, alliance, separation, distance, fear, tension, hostility, inequality, and so on. However, we seldom question those aspects of our environment that reinforce and foster practices of inclusion and exclusion. By looking at the meaning of spaces and acknowledging the various forms of power at play within any given space, it is then possible to think in terms of place and question taken-for-granted assumptions that we may consider as "naturally" occurring, and explore how certain places participate in the exclusion of particular individuals and groups. In this research, and as expressed in previous quotes, participants spoke of an interpersonal division (as opposed to a physical one) in the ED, one that took on the form of intolerance towards psychiatric patients. Here, participants spoke of an internal policy—zero tolerance to violence—as perpetuating violence, rather than eliminating it.

> We are a zero tolerance here now. You can only talk so much […] (Nurse).

> Provider violence takes place in the form of intolerance. There is intolerance towards psychiatry, its patients […](Nurse)

> […] Because it's not everyone that has the same tolerance towards psychiatric patients. … we have to be clear, there are people who don't like to work with psychiatric patients. So, when we give you a psychiatric patient and it's not your choice, you won't do your job the same way. (Nurse)

These participants suggest that such a policy justifies the actions to be taken in the face of disruption. But, as the following quotes suggest, psychiatric staff are portrayed as being more tolerant of intrusive/disruptive behaviors, which are often associated with psychiatric patients' mobility.

> I give them [patients] permission to be intrusive. I think that is what the main difference is. (Nurse)

> […] don't forget, when you work in psychiatry, you get used to the intrusiveness, you get used to that, people coming, coming … when you are not used to it, and you get a patient constantly asking, you just want to say: "Get over there!" Or people will just want to restrain them! Right there, you didn't address the problem, all you said [was]: "Get over there or else!" (Nurse)

In this situation, a zero tolerance policy proves to be a paradox. It both demonstrates a will to offer a safe work/care environment for nurses but also promotes intolerance and justifies controlling interventions against patients. Yet as Sibley (1995) argues, "power is expressed in the monopolization of space and in the regulation of weaker groups in society to less desirable environments" (p. ix). Here, Sibley (1995) describes a modern concern for socio-spatial separation in society and boundary maintenance between those individuals who embody certain societal ideals (pure) and those who do not (defiled). As we found in this research, virtual boundaries of intolerance reinforce a divisive culture in which both psychiatric nurses and patients lack a sense of belonging (being out of place). Psychiatric nurses identify with their patients and come to see them as not belonging and in need of a different environment.

> Of course, if I was in the hallway … sleeping with the lights on, with the noise, I would have a horrible character […] This is not ideal. Placing a patient in psychiatry here is not ideal. Containing them to a little room, giving them medication. If that doesn't work, use restraints. But that is because I don't want the situation to escalate in the ED. Because it's too risky for everyone. It has happened in the past where a situation was completely out of control and we had to evacuate everyone from the ED to protect them. If I had a closed section for psychiatric patients I would be in a better position to try other things. (Nurse)

Processes of exclusion are thus exemplified by the removal of undesirable individuals and subsequent purification of spaces (Sibley 1995). Of particular importance to our discussion on places of exclusion are the various practices that reinforce boundaries between individuals and groups. Using words that suggest "defilement," for example, participates in the symbolic representations and subsequent negative portrayal of the "Other"— representations that justify practices of exclusion (for example, maintaining a certain distance or building divisions between people). In our research, we see psychiatric nurses using a language of therapy, disruption, and the apparent dangers for other patients in the ED to justify the separation of a seemingly different group of people.

The divisive process described above may be referred to as an "Othering" process, one that establishes boundaries between groups: those who are labeled as 'different' and those who are deemed to belong to the mainstream (Johnson, Bottorff, Browne,

Grewal, Hilton, and Clarke 2004). Generally speaking, references to "Othering" in the health care literature highlight its negative connotation (Canales 2010); that is, the boundaries that are established between individuals evoke oppositional differences, whereby the Other is attributed a negative value (MacCallum 2002). In this sense, practices that are involved in dividing individuals and groups based on negative portrayals are inevitably rooted in power relations, where those who are viewed as being different are set out to be (socially, physically, geographically) distanced (Hellzén et al. 2004). Here, we may refer to *structural Othering* as the different institutional structures/dynamics that create or even reinforce divisive practices and the "stigmatic assumptions" that become embedded in policies and practices in the form of a risk discourse that identifies some groups as 'dangerous' and that legitimizes various forms of interventions (Bruckert and Hannem 2012: 5). Along with Johnson and colleagues (2004), we can envision those instances where individuals do not "easily fit into routines and the culture of efficiency that characterizes the mainstream health care system" (p. 266); a system that will, in turn, participate in the construction of these individuals as "being difficult to deal with and a burden on an already resource-strapped system" (p. 266).

In looking at the dynamics of place in this research, we are in a position to focus on those elements that may normally go unnoticed and with which any member of a dominant group may be unaware. In order to examine those elements that are implicit in the design/conception of spaces (both inclusionary and exclusionary), Sibley (1995) suggests we ask ourselves: "who are places for, whom do they exclude, and how are the prohibitions maintained in practice?" (p. x). By asking these questions, we are (re)locating practices into their context and addressing the complex set of relations that affect our everyday practice and that we have come to understand as being normal and true. In this research, nurses recognize both an inability to work to their full potential and the detrimental effects of the environment on their patients.

> I may have the capacity, but I don't have the environment to act in the same way [as I would on a psychiatric unit] because in the ED, I have to make decisions faster. I have to keep control given the environment. […] Because the space is so tight, he will scare the other patients […] So what do I do? Try to constrain him to his room, no? (Nurse)

One patient described problems associated with the PED in a particularly telling manner, qualifying it as an anomaly in the ED and a "necessary evil" in a patient's passage to the psychiatric ward.

> It's like, we can't screw around, there are patients here, trauma patients, there are patients here with other things. Psych patients who are in emergency rooms, I would call them necessary evils. They're there because they have to be, for whatever reason, the circumstances, they have to transit through there, the ER system. But they're definitely an anomaly within the overall ER structure. So in consequence,

> what I've perceived and what I've seen is that they use the big guns faster, to try and subdue, desist, put away. […] They don't dick around. They cut– move to the point, to control, because they know […] there's so [many] other things of critical importance taking place within an ER, from a medical point of view. There's no time to waste with the anomaly which is the psych patients. (Patient)

Reproducing the Biomedical Hegemony

In 1979, Jeffery spoke of illness as a "morally ambiguous condition" (p. 90), one that is negotiated within the medical encounter and inevitably bound to the context in which it is experienced. His analysis of ED patients reminds us of the fragile conception of belonging by exposing divisive practices that situate patients on opposite ends of a continuum—either good (interesting) or bad (rubbish)—and thus assigning them a "prognostic place" (Murray 2009: 8) in the vast healthcare infrastructure. As Jeffery (1979) notes, emergency departments tend to favor certain forms of illness over others. We quickly realize that with specialized knowledge also come specific forms of language, organization, spatial formation, and practices of differentiation and exclusion. The "smelly," the "dirty," and the "mentally ill" patients are often constituted through this knowledge, and are construed as being a difficult fit in medical emergency departments. This results in the subsequent production of boundaries (real and virtual) between patients of (dis)interest and the rest of the ED patients. Inadvertently, the ways by which we come to conceptualize patients end up defining us as health care providers—the way we define health and good practices. The implicit danger in the way we come to define "Others" is that we may experience these classifications as natural, necessary, and true—that is, they will constrain what we are permitted to think, say, feel, and do in any given situation (Murray 2009).

Along with Jeffery (1979), we may think of the ED as a place of biomedical hegemony. Evidently, psychiatric presentations (acute psychosis, odd behaviors, severe distress, and harm both to self and others) pose significant concerns to emergency department staff who often feel they lack the skills to address the needs of this clientele and, as a result, reinforce a divisive and controlling/coercive culture of care (Clarke et al. 2005, McArthur and Montgomery 2004). Uncertainty with psychiatric presentations, both in terms of validity of symptoms and of ways in which they can be dealt with in the ED, may foster frustration and hostility from staff towards patients (Jeffery 1979). We are thus inclined to think of the PED itself as *Other*, because psychiatric complaints, assessments, and treatment disrupt the normal flow of the ED as they do not fit within its dominant biomedical orientation (Clarke et al. 2005). As the results of this research indicate, there is a tension between the ED and PED in which psychiatric patients may be seen as taking up much needed space. In parallel, however, psychiatric staff are valued for their capacity to help secure the environment—a capacity we speculate contributes to reinforcing views that psychiatric patients need to be contained and restrained.

> The medical side often perceives psychiatry as taking up beds which could be used for their medical cases. Some lack knowledge regarding psychiatry. But when there's a code, they're happy that we're always there to fix the problem, from medication to restraints and securing the environment. (Nurse)

Despite clear distinctions between "ideal" ways of working with psychiatric patients in the ED, reproduction of the biomedical discourse within the PED remains pervasive. In response to a lack of alternative ways to work with psychiatric patients, nurses revert back to medication (and possibly other forms of restraints) in order to counter the negative environment of the ED and find a solution to the issue of mental illness—one that is dealt with internally (biochemically) rather than externally. In this sense, prevailing practices of control of illness within the ED carry on into the PED in the form of pharmacological management.

> We complement as much as we can […] we try to put people in different rooms. But when we can't, we use medication … it's not ideal but that's that. (Nurse)

The use of medication to deal with the busyness of the ED flirts with the notion of chemically restraining patients but fits with the necessity to control the environment and protect others.

> I keep them in chemical restraints all evening, perhaps. But at least, it's more livable for others. (Nurse)

This participant goes on to explain how medication becomes the tool of practice in the ED. The issue now becomes a problem of individual and internal struggle, one that is situated inside the person rather than recognized as a symptom of a non-therapeutic environment. The aggressive use of pharmacologic agents in the PED fits well with modern views of (bio)psychiatry whereby rapid tranquilization and control of signs and symptoms of acute psychiatric disturbances are desired. This view, however, should not be confused with using pharmacologic agents to compensate for a poor therapeutic environment—a reality that seems to be difficult to untangle at the point of care.

> […] but I find the chemical restraint … it's certain that I use it, and I use it often, given the situation in the ED, given the workload, given the level of stress in the ED. I don't only do it for my own benefit, but I also do it for the person's benefit, because a patient in psychosis, a patient who is anxious is a person who suffers[…] It's not only a question of restraints … it's also a question of relieving the person. (Nurse)

The results of this research indicate certain expectations from ED staff, in which psychiatric nurses who work there must control disruptive behaviors. At first glance, one may consider such expectations as falling within the psychiatric nurse's field of expertise, in that s/he is in a position to deploy an array of therapeutic techniques that would help manage problematic behaviors. What seems evident, however, are the many ways in which psychiatric practice is constrained by its location, both in terms of space and dominant medical functioning. This hinders the provision of mental health services and participates in the construction of psychiatric patients as disruptive and in need of containment. That is, the complexity of psychiatric presentations is oversimplified and made secondary to the maintenance of order in the (medical) ED. Individualized approaches are thus re-inscribed into a biomedical (biopsychiatric) model of care in which reliance on psychopharmacological treatment perpetuates the predominant medical ideology of the ED, whereby they offer quick and effective short-term solutions to disruptive behaviors. As this next excerpt shows, a consumerist view could form part of a counter discourse to prevailing ways of doing in the ED, in that it challenges the "quick" fix approach and embraces the complexity of psychiatric issues.

> But I would take it out of the context of the ER. I guess it's inappropriate to say one's more medical, you know, your heart, someone's had a heart attack, someone just got their leg shaved off by machinery at the factory, or, there are issues at hand that people who require treatment which are very different from psych patients who are in crisis. Um, this might sound crazy, what I'm about to say, but it is like the medicalization of the crisis […] what it would mean to me is that my crisis is being looked at like it could be dealt with simply with a pill, or some sort of medical intervention, uh, you know, a bypass or something like that. That's not what it's about. I need empathy, I need someone to listen to me. I need a soft approach to help me deal with my crisis. (Patient)

As this participant explains, an approach that is centered on symptom management with medication does not address the complexity of psychiatric emergencies and could be described as the medicalization of distress—one that may very well be exacerbated by the ED department. Such insights remind us of the contextual nature of psychiatric nurses' interventions, the need to take into account places of care and to give ourselves permission to question whether there may be other ways of addressing the situation.

Final Remarks

We wish to revisit Murray's (2009) characterization of two kingdoms, the kingdom of the well and the kingdom of the sick, to highlight the problematic system of binary identities that govern our ways of thinking. As we have seen throughout this chapter, being categorized as psychiatrically ill does not necessarily mean a safe transition into the kingdom of the sick, but rather highlights some important elements in the construction of psychiatric patients as disruptive and the subsequent reliance on psychiatric nurses to act as agents of control. In this case, place emerges as an actor in determining both patient and nursing subjectivities and practices. It further pushes our reflection on the mainstreaming of practices for the ED to the PED; practices that may prove to be detrimental rather than inclusive. As participants explain, there may be a need to shift the configuration of the PED to accommodate (not exclude) psychiatric patients' needs in the ED, rather than try to make them fit in an environment that positions them as an anomaly to be contained/controlled rather than cared for.

References

Andrews, G.J. 2002. Towards a more place-sensitive nursing research: An invitation to medical and health geography. *Nursing Inquiry*, *9*, 221–238.

Bruckert, C. and Hannem, S. 2012. Introduction. In S. Hannem and C. Bruckert (Eds). *Stigma Revisited: Implications of the Mark.* Ottawa: University of Ottawa Press, 1–5.

Canales, M.K. 2000. Othering: Toward an understanding of difference. *Advances in Nursing Science*, *22*(4), 16–31.

Clarke, D.E., Hughes, L., Brown, A.M., and Motluk, L. 2005. Psychiatric emergency nurses in the emergency department: The success of the Winnipeg, Canada, experience. *Journal of Emergency Nursing.*, *31*(4): 351–356.

Dorvil, H., and Guttman, H. 1999. *35 ans de désinstitutionnalisation au Québec 1961–1996. Défis de la reconfiguration des services de santé mentale.* [Online]. Available at: http://msssa4.msss.gouv.qc.ca/fr/document/publication.nsf/0/d1251d29af46beec85256753004b0df7/$FILE/97_155a1.pdf

Downey, L.V., Zun L.S., and Gonzales S.J. 2007. Frequency of alternative to restraints and seclusion and uses of agitation reduction techniques in the emergency department. *General Hospital Psychiatry*, *29*(6), 470–474.

Foucault, M. 1980. The politics of public health in the 18th century. In C. Gordon (Ed.). *Power/Knowledge and Selected Interviews and Other Writings 1972–77 by Michel Foucault.* New York: Pantheon Books, 194–210.

Foucault, M. [1975] 1995. *Discipline & Punish.* New York: Vintage Books.

Giddens A. 1991. *Modernity and Self-Identity: Self Society in the Late Modern Age.* Stanford, CA: Stanford University Press.

Goffman, E. 2002. *Asiles: études sur la condition sociale des malades mentaux.* Paris: Éditions de minuit.

Gordon C. 1991. Governmental rationality: An introduction. In G. Burchell, C. Gordon and P. Miller (Eds). *The Foucault Effect.* Chicago: University of Chicago Press, 1–51.

Hellzen, O., Asplund, K., Sandman, P.-O., and Norberg, A. 2004. The meaning of caring as described by nurses caring for a person who acts provokingly: An interview study. *Scandinavian Journal of Caring Sciences*, *18*, 3–11.

Holmes, D. and Gastaldo, D. 2002. Nursing as means of governmentality. *Journal of Advanced Nursing*, *38*(6), 557–565.

Jeffery, R. 1979. Normal Rubbish: deviant patients in casualty departments. *Sociology of Health and Illness*, *1*(1), 90–107.

Johnson, J.L., Bottorff, J.L., Browne, A.J., Grewal, S., Hilton, B.A. and Clarke, H. 2004. Othering and being Othered in the context of health care services. *Health Communication*, *16*(2), 253–271.

Kearns, R.A. 1993. Place and health: Towards a reformed medical geography. *The Professional Geographer*, *45*(2), 139–147.

Latour, B. 2005. *Reassembling the Social: An Introduction to Actor-Network Theory*. New York: Oxford University Press.

Lehoux, P., Daudelin, G., Poland, B., Andrews, G.J., and Holmes, D. 2007. Designing a better place for patients: Professional struggles surrounding satellite and mobile dialysis units. *Social Science and Medicine*, *65*, 1536–1548.

Lincoln, A.K., White, A., Casandra, A., Johson, P., and Strunin, L. 2010. Observing the work of an urban safety-net psychiatric emergency room: Managing the unmanageable. *Sociology of Health and Illness*. *32*(3), 437–451.

MacCallum, E.J. 2002. Othering and psychiatric nursing. *Journal of Psychiatric and Mental Health Nursing*, *9*(1), 87–94.

McArthur, M. and Montgomery, P. 2004. The experience of gatekeeping: A psychiatric nurse in an emergency department. *Issues in Mental Health Nursing*, *25*, 487–501.

McGrath, L. and Reavey, P. 2013. Heterotopias of control: Placing the material in experiences of mental health service use and community living. *Health & Place*, *22*, 123–131.

Murdoch, J. 2006. *Post-Structuralist Geography: A Guide to Relational Space*. Thousand Oaks: Sage.

Murray, S.J. 2009. Towards an ethic of critique. *Aporia*, *1*(1), 8–14.

Olsen J.C. and Sabin B.R. 2003. Emergency department patient perceptions of privacy and confidentiality. *Journal of Emergency Medicine*, *14*(3), 329–333.

Poland, B., Lehoux, P., Holmes, D., and Andrews, G. 2005. How place matters: Unpacking technology and power relations in health and social care. *Health and Social Care in the Community*, *13*(2), 170–180.

Rabinow, P. 1984. *The Foucault Reader*. New York: Pantheon Books.

Roberts, M. 2005. The production of the psychiatric subject: Power, knowledge and Michel Foucault. *Nursing Philosophy*, *6*, 33–42.

Sontag, S. 1990. *Illness as Metaphor and AIDS and its Metaphors*. NewYork: Picador.

Sibley, D. 1995. *Geographies of Exclusion*. New York: Routledge.

Vibha, P. and Saddichha, S. 2010. The burden of behavioral emergencies: Need for specialist emergency services. *Internal and Emergency Medicine*, *5*, 513–519.

Wilbert, M. and Kearns, R.A. 1999. *Culture/Place/Health*. New York: Routledge.

Chapter 9
When You Try to Speak Truth to Power: What Happens if the Powerful Turn Off Their Hearing Aids?[1]

Paula J. Caplan

These days, when I think of the American Psychiatric Association (APA), I remember Lily Tomlin's character Ernestine, an obstreperous telephone operator who was damned if she *really* wanted to help anyone. Emitting her snorting laugh, she said, "We don't care. We don't have to. We're the telephone company." The APA doesn't care. It doesn't have to. It is totally unregulated. That makes it even less regulated than the financial giants who have damaged the economy.

I write this chapter as part of a larger, ongoing public education effort, because people need to know how utterly unresponsive and cold-blooded this unregulated lobby group is. The APA's fortress protects 36,000 psychiatrists, and although some I know personally and consider great human beings and helpers, the organization's power and the cover of its so-called ethics standards provide protection for those who break the "Do no harm rule." In fact, the APA's motto could be, "We will allow no harm to be done to our members who do harm to those who come seeking help."

In summer, 2012, I coordinated the filing with the APA's Ethics Department of nine groundbreaking complaints about psychiatric diagnosis destroying people's lives, because the APA creates, markets, and profits from the *Diagnostic and Statistical Manual of Mental Disorders* while promoting the false beliefs that its contents are scientifically grounded, help reduce suffering, and carry no risks of harm (Caplan 2012a). The heart of each complaint was its writer's eloquent description of the staggering array of harms she had suffered. Each complainant requested action to redress the harm done to her and prevent future harm to others (I had filed the ninth complaint as an "interested party" who over decades had witnessed harm done by psychiatric diagnosis.) On November 11, 2012, I announced that the APA summarily dismissed the complaints without the slightest indication of having considered their merits (Caplan 2012b). They ignored our

1 This chapter was adapted from Caplan, Paula J. (2013). Psychiatric diagnosis as a last bastion of unregulated, rampant harm to the populace. In M. Dellwing and M. Harbusch (Eds). *Krankheitskonstruktionen und Krankheitstreiberei: Die Renaissance der soziologischen Psychiatriekritik*. Wiesbaden: Springer.

request that they bring in objective people from outside the APA to handle the complaints; we had noted that, because the APA itself was named as a respondent, it would be important to do this in order to avoid conflicts of interest. The November 11 essay contains Jenny McClendon's heartbreaking story: She was repeatedly raped while in the Navy, and when she sought help, was diagnosed first with Bipolar Disorder and later with Borderline Personality Disorder and told her mental illnesses were what caused her upset. The dismissals caused all of the complainants pain, rage, and feelings of yet again being treated as though their suffering did not matter … but what special irony that the news came to Jenny shortly before Veterans Day.

The APA's Notice of Dismissal

On October 22, 2012, the following brief, strange notice of the summary dismissal of the complaints had been sent from apace@psych.org to all complainants simultaneously:

> Dear Complainants:
>
> The APA Ethics Committee met and reviewed the complaints that you filed. After thorough discussion, the unanimous conclusion of the Committee is that none of the complaints filed comply with APA's procedures for filing and resolving ethics complaints, and in any event, none of the complaints state a violation of the Ethics rules against the respondents named in the complaints. Instead, the complaints reflect a fundamental misunderstanding on your part of the purpose and appropriate use of DSM-IV in diagnosing mental illness. Since you filed these complaints with the APA Ethics Committee rather than with a district branch, there is no further appeal from this Committee's unanimous decision and these cases are closed.
>
> Sincerely,
>
> The APA Ethics Committee

In that paragraph, they relied solely on spuriously interpreted and/or unclear procedural grounds.

Response to the Notice of Dismissal

I emailed the complainants to suggest that we consider how to proceed before publicly announcing the dismissal. Unfortunately, I unthinkingly hit "Reply All," and since the notice of dismissal had been copied to Linda Hughes, who appears to be head administrator of the APA's Ethics Department, it also went to her. In that message, I referred to a planned "November 12 action" and proposed that in addition to asking for an in-person meeting with the APA staff, we should also ask them to explain the grounds they cited for dismissal. You will see later how that may have become relevant.

On November 2, I emailed a response to the dismissal, challenging what the committee members had written, asking questions, and making six requests. To understand my questions, you need to know that we filed the complaints against a great many respondents, aiming to include all who had major responsibility for the *DSM* edition that had caused harm to the complainants. They included the top *DSM-IV* and *IV-TR* people who remain APA members, everyone who had been an APA president or member of the board of trustees from 1988 (when work on *DSM-IV* began) to the present, and the APA itself, because the organization publishes the manual, oversees its advertising, and reaps the massive profits (they were said to have made more than $100 million from those editions). We argued that each respondent knew or ought to have known the truth about the manual and could have reduced the harm by making the truth public. Instead, each either did nothing of the kind or made public statements that the manual is scientific and/or helpful and failed to warn of or try to document, prevent, or redress the harm.

The APA's description of complaints procedures includes a statement that a complaint can be filed with a district branch and that a complaint filed with the APA itself will be referred to the district branch of what they call the "Accused Member." We filed our complaints with the APA itself and asked that they be dealt with at the national level, both because the respondents live in many different districts and because the matters in the complaints are of national (even international) import. In the months after we filed, emails from Linda Hughes and APA General Counsel Colleen Coyle revealed that they were trying to find ways to dismiss the complaints without considering their merits, and in part by asserting that their procedures did not allow for consideration at the national level (Caplan 2012b). Coyle had stated that to be fair to previous complainants, they must use the same procedures with us that they have used with others, including assigning ours to district branches. I had responded to her that as an attorney, she would recognize that the history of the United States legal system shows that some circumstances warrant major changes and that if the courts had not considered such changes important, then slavery would still be legal, and she and I would not be allowed to vote. This argument carried no weight: The APA's determination to dismiss the complaints overrode their willingness to consider what really matters. How troubling that it was the APA's division charged with ensuring ethical conduct that made this determination.

Here is my November 2 email:

> Dear Colleen Coyle, Linda Hughes, and "Ethics Committee":
>
> On behalf of all nine of us complainants, I am writing to ask the following, and we hope you will do us the courtesy of sending replies:

(1)In the brief note you sent on October 22, 2012, you said it was "the unanimous conclusion of the [Ethics] Committee" that the complaints should be dismissed. We ask yet again that you tell us the names of the members of that committee. Does it not strike you as rather medieval for the committee members' names to be kept secret from the complainants, especially given that these are the people whom the APA entrusts with ensuring that its ethical rules are followed? In the absence of this information, you are telling all of these people whose horrible suffering is documented in their complaints that some undisclosed secret members have summarily decided the fate of their request for fair consideration.

(2)In the October 22 note, you allege that "none of the complaints filed comply with APA's procedures for filing and resolving ethics complaints." Only the sparsest guidelines for filing a complaint are given in the materials you make available online to people wishing to file complaints (at http://www.psychiatry.org/practice/ethics/resources-standards under "PROCEDURES FOR HANDLING COMPLAINTS OF UNETHICAL CONDUCT,") but all nine of us followed those guidelines. Therefore, we ask that you tell us specifically which procedures any of the complainants failed to meet.

(3)In the October 22 note, your statement that "none of the complaints state a violation of the Ethics rules against the respondents named in the complaints," is simply and patently untrue — Section 1 and the lengthy Section 3 in each complaint state precisely that — we ask that you tell us what basis you use for ignoring all of that material.

(4)In the October 22 note of dismissal, you allege that "the complaints reflect a fundamental misunderstanding on your part of the purpose and appropriate use of DSM-IV in diagnosing mental illness." That is a stunningly vague statement, and it is offensive to make that statement after you have read of the horrendous suffering described by the complainants as resulting from the use of DSM-IV. For you to make that statement in fact is yet another example, beyond the huge number cited in the complaints, of those in the APA who ought to act to prevent harm from your manufactured products actually turning icily away from evidence of harm and claiming it is not their fault. We remind you, as you wrote in your own materials about the APA's ethics, that the purpose of having and enforcing ethical rules is to reduce the frequency of unethical conduct. We request that you instead explain specifically and precisely what you mean by your statement.

(5)If you have a look at your own published guidelines and procedures for complaints (at the place cited here above), you will note that you made a serious error in your October 22 statement that since we "filed these complaints with the APA Ethics Committee rather than with a district branch, there is no further appeal from this Committee's unanimous decision and these cases are closed." In fact, your own guidelines (Section A.3.c) shall be addressed to the district branch of the accused member, but as you know, there were a great many accused members named in our complaints, and they reside in a great many of your districts. Your section A.3.c clearly allows for the filing of complaints with the APA rather than a district branch, because it specifies that "If [the complaint is] addressed to the APA, the complaint shall be referred by the APA to the Accused Member's DB." As you will recall, because the Accused Members (we called them respondents) reside in so many different districts, and also since the matters addressed in our complaints are of national and even international import, we requested that our complaints be heard at the national level. Ms. Coyle claimed in a letter that in order to be "fair," you would not want to use procedures that differed in any way from anything you have done in the past. I pointed out to her that had the United States judicial system used that kind of rationale, slavery would still be legal here, and neither she nor I would be allowed to vote. You will recall further that when it appeared that you were looking for ways to dismiss the complaints without considering their merits and were wanting to use the argument about the district branch for that purpose, we explicitly asked that you not use a decision to reject any part or parts of our requests in order to justify dismissing each complaint in its entirety. That, however, is exactly what you did. We request accordingly to know (A) whether any complaint has ever been filed with your Committee that involved members of more than one district branch, and if so, how you handled that; and (B) what you offer as justification for using the district branch argument for summarily dismissing every complaint in its entirety. You could, after all, have assigned each complaint to a district branch where the largest number of Accused Members resides, and of course you could have acknowledged that these were matters of more than district import and had them considered at the national level. To do so—and of course it is still not too late to do so, given that your invisible, protected committee members have all the power they want to take upon themselves—would still have allowed you to make whatever findings you wanted about the merits of each complaint. But to make twisted arguments about procedures, ignoring the complainants' requests that even if you decided not to hear them at the national level, reveals in yet another deeply troubling way how little you care about the suffering your products cause. It also reveals the serious dangers of allowing a lobby group like the APA to operate unregulated.

(6) I have twice requested a time and date the week of November 5 to meet with anyone from your Ethics Committee or Ethics Department. I would appreciate the courtesy of a reply with an appointment time. At this point, my November 5 schedule is full, but I can arrange to come to your office and meet with you any other day that week.

Paula J. Caplan Ph.D.

They did not respond to these questions.

Other Actions Taken

A week before the complaints were dismissed, I had emailed Linda Hughes and the APA's General Counsel Colleen Coyle, asking to meet with them in person during my then-upcoming trip to Washington, D.C. I wrote:

> Perhaps we can make more headway by talking in person than has been made so far. I am sure that you are as eager to get these matters dealt with as are those who have been harmed and who understandably feel that the APA is treating them as though they simply do not matter.

They did not respond. On October 29, I emailed APA's then-President Dr. Dilip Jeste, listed as based in San Diego, to ask to meet with him in his office to discuss some questions about the APA, and on November 14 I resent the message. He did not reply.

On November 13, 2012, four of us went to the building that houses APA headquarters in Arlington, Virginia. The aims were: (1) to request in person a meeting with Hughes and Coyle and (2) to deliver a document (one page on ordinary printer paper) called "The Need and The 9 Demands." The demands were some of the actions requested in the complaints, and the APA could take these actions despite dismissing the complaints. Here is the document:

> THE NEED
>
> Untold numbers of people will suffer harm from *DSM-IV-TR* between now and the time that *DSM-5* is published, and then the *DSM-5* will cause harm, and the American Psychiatric Association knows that. We demand that the APA act to stop the harm, preventing future harm and redressing harm already caused.
>
> THE 9 DEMANDS
>
> The APA must:
>
> 1. Announce that past editions of the *DSM* and the one scheduled for 2013 publication have almost no grounding in high-quality science, that use of *DSM* labels has not been shown to reduce human suffering and in fact often masks the real causes of suffering, and that their use is highly subjective and can cause a vast array of kinds of harm. This announcement should be issued as a press release and be published in every APA outlet, as well as sent to the heads of every mental health and related organization and training program, the Department of Health and Human Services, and the military and Veterans Affairs mental health departments.
>
> 2. Develop other ways to make widely known to the public and to professionals the serious limitations of the *DSM*'s scientific basis, including the poor reliability

and lack of predictive and other kinds of validity, and the risks of harm that getting a *DSM* diagnosis can carry.

3. Send an official letter to all training programs for psychiatrists and indeed all medical doctors—since many non-psychiatrist physicians also use psychiatric diagnosis, as well as the American Medical Association, and the Association of American Medical Colleges (AAMC), urging them to require all medical students to be intensively trained in thinking critically about research in general and about research about psychiatric diagnosis in particular.

4. Set aside a significant portion of the enormous monetary profits from the *DSM-IV* and *DSM-IV-TR* for APA-funded programs aimed to undo harm already done and programs aimed to prevent future harm. The APA as an entity, as well as the current president and trustees, should immediately begin collecting information about who has been harmed and the nature and extent of the harm, and then begin to redress that harm.

5. Disseminate widely such warnings as: ... *our diagnostic classification is the result of historical accretion and at times even accident without a sufficient underlying system or scientific necessity. The rules for entry have varied over time and have rarely been very rigorous. There is no scientifically proven, single right way to diagnose any mental disorder—and don't let any expert tell you that there is.* [1]

6. Post Black Box warnings on every *DSM* and *DSM*-related product and in advertisements of every kind related to the manual both currently and in the future, these warnings to include the statement that the products are not grounded in high-quality science, are not reliable or valid and thus have no predictive validity, and can be hazardous to the health and well-being of the persons to whom the diagnostic labels are applied. This might include the following description of the process by which the manual is compiled: "*DSM-IV* is the natural outcome of what is essentially a process of discussion and debate within a sociopolitical context. In the absence of more powerful scientific foundations, this was and is inevitable ... very few of the hundreds of diagnostic categories have been satisfactorily validated according to these criteria." [2]

7. Compile and distribute at no cost within the U.S. and internationally curriculum materials for teaching psychiatrists, residents, interns, and others in the mental health field how to minimize the harm from diagnosis, including but not limited to stating in the patient's chart and in a letter to the patient that whatever diagnoses they were given are not scientifically grounded and cannot legitimately be assumed to shed light on the patient's ability to be a good employee or parent or to make decisions about their medical and legal affairs.

8. Convene public hearings within six months of today's date, these hearings to be about the subject of harm that those given *DSM-IV* and *DSM-IV-TR* diagnoses have experienced as a result of receiving those labels, and hold annual hearings after the DSM-5 is published.

9. Ensure that beginning with the APA's 2013 convention, at every annual convention, those who have been harmed as a result of being given *DSM* labels be impaneled as speakers in a series of presentations about these kinds of harm.

[1] Frances and Widiger (2012).
[2] Guze, Samuel. (1995). Review of *DSM-IV*. *The American Journal of Psychiatry 152.*

Based on consultations with two Virginia lawyers, the plan was to try to record whatever transpired but turn off the recording device(s) if asked and depart if asked. We did not aim to get arrested, just to make a civil request for an appointment and deliver the "The Need and 9 Demands" in person to Hughes, Coyle, or anyone in authority.

It was important that Jenny McClendon was there, because she is a complainant who is a military veteran, because it was the day after Veterans Day (the APA was closed on Veterans Day), and up to then, no APA authority had had to look upon the face of a complainant and know how the *DSM* had tragically harmed them. Activist and videographer Leah Harris also attended and brought her video camera and social worker Debra Turkat attended for backup filming.

If I had it to do over again, I would have gone to the site before November 13 to learn the physical layout and make plans in case of inclement weather. Wanting the events to be filmed in the order in which they would occur, I suggested we meet outside the complex of buildings that houses the APA, where Leah would record us saying what we were about to do and why, after which we would unscroll a 24 × 33-inch, laminated version of the "The Need and 9 Demands" and read it aloud before heading to the APA office.

The morning of November 13 was too cold and rainy to allow us to film outside. Around 10:30 a.m., I headed to the APA offices to see whether we would need to be buzzed, so that Leah and Debra would know where to stand to do the filming. On the main floor, two men were at the concierge desk. A nearby directory listed the APA office as in "2000." The concierges and I chatted amiably, and I asked if 2000 was on the second floor. "No, it's on the 20th," they said, pointing toward two sets of elevators and instructing me to take the ones on the right. No sign-in book, no visitors' badges were visible, and they did not ask who I was. I entered the elevator with numerous other people, some of whom wore badges, and the concierges questioned no one.

When the elevator door opened on the 20th floor, I saw that the APA appears to occupy the entire floor. I needed to throw away a food wrapper, and as I walked about 15 feet past the door to a trash can, I heard a voice not inquire politely but demand, "May I help you?" I headed back to the elevator, and as I did so, the tall man who had spoken, who wore an ID card, came within inches of me and repeated his question more urgently. I smiled and continued to the elevator, saying, "No, thank you. I'm supposed to meet somebody, but she's probably downstairs."

Back on the ground floor, we decided to begin filming in the hallway, which was filled with natural light. If we went far from the concierge's desk, it was too noisy, so about 30 feet from that desk, on camera, Jenny and I began our explanation of where we were and what we were about do. We unfurled the large version of the "The Need and 9 Demands" and began to read it aloud but not loudly. When we got about two-thirds of the way through, a security guard approached and said we could not film there, because the building is privately owned. I said we would stop filming immediately. I asked who owns the building, and he said "Monday." (A later internet search showed that Monday Properties Securities owns it.) I asked whether it was Monday's or the APA's no-filming rule, and he said, "Both."

In a non-confrontational conversation, I said we would do no further filming but had a document to deliver to the APA office. He asked to whom we wanted to deliver it, and I said, "Linda Hughes in the Ethics Department and Colleen Coyle, General Counsel." He asked if I had been in touch with them, and I replied that we had emailed each other for months. He asked if I had their phone number, and I said that I did and started to look it up on my phone. He smiled and said that he just needed the number so he could be sure that I had truly been in touch with them. When I gave him the number, he dialed and walked away. I also dialed it but was put on automatic hold. Soon, several other people, including others dressed in security guard uniforms and a woman in brightly colored business attire (was she from the security company or APA?) were conferring with "our" guard. Then he told us we had to leave and said that neither Hughes nor Coyle was in. I said we could leave the document we had brought them, but he refused to allow that. I asked to meet with someone else in the APA, and he refused. I introduced Jenny and briefly told him her story and said that she was one of nine people harmed by the diagnostic handbook the APA produces who had filed ethics complaints with the APA, that the APA had dismissed them, and that they had ignored our requests simply to meet with them. I suggested we leave the documents with the concierge for Hughes and Coyle, but he said the concierge is not allowed to accept documents. We asked if security is always this tight, and he said that it is. I would love to know if others trying to leave a document for the APA would be refused.

Jenny, speaking gently but matter-of-factly, said to our guard that she can walk into her Congressman's office any time and that that was totally different from her experience trying to go upstairs to ask the APA ethics people for an appointment.

A woman who had by then taken over at the concierge desk and rarely looked up. People with and without badges walked past her to elevators without being stopped or even noticed.

Two guards escorted us out, while I told them we understood that they have rules they have to follow and thanked them for being gracious. I explained to the first guard what the *DSM* is and that it has hurt many people, including in ways that are racist, sexist, and classist. I said that my work involves trying to reduce some of that harm and gave him the psychdiagnosis.weebly.com address in case he might know anyone who needs our help.

Is the APA always so vigilant about keeping people without prearranged appointments from even appearing in their reception area? Because I, a 5′1″ woman with white hair and not wearing an APA ID badge had appeared in their office space for about 20 seconds a few minutes before? Had they read the November 11 essay I posted and seen at the end of it or under How You Can Help at psychdiagnosis.weebly.com, where people were urged to contact Hughes, Coyle, and the APA president to ask them to overturn the dismissals?

These events reflect the APA's lack of care and concern for those for whom the *DSM* was the "first cause" of so much suffering. Who knows what occurred on November 13 in the APA offices? Perhaps they were on alert because of my error in copying Linda Hughes when I emailed about a November 12 action. But I have never done anything violent, destructive, or menacing with regard to the *DSM*, only spoken the truth. So if they were on alert in some way, why was that? Not wanting to be held accountable for ignoring the harm they do? After reading a draft of this essay, survivor movement activist Amy Smith wrote to me:

> It is worse, much worse, than I had imagined it could be. It truly reads like a bad dream, a descent into the bowels of the beast (even though it was on the 20th floor!). … how arrogant, paranoid and cold they are. I'll tell you, if I or any of my friends behaved in such a manner, you can believe we would be immediately smacked with multiple labels from the *DSM* ourselves.

At some level, some people at the APA must surely care about harm they do. So on November 14, I sent the following email, with "The Need and 9 Demands" document attached, to Hughes and Coyle:

> Hello, Linda and Colleen,
>
> You are no doubt aware that Professor Jenny McClendon, who is the military veteran who filed one of the complaints you dismissed, and I came with two other people yesterday to deliver the attached document to you. You will see in this Need and 9 Demands some of the actions the complainants had requested of you. The APA could take these actions despite having dismissed the complaints. To act on even one of these demands would be to give the first indication in this entire process that the APA has any interest in redressing past harm and preventing future harm from your diagnostic manual. In vain have we searched your communications—and failures to communicate—for signs of concern about the human beings your organization's product and the respondents' actions and inactions have harmed. It would have been in the APA's interest and your interest as APA employees if you had allowed us to meet with you yesterday, for once you meet one of the complainants in person, you will find it harder

to disrespect them, harder to act as though they do not deserve an adequate, reparative response. Linda and Colleen, your concern for the suffering of others, which one tends to believe must reside in the hearts of most people, must surely have plagued you as you have carried out the wishes of your bosses at the APA. Their wishes must be hard to reconcile with compassion and empathy. I speak for all nine complainants when I say that we do not assume that you are bad people but that it seems that, like pilots of drones who send death to people thousands of miles from where they press the buttons, you can only do your work by acting as though your targets are less than human. When the humanness of the drones' targets breaks through to the pilots, they crack. We hope that for your sakes and the sakes of the complainants and the countless others your organization harms, you will confront their humanity, ask the Ethics Committee to reverse its dismissals, and give the complainants' suffering the respect and consideration that you must know they deserve.

Paula

New Developments

As this chapter underwent final readiness for publication, important new developments took place. The APA's dismissal of the nine ethics complaints made it clear, in case there had been any doubt, that the APA would not monitor or rectify the effects of its actions or the actions of its officers and many of its members with regard to psychiatric diagnosis. Attorney Wendy Murphy proposed that complaints be filed with the Office of Civil Rights in the U.S. Department of Health and Human Services (OCR/HHS). That federal department is the most obvious one that should regulate psychiatric diagnosis, but it currently does not do so.

On April 8, 2013, five of the nine people who had filed APA complaints also filed complaints with the OCR/HHS. I did not file one, because OCR guidelines allow only the direct subjects of discrimination to do so. The grounds on which the complainants filed were that they had been discriminated against pursuant to the Americans with Disabilities Act (ADA). According to the ADA, one type of discrimination is being treated as though one has a disability when one does not, and these complainants had been having understandable reactions to life events that were instead classified as mental illnesses, and they were treated—and harmed—as a result. The complainants named the same respondents as in the APA complaints and also added *DSM-IV* and *DSM-IV-TR* head Allen Frances. (He had been excluded from the APA complaints, because he is no longer an APA member and thus was not subject to APA procedures.) At this writing, it is too early to know whether the OCR/HHS will consider the merits of the complaints or will find procedural grounds on which to dismiss them. It seems highly doubtful that complaints like these have been filed with them before. If they consider the merits, that would be an important step forward. If they dismiss them, that will be another powerful piece of evidence that no one regulates psychiatric diagnosis, not even the federal department that ought to be doing so.

New York Times' Sunday Dialogue about Psychiatric Diagnosis[2]

Further reflecting the failure of those in power to listen to the truth were portions of *The New York Times'* March 24, 2013, Sunday Dialogue. *The Times* invited psychiatrist Ronald Pies' to write the opening statement about psychiatric diagnosis and sent it out ahead of time with invitations for others to respond. Some responses would be published right below Pies' piece, and Pies' answer to those responses would wind up the section.

Pies was an interesting choice. He wrote his Sunday Dialogue statement as though psychiatric diagnoses were as scientifically grounded as are clearly medical problems such as migraines—he says that psychiatric diagnoses are made like diagnoses of migraines, based on patients' history, symptoms, and observations—and that such diagnoses can be humanizing, because patients are relieved to have their suffering given these labels. He wrote that it is important to tell one diagnosis from another but neglected to mention that the scientific research has shown conclusively that psychiatric diagnostic categories overlap hugely with each other as well as with clearly non-pathological behavior and feelings. It is reprehensible that he failed to disclose the now well-established facts that psychiatric diagnosis is unscientific, does not reduce human suffering, and causes many kinds of serious harm. What is downright weird is that just over a year ago, he published a strong critique of psychiatric diagnosis (Pies 2012) called "Why Psychiatry Needs to Scrap the *DSM* System: An Immodest Proposal," advocating doing away with that system in favor of carefully listening to the patient and trying to understand rather than label them.[3]

After his *Times* piece appeared, I drew the attention of the newspaper staff to his striking and total inconsistency, and I asked if they publish letters to the editor about Sunday Dialogue so that this could be made known. They responded that they do not publish letters about that column but in any case would not do were the letter "mainly to attack the credibility of the writer; we prefer that the focus stay on the issue." How strange to cast my query as attacking the credibility of

2 The following is reprinted from Paula J. Caplan. How the NY Times Portrays Psychiatric Diagnosis: Thinking Critically About "Sunday Dialogue" about Defining Mental Illness March 30, 2013 by Paula J. Caplan, Ph.D. @ https://my.psychologytoday.com/blog/science-isnt-golden/201303/how-the-ny-times-portrays-psychiatric-diagnosis

3 One had to wonder why in that article, Pies cited Allen Frances, who as head of the current edition of the *DSM* was responsible more than any human being in history for the diagnosing of millions more people than ever before as mentally ill. Frances is a johnny-come-lately to a critique of psychiatric diagnosis, and his is minimal compared to its enormous and numerous flaws, as well as being strikingly inconsistent.

the writer rather than as making the point that readers have a right to know when someone given the prominent authorship of the lead piece in their special feature totally contradicts himself, because that surely sheds light on the way the issue is addressed.

The first "reader's" reaction printed was by Allen Frances, hardly an average reader, given that he headed the group that wrote the current and previous editions of the diagnostic manual. Frances, whose manuals are responsible for millions more people being pathologized than at any time in history, actually complained in his *Times* response that "the realm of normal is shrinking." Less than anyone on earth should he be surprised. He added 77 categories to the 297 in the edition that had been published just seven years before (Caplan 1995).

When at his invitation I served on two of his committees and repeatedly sent evidence of the abysmal quality of the "science" he was using to create and justify diagnoses and of the devastation they caused people, he not only ignored but actually publicly denied that that was true. (I resigned from his committees, considering it unethical and unprofessional to participate.)

In the *Times* piece, Frances called diagnosis "the essential prelude to effective treatment," though he more than anyone has seen ample evidence that this is untrue. In fact, the chances that two therapists simultaneously meeting with the same person will even assign that person the same label are poor, which of course means that diagnosis is not helpful in choosing treatment or improving outcome (Caplan 1995).

Frances is a Johnny-come-very-lately when in 2013 in the *Times* he presents as his own, new idea that Congressional action is needed. I had initiated in 2002 two Congressional briefings. During that time and for years afterward, he continued to defend uncritically his diagnostic empire. He seems to love my ideas, though, because also very recently, without attributing this one to me either, he suddenly proposed that the *DSM* carry a black box warning, one of the points in "The Need and the 9 Demands" document about which I had written in November, 2012 (Caplan 2012b). One can only hope that soon he will act on the pleas some of us issued to him more than a quarter of a century ago, that he act to prevent future harm and redress harm that his editions have caused. Instead, his emphasis is on trashing the next edition of the manual, and it will indeed be terrible, but that is in large part (though not entirely) because it is likely to include so much of the content of Frances' editions.

The next response in the *Times* feature came from Sera Davidow, writing as one who was diagnosed but who now directs "a recovery community for others who have been so labeled." She decimated Pies' absurd attempt to draw an analogy between psychiatric categories and migraines by saying that no one "attempted to hospitalize or medicate me against my will for [migraines]," and she describes how a person's psychiatric label often becomes their sole and demoralizing identity.

The New York Times includes in its print edition only some of the responses they post online. My own did not appear in the print edition but did appear online. I have no idea how they choose which ones will appear in print, but it troubles me that only one response in the print version was from a woman.[4] This is the version, slightly shortened from what I submitted, that appeared online:

"Surprising though it may seem, psychiatric diagnosis is not scientifically grounded, does not reduce human suffering, and carries risks of a wide array of serious kinds of harm. Even more disturbingly, it is totally unregulated, making it even less regulated than the financial institutions in this country.

"I served for two years on two committees that wrote the current DSM but had to resign on ethical and professional grounds when I saw the way they ignored or distorted what high-quality research showed but presented junk science as though it were good when it suited their purposes.

"The potential damage caused by a diagnosis is virtually limitless, including loss of custody of a child, loss of employment, skyrocketing insurance premiums, and loss of the right to make decisions about one's medical and legal affairs."

Omitted from my list of kinds of harm was the ultimate one: The physical death that too often results from various consequences of psychiatric diagnosis, sometimes caused by the unwanted effects of psychiatric drugs (and their interactions with each other) and sometimes from other causes, with the diagnosis always as the first cause.

Another response appearing only online came from psychiatrist Michael F. Grunebaum, who argued that psychiatric diagnosis is a work in progress "with the shortcomings of any human endeavor in which scientific knowledge is incomplete." He apparently is entirely unaware that the *DSM* is not based on solid scientific knowledge, in contrast to being simply incomplete, and that difference matters enormously. Just ask the people whose lives have been ruined because of the mistaken belief that the labels they were given were scientifically supported and would lead to better things.

In Pies' response (appearing both in print and online) to a few of the comments, he unsurprisingly claimed that diagnosis leads to effective treatment, despite the absence of data supporting that claim. He took offense at Ms. Davidow's comments, claiming that it is "unfair" to blame psychiatric labels for the abridgement of civil liberties and excesses of the drug companies and that instead one must blame Pharma. It is unconscionable for him or Frances or anyone else to try to steer the blame away from diagnosis, because *psychiatric diagnosis is the first cause of virtually everything bad that happens in the mental health system.* Few, if any, people have been deemed psychiatrically normal but then had terrible things done to them in the name of treatment or protection of themselves or others.

---

4 A cartoon I saw years ago showed a great many men and one woman sitting around a boardroom table, and the caption, spoken by the Chair of the Board, was something like, "Thank you for that excellent suggestion, Ms. Jones. Now, just as soon as one of the men makes it, we can act on it."

The Rewriting of History

Those responsible for causing harm to others ought to be held accountable, and it is alarming when such people take it upon themselves to rewrite history to cover up their role in causing harm. I am as quick to repudiate much of what the *DSM-5* heads have done as what editors of previous editions have done; but the virulent attacks by Spitzer and especially Frances on the *DSM-5* heads has been wildly successful in shifting the attention of the public and professionals away from the harm they themselves caused. Spitzer and even more, Frances, oversaw the ballooning of numbers of diagnoses in *DSM-III, III-R, IV,* and *IV-TR* and thus of people classified as mentally ill on a scale far beyond anything anyone else had ever done. But to look at most of the written and broadcast material since Spitzer and Frances mounted their anti-*DSM-5* campaign, one would think that they, and especially Frances, are heroes for warning of the harm that *DSM-5* would cause. It has gone almost totally unnoticed that nearly every criticism they have made had been made about their own editions for decades—and that for decades they largely ignored or even denied that the criticisms were legitimate—until *DSM-5*'s publication became imminent. Consider just one major example of how this has worked.

One of Frances's attacks provoked a tremendous outcry about the *DSM-5* and reflects how many powerful professionals and media people failed to examine the truth about diagnosis deals. It is about the "bereavement exclusion," which is an instruction not to diagnose someone as mentally ill if bereavement caused their suffering. In the leadup to *DSM-5,* a myth created by Frances spread like wildfire. Frances claimed that *DSM-5* would "eliminate the bereavement exclusion" that, he implied, appeared in his own editions. His claims were so furious that I was worried: Since *DSM-IV* appeared in 1994, every time I had lectured about the manual and in my playwriting, I had given Major Depression as one of the most dangerous labels and stated that "If someone close to you dies, and you are 'still' grieving two months later, you qualify for Major Depression!" In the face of Frances' statements that his "bereavement exclusion" would be eliminated, I went back to look at *DSM-IV* and *DSM-IV-TR*, doubting my own memory, but what I saw there was even more frightening than I remembered. For anyone who reads the entire listing for Major Depressive Episode (MDE)—and almost no one ever does—one must get four pages into the dense text to find even the first time that bereavement is mentioned, and at first, it might look promising, for there is the statement that MDE should not be diagnosed if someone has been bereaved within the past two months. That is alarming enough, because bereavement does not end or, often, even diminish very much after 60 days, nor should we expect it to do so, and thus it is hard to think what would justify the intensity of Frances' outrage about (as per discussions about *DSM-5*) diagnosing a depressive "disorder" immediately or after two weeks rather than two months. But it gets worse. In *DSM-IV-TR* the instruction not to diagnose a disorder if the "symptoms" arose less than two months after loss of a loved one is followed by a comma and the following words: "unless they are associated with marked functional impairment or include morbid preoccupation with worthlessness, suicidal ideation, psychotic symptoms, or psychomotor retardation" (American Psychiatric Association 2000: 352). Note especially the word "or" in the foregoing. One need meet only a single criterion in that list to qualify for MDE even as soon as the first day of bereavement. It is hard to think of anyone who has lost a loved one and not met at least one of those. It is absolutely clear that Frances' editions of the manual actually have *no* bereavement exclusion. Has no one who published his diatribes bothered to fact-check what he writes?

Indeed, a BBC radio employee contacted me about a show they were planning about the bereavement matter, and I told her all of the above. I had assumed the BBC would have high standards for fact-checking, but the broadcast, which remained on the BBC website only for a matter of days after it went out over the airwaves,[5] was based on the totally false notion that there had been an actual bereavement exclusion all these years, and it valorized Frances for warning of the allegedly far worse listing in the first *DSM* edition that he would not have overseen since his editions.

This is just more of the same pulling of the wool over the eyes of the public that had led me in 1991 to describe the head of the *DSM* enterprise as like the Wizard of Oz, who, when revealed to be nothing more than a human being masquerading as superhuman, told Dorothy and her companions that they did not know what they were looking at.[6] To draw on another fairy tale, Frances and Spitzer are unclothed emperors who draw attention away from their own nakedness by crying out about the nakedness of the emperor who has replaced them.

References

American Psychiatric Association. 1994. *Diagnostic and Statistical Manual of Mental Disorders-IV*. Washington, D.C.: American Psychiatric Association.

American Psychiatric Association. 2000. *Diagnostic and Statistical Manual of Mental Disorders-IV-TR*. Washington, D.C.: American Psychiatric Association.

Caplan, P.J. 1995. *They Say You're Crazy: How the World's Most Powerful Psychiatrists Decide Who's Normal*. Reading, MA: Addison-Wesley.

Caplan, P.J. 1996. CALL ME CRAZY (stage play). Available on request from the author at paulacaplan@gmail.com.

Caplan, P.J. 2011. *When Johnny and Jane Come Marching Home: How All of Us Can Help Veterans*. Cambridge, MA: MIT Press.

5 http://www.bbc.co.uk/programmes/b01rl1q8 was the URL while the broadcast remained posted

6 Caplan, Paula J. Response to the DSM wizard. *Canadian Psychology*, *32*(2), 1991, 174175.

Caplan, P.J. 2012a. Psychiatry's bible, the DSM, doing more harm than good. *Washington Post*. [Online]. Available at: http://www.washingtonpost.com/opinions/psychiatrys-bible-the-dsm-is-doing-more-harm-than-good/2012/04/27/gIQAqy0WIT_allComments.html?ctab=all_&#comments [accessed: April 27, 2012].

Caplan, P.J. 2012b. "Will the APA Listen to the Voices of Those Harmed by Psychiatric Diagnosis?" http://www.madinamerica.com/2012/10/p20137/.

Caplan, P.J. and Cosgrove, Lisa (Eds). 2004. *Bias in Psychiatric Diagnosis*. Lanham, MD: Rowman and Littlefield.

Caplan,P.J.ResponsetotheDSMwizard.*CanadianPsychology*,*32*(2),1991,174175.

Pies, R. 2012. Why psychiatry needs to scrap the *DSM*: An immodest proposal. *PsychCentral*. [Online]. Available at: http://psychcentral.com/blog/archives/2012/01/07/why-psychiatry-needs-to-scrap-the-dsm-system-an-immodest-proposal/ [accessed: January 7, 2012].

Chapter 10
Mainstreaming the Mentally Ill

Jem Masters, Trudy Rudge and Sandra West

Introduction

The concept of mainstreaming health services for patients with mental health issues has different meanings globally, with a range of services available across various health care environments. However, in general, mainstreaming is assumed to provide these patients with access to services without stigma and prejudice and in a health care system that is changing its perspective to meet these needs. A basic assumption of this process is that services (psychiatric, physical, and emotional) are coordinated in order to provide integrated care. As part of this integration, psychiatry is perceived to be an equal partner/service provider with other medical specialties (Lykouras and Douzenis 2008). Mainstreaming has been presumed to support parity between mental and physical illness, especially when emergency care for mental health clients is provided through emergency departments or rooms (EDs)[1] where physical and mental health can be monitored simultaneously. Yet, problems associated with integration of services and funding remain (Frank and Giled 2007, Mechanic 1998).

In this chapter we consider the mainstreaming of mental health services in order to understand its impact on treatment for individuals in EDs. We undertake this, as well, to analyse philosophical and social underpinnings of this policy, which was implemented to overcome historical and social outcomes of separation of mental health treatments and services from other forms of health services. The policy and social analysis that follows was also necessary to establish what the situation was in EDs and emergency practice so as to inform an Australian-wide, qualitative study into the impact of mainstreaming on nursing practices in EDs. As the study was using situational analysis, a key part of such a study was to map the context in which the study is located. Therefore as part of this mapping, we outline some of the history of mainstreaming and its effects on psychiatric services, tracing how the treatment of mental health patients has changed over the past 20 years. We focus on the dividing practices operationalized where ED services were mainstreamed for people with mental health problems. An historical perspective on the healthcare provided for those with mental health and psychiatric conditions

1 ED throughout this chapter refers to accident and emergency (A&E) departments or rooms, terms used by different countries for access points to hospitals for patients requiring immediate care without prior treatment or booking.

explains why mainstreaming benefit individuals physically and mentally and illuminates the thinking behind healthcare policy changes that influenced the transition to the provision of mental health care within generalist EDs.

Hence, this chapter draws on the previous studies of psychiatric segregation that provided evidence of how people with a mental illness were deemed outsiders to normal society and were stigmatized and excluded. It is important to do this as one of the central aims of mainstreaming the care of the mentally ill is predicated on a belief that bringing the care of those with a mental health conditions into 'the mainstream' would break down the barriers that stigmatize these people who are mentally ill and reduce the prejudice that they have encountered. Consistently throughout history and across cultures, beliefs that people with mental health issues are to be feared, are social deviants, or are violent and/or vulnerable, have plagued the provision and delivery of their mental health care (Morant 1995, Pilgrim and Rogers 1999). These beliefs have contributed to a lack of policy direction as well as reduced funding for mental health services, which, paradoxically, led to this change in policy direction (Frank and Giled 2007). Morant states that "while the medical model of psychiatry provides a dominant and much used way of anchoring mental illness into medical theory and practices, this conceptualization does not go unchallenged" (1995: 5). Moreover, it is our case that the medical model of psychiatric practice has only increased the fear of people with mental health conditions, and has caused non-psychiatric health professionals to stigmatize both these patients and the mental health professionals who attempt to care for them – practices we trace in the sections exploring the mainstreamed ED. Our aim is to expose, through an analysis of the research and the thinking behind mainstreaming policy and its implementation, the impact of the situation "when sick is not sick", and how this can be traced to social, political and other changes in health care throughout the latter part of the twentieth century.

The Derivation of Mainstreaming

Mainstreaming first became necessary to overcome the historical separation and isolation of people suffering with psychiatric and mental health conditions from the general community, particularly following the establishment of large lunatic asylums, which occurred simultaneously with the decline and eradication of leprosy during the Middle Ages in Europe and Great Britain. It was Foucault's (1965) thesis that as leprosy declined a means and a space was found to exclude those whose reason was in question. Prior to the Middle Ages, it was more likely to be the physically sick and infectious rather than the mentally ill who were shunned, locked away, or stigmatized; however, it is Foucault's argument that as society came to value reason above all else, the mad gradually came to be perceived as society's waste to be located outside of "city walls". Foucault argued that the "ship of fools" symbolized the ultimate abandonment of these people, and indicated a heightened awareness of the interplay between sin and evil in insanity as it was framed in the medieval mindset and its correlate imaginative landscapes in the Renaissance. Foucault also pointed out that confining madman either on board a ship or outside the city walls removed the problem of waste people for the governments of the medieval city (Foucault 1965: 11).

The fundamental exclusionary site for people who were defined as mad during the Victorian era became the large psychiatric hospitals or lunatic asylums developed in Britain, its colonies and in the USA. Bassuk and Gerson state argued that in America by 1840 there were 25 specialist hospitals established to care for the mentally ill who had formerly resided in squalid conditions in poor houses, almshouses, or jails (1978: 47). Authors such as Goffman (1987) continued to assert how these large psychiatric hospitals were perceived as sites for "society's waste". He further claims that asylums functioned merely as "storage dumps for inmates" (p. 74). Indeed, the classical, societal perception of the mentally ill was portrayed through "Bedlam" – the Bethlem Royal Hospital – which was identified as both a place of horror and fascination. Bedlam and in some cases the horrific treatment meted out to its inmates (patients), is iconic of madhouses, so much so that if one is to Google for images of mental illness, sketches of "Bedlam" are never far from the top of the list as well as portrayals of sane, middle class visitors viewing the mad as entertainment.

Nonetheless, McMillian (1997), in his history of Bedlam, clearly articulates how these institutions were cloaked in myths and misrepresentations fuelled by the very separation that was used to house the mentally ill in their confines. As Goffman (1987) found in his much later ethnography of such asylums these organizations operated as what he termed "total institutions", efficiently undertaking the task assigned to them by society to confine their inmates, to act as both protector and governor of the mental ill in separate organizations that controlled the daily lives of inmates and staff who lived in the institution supported through the inmates' work and labour, supervised by staff.

These large institutions, lunatic asylums, or psychiatric hospitals were a means of controlling and detaining people legitimately against their will so that society did not have to deal with "madness". However, such a separation not only segregated society from madness but separated mental health services as well (Wallace 1992). Wallace, in his history of mental health hospitals and services in Australia, contends that "Lunacy was regarded as an extension of benevolence in the early years of the Colony" (1992: 1). Such attitudes were common throughout the British Empire and other places in the Western world where containment of madness was during this time under the auspices of charity or social services. Thus, mental health practices were governed by the principle of benevolence, in harmony with, and derived from, the "old English poor law" practices of the eighteenth and nineteenth centuries. Accordingly, lunacy was not included in the administration of the Colonial Medical Service (Wallace 1992) but was viewed as part of welfare support provided by the colonial government.

Influenced by these approaches to the mentally ill and psychiatric service delivery, since colonization the Australian mental health services followed the trajectories of western trends in service delivery. Institutionalization initially began with the opening of the Lunatic Reception House in Sydney, followed by other larger facilities throughout Australia. This system remained in place with minimal changes until the 1960s when an Australian Royal Commission investigated the treatment of its "inmates" (Sainsbury 2005). After this investigation a process of deinstitutionalization commenced with hospitals discharging patients into community care. This development coincided with the advancement of medications and the availability of more effective, antipsychotic and other psychotherapeutic drugs (Bassuk and Gerson 1978). In addition to the advances in medication, more effective forms of therapeutic interventions gained in popularity and effectiveness, also supporting individuals living in the community. Societal expectations and particularly a reassessment of the delivery of psychiatric services to World War II and Korean War veterans with significant mental health conditions meant segregation became less well tolerated. A further change occurred when governments sought efficiencies by bringing together the mental/psychiatric and general health systems to function effectively as one healthcare system. Linked to these reforms and re-evaluation of service delivery were investigations into the human rights of mental health patients which exposed entrenched inequities of care especially among the severely mentally ill living in the community even after processes of de-institutionalization.

Human Rights of the Mentally Ill

After the Second World War, individual human rights became another driver for mainstreaming health care for mentally ill people. Just as the World Health Organization (WHO) and government policies sought to integrate services to benefit the physical and mental health needs of the entire population, the various WHO health charters (Ottawa Charter 1986) have encouraged national health services to overcome treatment and care silos. Investigations under both the WHO and the Human Rights Conventions of the United Nations showed that there were inequities in the health care provision for people with severe mental illness when compared to those of the general population with physical health needs (Lawrence and Kisely 2010). These inequities maintained the mentally ill in positions of vulnerability and uncertainty through lack of funding for services and failures to preserve their human rights, in particular those related to the provision of integrated care. Similarly, primary health care principles that are built on the removal of care silos proved to be insufficient to deliver equitable care for those who are considered to be mentally ill, or for their carers and families.

Human rights discourse has become a powerful voice to improve the health needs of people with mental health issues. Over the past 70 years following the adoption of the Universal Declaration of Human Rights (United Nations 1948), human rights principles have been used to guard against coercion and forced treatment of those detained in institutions and to promote positive rights such as the right to fair and equitable treatment in society (Arboleda-Florez 2008, Cobigo and Stuart 2010). Following establishment of the United Nations Commission on Human Rights, there was a move to explore human rights of vulnerable populations such as the mentally ill or displaced or refugee groups. In this situation, several governments undertook under the umbrella of national human rights commissions, investigations into the rights of the severely mentally ill (for instance in Australia, a human rights commissioner and judge, led a investigation into the rights of the severely mentally ill, see Burdekin, Guilfoyle, and Hall 1993). In this report called the Burdekin Report, (1993: 3), the commissioners claimed that there was "serious failure by governments to provide sufficient resources to protect the fundamental rights of many thousands of Australians affected by mental illness or psychiatric disability". Significantly, stigma and discrimination were major issues highlighted in the report. De-institutionalization and mainstreaming became central planks of the National Mental Health Plan developed by the Australian government through its health ministers at both Commonwealth and state levels of service (Australian Health Ministers 1992). These action plans were premised on principles of human rights and equity as well as principles of primary health care for integrated acute mental health and community services for people with mental illnesses. These principles were seen as contributing to prevention of illness, promotion of emotional health and well-being and the reduction of experiences of stigma for those with a mental illness (Kalucy, Thomas, and King 2005).

However, over the last two decades, there is growing global concern because of what Cooper et al. (2010) view as a mere rhetoric of human rights when associated with treatment of mental illness. Stigma and discrimination continue to impact on the human rights of mental health patients particularly in relation to a lack of change to mental health legislation that focuses on containment and control of the mentally ill rather than on their rights to care, dignity and rights to many valued aspects of living. Such a continued focus on legislation to exclude was noted tellingly by Douglas (2002) that "once a person is admitted to a mental hospital tolerance by society is withdrawn" (p.121). However, we would add that such a separation not only occurs once admitted but we would suggest that once diagnosed, people are marginalized and suffer the consequences of stigmatization/discrimination. Fisten, Holland, Clare, and Gunn (2009) compared Commonwealth jurisdictions (countries such as Canada, United Kingdom, New Zealand, Australia), pointing out that a significant part of mental health legislation is concerned with depriving people of their freedom, mainly due to risks of harm to self or others. They assert that this emphasis reinforces the perception that mentally ill people are violent. Instead, Fisten et al. (2009) suggest that the spirit of mental health legislation should be to promote the health and wellbeing of people with mental health issues by ensuring access to services across a variety of facilities wherever they are located. Fisten et al. (2009) assert that change is difficult to bring about while such legal frameworks based on containment contradict human rights discourse and continue a singular policy focus on the mentally ill as dangerous. Mental health legislation that informs and/or reinforces global health policy and human rights reforms, rather than maintaining constraint of those diagnosed as mentally ill is required and such a reform is the practice of mainstreaming of mental health care in an integrated health care system.

The Mainstreamed Emergency Department

While, Glasper (2011) along with Goldman, Glied and Alegria (2008) suggest that integration and mainstreaming of services post-deinstitutionalization has provided many benefits to people experiencing mental illness, Taylor, Bennett and Cameron (2004) claim that patients have not always been helped by the paradigm shift in care provision for people with acute or long term mental health needs. These changes have had a particular impact on emergency care. Often brought about by a closure of other services, mainstreaming has meant an increasing number of mental health patients presenting to EDs in general hospitals (Heslop, Elsom, and Parker 2000). This phenomenon has been observed in the USA, Canada, UK, New Zealand, India, and Australia, where deinstitutionalization and mainstreaming is current policy (Bassuk 1980, Heslop et al. 2000, Wellin, Slesiner and Hollister 1987). The increasing number of presentations to ED for those unfortunate people who have to use the only place available now for emergency care, has resulted in resentment by ED staff in some cases, which in turn has compounded the discrimination of the mentally ill (Broadbent, Moxham, and Dwyer 2010, Camilli and Martin 2005). EDs were ill-prepared for this onslaught, and mental health clients were caught up in the struggle to provide for their needs in mainstream health care services.

Developments in civil society, greater democracy, and the plurality of views in mental health provided the impetus for more transparency in the creation and evaluation of policy options (Jenkins 2008: 399). However, even in such a civic policy milieu, policy and strategies for the provision of mental health care in an integrated system were not linked. Reasons for bringing mental health into an integrated system to overcome inequities for people with severe mental illness were not made obvious at all levels (Lawrence and Kisely 2010). The consequence of this is that ED staff remain steadfastly ignorant of reasons for the integration or mainstreaming of mental health services as a means to promote quality physical and psychological health care for all citizens (Australian Health Ministers 1992).

The implementation of policies of deinstitutionalization influenced the readiness of those with a mental illness to access mental health services through EDs (Wong, Sands, and Solomon 2010, Morphet et al. 2012). However, the mainstreaming of mental health services failed to discuss the economics of healthcare provision, the societal costs of mental illnesses or the consequences of care provision in EDs where treatment of mental illness came up against the flow through model of care dominating the funding models of contemporary ED health care.

EDs face many challenges as Health Departments expect both cost-effective and efficient treatment for all patients presenting to each ED. Many governments have recently implemented "Access Target" to reduce waiting times and blockages occurring in EDs (Handel et al. 2010, Paul and Lin 2012). National Emergency Access Targets have been implemented in Australia, New Zealand, and the United Kingdom, but there is minimal recognition of the different needs of those with mental health issues, particularly when there are co-morbidities such as substance misuse. Mason, Weber, Coster, Freeman and Locker (2012) claim that while EDs were meeting targets, they were losing focus on the actual needs of patients and the optimal balance among safety, quality, and timeliness of emergency care. Also, they found that emergency care was abruptly halted during the last 20 minutes of the set four-hour targeted time as staff work to discharge or transfer the patient. This had significant consequences for patients with mental health issues where rapport and engagement in order to obtain much needed information need to be developed over time. EDs are designed to function within a set of rules, making it difficult for situations that fall outside these parameters. Health professionals can follow specific pathways for patients with physical trauma and life threatening events but these pathways were challenged by mentally ill patients who did not have such clear-cut care trajectories. The unpredictability of those with mental illness was considered to interfere with the smooth flow of the ED that is more geared towards treating those with physical emergency conditions. Therefore, a person with a mental health condition is made more vulnerable when staff are unable to adjust to an alternate process, which may not take any longer than the complicated treatment of multiple trauma but which was not accorded the same priorities even now in the mainstreamed ED. Government policies may have shifted toward making the health needs of people with mental health issues a priority, but EDs were forced to find solutions to what they continued to define as the "problem" of the mental health client.

Relations of trust and communication with mental health patients were made all the more difficult due to suspicion, fear and anxiety on the part of the professional health care staff in EDs. These problems were asserted as the result of the mind and body split in regards to the provision of care, although were more likely due to the perceptions of nurses and their frustrations in providing care for those who are perceived not to be worthy of their time and energy. Almost 30 years ago, research by Jones, Yoder and Jones' (1984) clearly demonstrated that ED nurses were unwilling to see mental health/psychiatric patients as "sick".

> At times they were frustrated because they considered these patients to be unreasonable, resistant to treatment, having poor prognosis, to be non-emergencies who took time away from the more acutely ill patients, or to be persons who did not take care of themselves. (Jones et al. 1984: 96)

From the on-going difficulties and challenges of mainstreamed care, clearly little has changed in the 27 years since Jones' research.

More guidance for a mainstreamed ED would result from a clearer definition of what constitutes "sick" or "acutely ill" in mental illnesses. Hunt (1993) theorized that ED nurses react to psychiatric patients in terms of the differences between the physically and mentally ill, where the mentally ill were categorized as mysterious, unpredictable, undesirable, and hopeless (p.375). People presenting with life-threatening conditions 'trumped' those with mental health issues – cardiac arrest, acute trauma, or fulminating septicaemia were first priorities. Suicide attempts trump 'suicidal ideation', acute trauma overrides 'profound' depression arising from ongoing trauma (PTSD or physical symptoms), florid behavioural issues associated with psychosis or the person in fear of their life with schizophrenia are more likely to be dealt with as dangerous rather than as ill. What was also clear was that patients presenting with symptoms of a mental illness often had their physical symptoms overlooked. While there is no clear rationale for the overlooking physical conditions it could relate to stigmatization of the mentally ill and the associated belief that physical complaints are delusional or part of the patients' condition. When such rules govern ED staff behaviour, it is easy to see how the needs of mental health clients were not met.

The systems in EDs govern when and who will provide care and not understanding patients with symptoms of mental illness impacted from the point of entry (triage) and throughout the assessment and treatment stages. The codes for triage numbering systems themselves worked against the acutely mentally ill, fostering inadequate triaging or downplaying the severity of symptoms and resulting in frustratingly longer waiting times for those who are already emotionally unwell. The new distinct mental health triage scales could have introduced less confusion and provided the appropriate amount of time but this scale is not yet considered to be a reliable tool (Broadbent et al. 2010). Such a triage system is also subjective and only as good as the person administering it and the respondent's ability to provide a history, as with any assessment system. Broadbent, Moxham, and Dwyer (2010) highlighted how language used by triage nurses influenced the application of the triage scales and added to the potential for discrimination. Bullard, Unger, Spencer and Grafstein (2008) found similar issues in the Canadian health care system, suggesting the need to revise the triage system to improve the understanding of emergency nurses and physicians about the urgency of mental health conditions.

Bauman (2004: 31) suggests that orderly, streamlined spaces are ruled-governed spaces where rules forbid and exclude. The ED is such a streamlined space that contains and suppresses variation and uncertainty. In orderly spaces, vulnerability and uncertainty are the two qualities of the human condition which mould "official fear" (Bauman 2004). To understand how people with mental illnesses are dealt with in the streamlined ED, it could be asserted that official fear positions both the ED staff and mental health patients. Patients' vulnerability is increased when uncertain behavioural traits cause staff to be 'officially fearful' of these outsiders to ED nurses and doctors. This suggests that while policies act to integrate care, such integration has not occurred at the implementation level, where official fear shapes practices. Clearly, and additional and on-going education of health professionals in EDs was needed to overcome the uncertainty and vulnerability bred in such situations. However, alongside such implementation failures, mental health professionals who were employed to work in EDs who may provide such education are equally stigmatized in the emergency care environment. Mental health professionals, due to their close connection with patients, are perceived to be less skilled, idle, and illogical and are generally disrespected when compared with ED nurses (Halter 2008). Also mental health professional working within ED are perceived as guests within the department, because they are less "hands on" than ED staff.

Several solutions have been tried to overcome the considerable difficulties experienced in EDs where patients with mental illness are now "mainstreamed". Many EDs now employ nurses who have specialist education in, or have experience with patients with mental health issues. In some instances, space is set aside in the ED to care for mentally ill patients. Many health jurisdictions have made it a priority to build Psychiatric Emergency Care Centres (PECCs), staffed by mental health professionals who care for these patients on a collaborative basis (Frank, Fawcett and Emmerson 2005). Opening of these centres has not been without controversy, since many feel that they re-institute the segregation of mental health care within the EDs themselves (Wand 2005). This also means that ED health care staff can maintain their practices and continue to remain secure in their knowledge area despite their inability to know or deal with those with a mental illness, a significant form of illness in contemporary society.

Limits to Change in Mental Health Care through Policy?

Global mental health policies have drawn attention to the neglected health needs and social policies that support people with mental health issues (Dhanda and Narayan 2007). A significant part of this drive to improve the health needs of those with mental illness and/or disorders has been the integration of health care services. Similarly, changes to policies and development of systems that decreased the segregation of mental health from the general health care system are concerned to equalize care and access to it.

Over the time of these developments, mental health and emotional wellbeing has become politicized with advocates demanding equity for all, which in turn has driven policy activities such as mainstreaming. Advocates, by raising the profile of the social and emotional effects of mental illness, have emphasized needs within the general population, highlighting how mental health issues affect everyone in the population at some time in their lives using statistics about occurrence of mental illness in populations to illustrate how we may all be vulnerable. The WHO acknowledged that mental health and psychiatric conditions will be some of the leading health issues affecting both the developed and developing countries (World Health Organization 2008). In collaboration with WHO, the World Bank (2008) reports that currently Unipolar Depressive Disorders are the leading cause of disability adjustment life-years (DALY) in the Americas and the third leading cause of health issues in Europe. Depressive disorders are to become more prevalent in lower income countries (Das, Do, Friedman and McKenzie 2008). While the WHO (2008) identified that mental health and psychiatric conditions were leading health issues affecting the developed world and the developing countries, the World Bank, with its focus on global productivity, predicted that these conditions were likely to affect the productivity of both developed and developing economies, arguing that the costs related to DALY were particularly significant for the global economy when mental health care does not bring about recovery and rehabilitation of persons with major illnesses. From this perspective, Glasper (2011: 250–251) identifies six possibilities for improving life outcomes through policy developments such as mainstreaming.

1. More people will have good mental health;
2. More people with mental health problems will recover;
3. More people with mental health problems will have good physical health;
4. More people will have a positive experience of care and support;
5. Fewer people will suffer available harm;
6. Fewer people will experience stigma and discrimination.

Over the last 20 years, people with a mental illness have benefitted from the advocacy of the WHO and the consumer movement that has helped to introduce new government policies on health care (Glasper 2011). Mainstreaming of health care was designed to help those who had previously not been given any priority – who had been deemed “unworthy”, or who had failed to fit the general definition of being “unwell” (Lawrence and Kisely 2010). Nonetheless, research has demonstrated a significant mortality and morbidity ‘gap’ for those with a mental illness, with a 15 to 25 year mortality rate difference between the mentally ill and that of the ‘normal’ population (Collins, Tranter, and Irvine 2012, Druss 2007, Kisely et al. 2007). However, Collins et al. (2012) assert that due to persistent inequities in the health care system the provision of optimal physical health care for those with mental health issues remains under challenge. The rates of some physical illnesses remain higher in those with severe mental health conditions, due not only to the side effects and toxins from prescribed medications and substance misuse, but also through the failures of mental health practitioners to bring health education, health promotion other primary care health activities in their practices and services (Lawrence and Kisely 2010).

Lawrence and Kisely (2010) report that there are higher death rates from cardiovascular disease in people with schizophrenia, yet this group have lower rates of coronary surgical interventions than in the general population. This finding is supported by Brown, Kim, Mitchell, and Inskip (2010) who conducted a longitudinal study, which identified that mortality rates from natural causes were higher in those with severe mental health conditions, such as schizophrenia. Yet, those with a mental illness who do access physicians and other health care professionals experience stigma, prejudice, and at times disbelief in their physical complaints, thus limiting the kind of care they received. Indeed it is findings such as this that offer support for the study we propose to explore the impact of mainstreaming on contemporary EDs and the nurses who work there. Similarly, people with severe mental health conditions are less likely to be screened and treated for cancer and diabetes even though such conditions are recognized side effects of prescribed medications (Collins et al. 2012). From research studies such as this it appears that the effective provision of integrated care for those suffering with mental illness may not only rely on bringing their care to mainstream hospitals but it also requires other changes in the attitudes of ED and other staff to improve total health care for such clients.

Whilst there has been some change in the provision of health care for those with mental health issues, stigmatization coupled with the concept of strangeness continues to affect what can be done. The failure of mainstreaming policies to address historical conditions of stigma and discrimination has contributed to on-going failures in the provision of a fully integrated care system for people who are still perceived as unworthy of care. The imperatives for integrated care could not be clearer, yet it remains that people with co-morbid physical and mental health conditions did not have their physical care needs met. Douglas (2002) and Bauman (2004) provide some understanding of how the legitimacy of people with a mental illness is socially discredited and how their 'strangeness' excludes them from access to healthcare that society considers typically a natural right. Bauman (2004) suggests that such people are determined to be 'waste' when they are no longer considered players in society. Moreover, Douglas (2002) asserts that objects and people are assigned to the category of "waste" by human design, not by "nature". Such a conceptualization fits with Jeffery's (2001) observational study of triage and emergency care, where those identified as mental health patients and/or drug users were termed "rubbish patients" who wasted resources and staff time. Such judgements echo Foucault's arguments about the practices and belief systems that contribute to those defined as mad being excluded or exiled from "normal" society.

From Jeffrey's research, ED nurses, as members of the general population, are prone to see mental health clients as having deficits of character, rather than just a troublesome diagnosis, because they are encouraged to take a moral stance against their spoiled identity (Goffman 1986: 5). Such a marginalization of people with mental health issues suggests how differences between people defined as physically or mentally sick play out, and why the failure to address discrimination in the practices of health professionals continues to have the effects it does. Clearly, the major issues faced by those people within the western and developing world who are suffering from mental health issues or psychiatric conditions are prejudice and bias with stigmatization impacting on their ability to receive appropriate, effective and timely care for all their health needs (Sartorius 2007a, 2007b).

In contemporary society, both death and madness are identified as seen as "strangeness" or the uncanny. This idea of the stranger and their strangeness also ties in with Bauman's (2011) argument about effects from this in society. This focus on the strangeness of the mentally ill leads those seen as strange or as an outsider to be viewed as untrustworthy, and has a consequence for those thought of this way by ED nurses. He says,

> Perhaps the most pernicious, seminal and long-term effects of security obsession (the collateral damage it perpetrates) is the sapping of mutual trust and the sowing and breeding of mutual suspicion. … The deficit of trust inevitably leads to a wilting of communication; in avoiding communication, and in the absence of interest in its renewal, the strangeness of strangers is bound to deepen and acquire ever darker and more sinister tones. (p.70)

Goffman (1986) in his study of spoiled identity saw similarities in the way that the concept of stigma operated in contemporary society was similar to that of early Greek society. In classical Greek society, a person with physical marks or visible physical difference was treated as outcast, while the modern form of stigma related most strongly to that of a spoiled identity, a deficit of character rather than a physical deficit. The effects of this difference means that stigma, and its operations of discrimination results in taking a moral stance towards those identified as having spoiled identity.

Many claim that combining or mainstreaming mental health services within the ED is of greater benefit to patient outcomes (Browne et al. 2011, Garling 2008, Shafiei, Gaynor, and Farrell 2011) despite the obvious difficulties. They argue that patients have better access to medical screening/investigations with the hope that the gap in mortality rates between the mental health population and the general population reduces over time. The hope is too, that the presence of mental health nurses within the ED will encourage all of the staff to develop the skills knowledge and compassion to care for all patients who enter the ED. Moreover, it was clear that research is required into the situation for ED nurses and the impact access by mental health patients to the mainstreamed ED has had on their ability to provide care.

Conclusion

The unwillingness to see people with a mental illness as "sick" can be due to lack of knowledge or poor implementation of integration policies in health care systems. Where physical care dominates, sufferers of mental health issues remain stigmatized despite moves to break down walls erected between the differing paradigms of care. Hofman (2008) argues that education and increased awareness have de-stigmatized mental health issues, yet inequality in treatment between physical and mental health problems remained. Funding still continues as an issue, as does recognizing the many physical effects that mental illnesses have on patients. Lawrence and Kisely (2010) and Saxena, Thornicroft, Knapp, and Whiteford (2007) emphasize the global inequities in the provision of mental health care and the tragic results from poor access to total health care that results from stigmatizing mental illness.

Although disparities in care continue throughout the health care system, they are particularly obvious in EDs where the human rights of the mentally ill are still flouted due to poor implementation of mainstreaming policies. For these reasons, mainstreaming has had mixed effects, with patients able to access the general health care system but experiencing limited effectiveness of care in EDs due to stigma and prejudice. True mainstreaming requires more than changes to the architecture of EDs, or more than employment of mental health professionals that maintain separation in the mainstream system. Mainstreaming requires the support of all health professionals working in EDs to ensure that all of the needs of mental health patients are met.

References

Arboleda-Florez, J. 2008. Mental illness and human rights. *Current Opinions in Psychiatry*, *21*, 479–484.

Australian Health Ministers. 1992. *National Mental Health Plan*. Canberra: Australian Government Publishing Service.

Bassuk, E.L. 1980. The impact of deinstitutionalization on the general hospital psychiatric emergency ward. *Hospital & Community Psychiatry*, *31*(9), 623–627.

Bassuk, E.L. and Gerson, S. 1978. Deinstitutionalization and mental health services. *Scientific American*, *238*(2), 46–53.

Bauman, Z. 2004. *Wasted Lives*. Cambridge: Polity Press.

Bauman, Z. 2011. *Collateral Damage*. Cambridge: Polity Press.

Broadbent, M., Moxham, L., and Dwyer, T. 2010. Issues associated with triage of clients with a mental illness in Australian emergency departments. *Australasian Emergency Nursing Journal*, *13*, 117–123.

Brown, S., Kim, M., Mitchell, C. and Inskip, H. 2010. Twenty-five years mortality of a community cohort with schizophrenia. *The British Journal of Psychiatry*, *196*, 116–121.

Browne, V., Knott, J., Dakis, J., Fielding, J., Lyle, D., Daniel, C., and Virtue, E. 2011. Improving the care of mentally ill patients in atertiary emergency department: Development of a psychiatric assessment and planning unit. *Australasian Psychiatry*, *19*(4), 350–353.

Bullard, M.J., Unger, B., Spencer, J., and Grafstein, E. 2008. Revisions to the Canadian Emergency Department Triage and Acuity Scale (CTAS) adult guidelines. *Canadian Journal of Emergency Medicine (CJEM)*, *10*(2), 136–142.

Burdekin, B., Dame Guilfoyle, M. and Hall, D. 1993. *Human Rights And Mental Illness: Report of The National Inquiry Into The Human Rights Of People With Mental Illness*. Canberra: Australian Government Publishing Service.

Camilli, V. and Martin, J. 2005. Emergency department nurses' attitude towards suspected intoxicated and psychiatric patients. *Topics in Emergency Medicine*, *27*(4), 313–316.

Cobigo, V. and Stuart, H. 2010. Social inclusion and mental health. *Current Opinions in Psychiatry*, 23, 453–457.

Collins, E., Tranter, S., and Irvine, F. 2012. The physical health of the seriously mentally ill: an overview of the literature. *Journal of Psychiatric and Mental Health Nursing, 19*, 638–646.

Cooper, S., Ssebunnya, J., Kigozi, F., Lund, C., Flisher, A., and The MHAPP Research Programme Consortium. 2010. Viewing Uganda's mental health system through a human rights lens. *International Review of Psychiatry*, *22*(6), 578–588.

Das, J., Do, Q., Friedman, J. and McKenzie, D. 2008. *Mental Health Patterns and Consequences: Results from Survey Data in Five Developing Countries: Development Research Group*. The World Bank.

Dhanda, A. and Narayan, T. 2007. Mental health and human rights. *Lancet*, *370*, 1197–1198.

Douglas, M. 2002. *Purity and Danger: An Analysis of Concepts of Pollution and Taboo*. Abingdon: Routledge.

Druss, B.G. 2007. Improving medical care for persons with serious mental illness: Challenges and Solutions. *Journal of Clinical Psychiatry*, 68(Supplement 4), 40.

Fisten, E.C., Holland, A.J., Clare, I.C.H. and Gunn, M.J. 2009. A comparison of mental mental legislation from diverse Commonwealth jurisdictions. *International Journal of Law and Psychiatry*, 32, 147–155.

Foucault, M. 1965. *Madness and Civilization; A History of Insanity in the Age of Reason*. New York: Vintage Books.

Frank, R.G., Fawcett, L., and Emmerson, B. 2005. Development of Australia's first psychiatric emergency centre. *Australasian Psychiatry*, *13*(3), 266–272.

Frank, R.G. and Giled, S.A. 2007. Mental health in the mainstream of health care. *Health Affairs*, *26*(6), 1539–1541.

Garling, P. 2008. *Final Report of the Special Commision of Inquiry: Acute Care Services in NSW Public Hospitals Sydney*. [Online]. Available at: http://www.lawlink.nsw.gov.au/acsinquiry.

Glasper, A. 2011. Mainstreaming mental health issues within the NHS. *British Journal of Nursing*, *20*(4), 250–251.

Goffman, E. 1986. *Stigma: Notes on the Management of Spoiled Identity*. New York: Simon & Schuster Inc.

Goffman, E. 1986. *Asylums: Essays on the Social Situation of Mental Patients and Other Inmates*. London: Penguin.

Goldman, H.H., Glied, S.A., and Alegria, M. 2008. Mental health in mainstream of public policy: Research issues and opportunities. *American Journal of Psychiatry*, *165*(9), 1099–1101.

Halter, MJ. 2008. Perceived characteristics of psychiatric nurses: Stigma by association. *Archives of Psychiatric Nursing*, *22*(1) 20–26.

Handel, D.A., Hilton, J.A., Ward, M.J., Rabin, E., Zwemer, F.L., and Pines, J.M. 2010. Emergency department throughput, crowding and financial outcomes for hospitals. *Academic Emergency Medicine*, *17*, 840–847.

Heslop, L., Elsom, S., and Parker, N. 2000. Improving continuity of care across psychiatric and emergency services: Combining patient data within a participatory action research framework. *Journal of Advanced Nursing, 31*(1), 135–143.

Hofman, A.O. 2008. Mental health parity: Reconnecting the mind and body. *OT Practice, 13*(11), 16–19.

Hunt, E. 1993. On avoiding 'psych' patients. *Journal of Emergency Nursing, 19*(5), 375–376.

Jeffery, R. 2001. Normal rubbish: Deviant patients in casualty departments. In B. Davey, A. Gray, and C. Seale (Eds). *Health and Disease: A Reader* (3rd ed.). Buckingham: Open University Press.

Jenkins, R. 2008. Mental health policy. *Mental Health Policy*, 393–406.

Jones, S., Yoder, L., and Jones, P. 1984. Implications for continuing education. *The Journal of Continuing Education in Nursing, 15*(3), 93–98.

Kalucy, R., Thomas, L., and King, D. 2005. Changing demand for mental health services in the emergency department of a public hospital. *Australian and New Zealand Journal of Psychiatry, 39*, 74–80.

Kisely, S., Smith, M., Lawrence, D., Cox, M., Campbell, L.A., and Maaten, S. 2007. Inequitable access for mentally ill patients to some medically necessary procedures. *Canadian Medical Association Journal, 176*(6), 779–784.

Lawrence, D. and Kisely, S. 2010. Inequalities in healthcare provision for people with severe mental illness. *Journal of Psychopharmacology, 24*(11), 61–68.

Lykouras, L. and Douzenis, A. 2008. Do psychiatric departments in general hospitals have an inpact on the physical health of mental patients? *Current Opinions in Psychiatry, 21*, 398–402.

Mason, S., Weber, E.J., Coster, J., Freeman, J., and Locker, T. 2012. Time patients spend in the emergency department: England's 4-hour rule- A case of hitting the target but missing the point? *Annals of Emergency Medicine, 59*(5), 341–349.

McMillian, I. 1997. Insight into Bedlam: One hospital's history. *Journal of Psychosocial Nursing & Mental Health Services, 35*(6), 28–34.

Mechanic, D. 1998. Emerging trends in mental health policy and practice. *Health affairs, 17*(6), 82–98.

Morant, N. 1995. What is mental illness? Social representations of mental illness among Bristish and French mental health professionals. *Papers on Social Representations, 4*(1), 41–52.

Morphet, J, Innes, K, Munro, I, O'Brien, A, Gaskin, CJ, Reed, F., and Kudinoff, T. 2012. Managing people with mental health presentations in emergency departments – A service exploration of the issues surrounding responsiveness from a mental health care consumers and carer perspective. *Australasian Emergency Nursing Journal*, 15, 148–155.

Morris, R., Scott, P.A., Cocoman, A., Chambers, M., Guise, V., Valimaki, M., and Clinton, G. 2012. Is the community attitudes towards the mentally ill scale valid for use in the investigation of European nurses' attitudes towards the mentally ill? A confirmatory factor analytic approach. *Journal of Advanced Nursing, 68*(2), 460–470.

Paul, J.A. and Lin, L. 2012. Models for improving patient throughput and waiting at hospital emergency departments. *The Journal of Emergency Medicine, 43*(6), 1119–1126.

Pilgrim, D. and Rogers, A. 1999. *A Sociology of Mental Health and Illness.* Buckingham: Open University Press.

Sainsbury, M. 2005. *Richmond Revisited.* Paper presented at the Medico-Legal Society of NSW Inc: New South Wales.

Sartorius, N. 2007a. Stigma and mental health. *Lancet, 370*, 810–8111.

Sartorius, N. 2007b. Stigmatized illness and health care. *Croatian Medical Journal, 48*, 396–397.

Saxena, S., Thornicroft, G., Knapp, M., and Whiteford, H. 2007. Resources for mental health: scarcity, inequity, and inefficiency, *Lancet, 370*, 878–889.

Shafiei, T., Gaynor, N., and Farrell, G. 2011. The characteristics, management and outcomes of people identified with mental health issues in an emergency department, Melbourne, *Austalia Journal of Psychiatric and Mental Health Nursing, 18*, 9–16.

Taylor, D.M., Bennett, D.M., and Cameron, P.A. 2004. A paradigm shift in the nature of care provision in emergency departments, *Emergency Medicine Journal, 21*, 681–684.

United Nations. 1948. *Universal Declaration of Human Rights*. Geneva: OHCHR.

Wallace, D. 1992. A history of the lunatic reception house, Darlinghurst. *Austalian and New Zealand Journal of Psychiatry, 26*(2), 307–315.

Wand, T. 2005. Psychiatric emergency centres, reinforcing the separation of mind and body. *International Journal of Mental Health Nursing, 14*(3), 218–219.

Wellin, E., Slesiner, D.P., and Hollister, C. D. 1987. Psychiatric emergency services: Evolution, adaption and proliferation. *Social Science and Medicine, 24*(6), 475–482.

Wong, Y.I., Sands, R.G., and Solomon, P.L. 2010. Conceptualizing community: The experience of mental health consumers. *Qualitative Health Research, 20*(5), 654–667.

World Health Organization. 1986. *Ottawa Charter for Health Promotion-World Health Organization.* [Online]. Available at: www.euro.who.int/__data/assets/pdf_file/0004/ … /Ottawa_Charter.pdf.

World Health Organisation. 2008. *mhGAP Mental Health Gap Action Programme.* Geneva: WHO.

Chapter 11

Legally-coerced Consent to Treatment in the Criminal Justice System

Jennifer A. Chandler

Introduction

The Canadian criminal justice system pressures offenders to consent to rehabilitative treatment by granting legal advantages in exchange for consent. Judicial dispositions do not, however, specify the treatments to be followed. Instead, they order offenders to follow the treatments recommended by their physicians. This makes sense given judicial lack of medical expertise, as well as the remoteness of judges from issues of resource availability and the evolution over time of an offender's condition. However, this system allows judges to avoid questions of what particular treatments an offender may be legally coerced into accepting, and it allows physicians to distance themselves from the coercion and more easily regard an offender's consent as voluntary. Neither judges nor doctors are clearly confronted with the over-arching system of legally coerced consent to rehabilitative treatment, with the consequence that critical reflection on the whole system is obscured and responsibility for it is diffused.

This chapter explores the nature and significance of the splitting of the judicial and medical roles within the overall practice of criminal rehabilitation. It draws inspiration from several themes introduced by Michel Foucault regarding the manner in which individuals are formed and their behavior governed in modern liberal states. Foucault's concept of the "apparatus" directs attention to the complexity and diversity of systems of governance, which may include "discourses, institutions, architectural forms, regulatory decisions, laws, administrative measures, scientific statements, philosophical, moral and philanthropic propositions—in short, the said as much as the unsaid" (Foucault 1980: 197). Foucault also emphasized the manner in which the government of individuals proceeds not just "from above" the governed individuals, but also by encouraging and channeling the active self-government of individuals (Foucault 2003, Peterson 2003). These themes emerge clearly in the "medico-legal apparatus" in which the fragmentation of judicial and medical roles allows judges to issue a sort of "coercive blank check" and physicians to fill in the details, while simultaneously adhering to their governing ideologies and professional ethical codes. The power of the system to encourage "self-government" is reflected not just in offenders' consent to the therapies proposed by physicians but also in the fact that some offenders seek and obtain treatments, such as surgical castration, that courts could not legally coerce them to accept.

The ultimate picture is of a system in which power is dispersed among three poles— judicial actors, physicians, and offenders—such that no one pole can be said to be responsible for the whole system. Instead, they work together in a web of mutual pressure and constraint. The purpose here is not to stake out a firm normative position on whether this system is right or wrong, but instead to inquire into how it functions and what might be its unintended consequences.

Legally-coerced Consent to Rehabilitative Treatment

The Legal Importance of Consent to Treatment

People accused or convicted of crimes come under pressure to consent to rehabilitative treatment at various stages of their transit through the criminal justice system. The pressure takes the form of legal benefits (e.g. the avoidance or shortening of terms of incarceration) which may be granted if an accused person or convicted offender consents to treatment. The rehabilitative treatments may include forms of counseling as well as biological treatments including medications, such as anti-androgen drugs (colloquially, "chemical castration"), and drug and alcohol addiction treatments.

The pressure to consent to treatment may begin prior to conviction where those who comply with the prescribed treatments may be diverted from the criminal legal process (Klag et al. 2005). For example, in the case of less serious offences a person may avoid sanctions if they agree to treatment conditions imposed by specialized "problem-solving" drug treatment or mental health courts (Amory Carr et al. 2011, Sirotich 2006). In this model, "the role of the court team, consisting of judge, defender, prosecutor, and clinical staff, is to maintain engagement with the offender while relying on the court's authority, and often the influence of the judge, to enhance motivation and adherence to recommended treatment" (Amory Carr et al. 2011). This close proximity of judicial and medical roles is not, however, present in the standard operations of the criminal courts, and certainly not in the context of dangerous offenders.

Consent to rehabilitative treatment is extremely important in the case of dangerous offenders, who may be sentenced to indefinite preventive detention (Criminal Code s.753(4)). This designation "dangerous offender" is reserved for serious repeat offenders, and the court may impose indefinite detention where it concludes that there is no reasonable prospect for the management in the community of the risk posed by the offender using a "long-term supervision order" (*R. v. Johnson* 2003, *R. v. P.G.* 2013, Criminal Code s.753 (4.1) and 753.2). Where treatment is a key component of risk management strategies, evidence of an offender's willingness to undergo treatment is thus central to avoiding indefinite detention as a dangerous offender. For example, in *R. v. McDonald*, the Court accepted that it would be possible to control the offender's risk in the community subject to a long-term supervision order, in part because he was "agreeable to participating in psychological and pharmacological therapy including the taking of Antabuse for his alcohol disorder and a medication, like Lupron, for his coercive sexual preference disorder." (*R. v. McDonald* 2013: para. 74) If a court decides to issue a long-term supervision order, it may recommend that the Parole Board of Canada impose a condition that the offender comply with treatments recommended by his physician, as discussed further below. If the offender subsequently refuses to comply with the treatment, he is exposed to arrest and suspension of the order, and possibly to conviction for breach of the condition where there is no reasonable excuse for failing to take the prescribed medication (*Corrections and Conditional Release Act* s.135.1, *Criminal Code* s.753.3(1), *R. v. R.B.* 2011: para. 13, *R. v. Ramgadoo* 2012: para. 53, *R. v. Payne* 2001: para. 138).

A demonstrated unwillingness or lack of interest in treatment may work against an offender, just as demonstrated enthusiasm for or success in treatment may work for the offender. In *R. v. K.W.B.*, the court declared the offender to be a dangerous offender and sentenced him to indeterminate detention. The Court noted that

> [t]he evidence of K.B.'s lack of motivation for treatment, linked to the potential obstacle to treatment from his denial of the offence, if this denial is the product of a psychologically entrenched belief, are factors to be considered when assessing the appropriate sentence to be imposed. Long-term offenders who are supervised in the community will continue to pose risk of harm to the public by reoffending if they have not been successfully treated and maintain those treatment benefits following their release into the community. There is no evidence of any specific willingness in K.B. to engage and participate in any treatment of his sexual offending behaviour. (*R. v. K.W.B.* 2013: para. 50)[1]

The significance of consenting to treatment is not lost on offenders. In *R. v. K.O.*, the defense psychiatric expert testified that "he informed [K.O.] that because K.O. was not willing to take anti-androgen medication, he would recommend that he be designated a dangerous offender" (*R. v. K.O.* 2013: para. 169) As a result of this, "K.O. then reconsidered his position and told Dr. Fed[o]roff that he was prepared to take Lupron" (*R. v. K.O.* 2013: para. 170) This particular sequence of events did not work to K.O.'s advantage, as the court concluded that K.O.'s history of deception and of non-compliance with court orders, among other things, suggested he would not comply with conditions such as continued anti-androgen therapy, and designated him a dangerous offender subject to indeterminate detention.

R. v. Ramgadoo offers an example that demonstrates how the defense may attempt to make use of the existence of legal coercion to obtain legal benefit. Ramgadoo was sentenced to indeterminate detention as a dangerous offender in

---

1 Along similar lines, see *R. v. Ominayak*, 2012, para.34; *R. v. Ramgadoo* 2012, para. 40; *R. v. Côté* 2012, para. 117 ; *R. v. P.G.*, 2013, para. 42–64.

part because of his unwillingness to accept treatment. He appealed, arguing that the court ought to have considered whether he would have accepted treatment in the context of a long-term supervision order, where the threat of conviction for breaching the order would have encouraged his compliance (*R. v. Ramgadoo* 2012: para. 48–59). In essence his argument was that the sentencing judge erred in extrapolating from his non-cooperation when treatment was voluntary, to his behavior under a long-term supervision order (*R. v. Ramgadoo* 2012: para. 52). This argument was ultimately unsuccessful, as the Court of Appeal stated that a long-term supervision order is meant to offer a "backstop or assurance that the appellant will continue his initial willingness to comply with treatment as required" (*R. v. Ramgadoo* 2012: para. 58). Given that this offender lacked the necessary commitment to treatment, there was no error in the sentencing judge's approach.

Courts and forensic psychiatric experts are also well aware that an offender's professed interest in treatment may be driven by the desire to avoid being designated a dangerous offender and sentenced to indefinite detention. For example, the Court in *R. v. M.B.* noted that the offender had indicated an interest in anti-androgen drugs "if it would save his neck and avoid the dangerous offender designation" (*R. v. M.B.* 2000: para. 233). In *R. v. K.J.B.*, a case where an offender sought and obtained physical castration, the judge mentioned the expert witness's acceptance of the possibility that "the offender was somewhat influenced or motivated with the possibility of being found a dangerous offender" (*R. v. K.J.B.* 2003: para. 78).

In sum, it is particularly important for offenders facing a dangerous offender application to make a credible commitment to rehabilitative treatment that may reduce the risk of recidivism. Indeed, it is preferable that they start treatment prior to the hearing so that any concerns about whether, for example, they can tolerate treatment such as anti-androgen drugs, can be met.

The Separation of Legal Coercion from Medical Decision-making

Canadian courts tend not to specify the treatments that offenders are required to follow. Instead, in the case of probation orders, they direct offenders to comply with such treatment as may be recommended by their physicians, and, in the case of long-term supervision orders, they recommend that the Parole Board of Canada order offenders to comply with such treatment as may be recommended by their physicians. This makes sense given that any treatment that might be ordered by the court following expert medical testimony at the time of the hearing may turn out to be medically inappropriate or ineffective later. On the other hand, this practice separates the judicial and medical roles, such that the court supplies a kind coercive "blank check," to be filled in later by the medical team without judicial oversight.

An example of a treatment term in a probation order is provided in *R. v. Simmons* (2010), which included terms requiring him to accept treatment as recommended by his physician, including injection of sex-drive reducing medication, to provide proof of compliance with the treatment orders, and to waive medical confidentiality so that probation services could verify compliance.

The courts may impose long-term supervision orders of up to 10 years in the case of dangerous and long-term offenders (*Criminal Code* s.753(4), s.753.1(3)). While they may recommend specific terms of the order, the responsibility of setting the terms is left to the Parole Board of Canada (*Corrections and Conditional Release Act* s.134.1). The courts retain the power to convict an offender of a breach of the long-term supervision order, an offence that may attract up to 10 years of imprisonment (*Criminal Code* s.753.3). The Parole Board cannot order an offender to take medication, but it may order an offender to follow treatment recommended by his physician, which may include medication (*R. v. Taylor* 2012). In *R. v. Weigel*, the Court recommended that the Parole Board direct the offender generally to comply with the recommendations of his treating physician as approved by his supervisor, and, more specifically, to take "sex-drive reduction medication" as recommended by the treating physician and to submit to regular blood testing to ensure compliance where the drug was not injected by a medical professional (*R. v. Weigel* 2010: para. 105).

Occasionally, courts are uncomfortable with the splitting of the judicial and medical roles, with courts supplying the legal pressure to consent to unspecified treatments and physicians choosing and applying the specific treatments where consent is given. In deciding whether to release a high-risk offender as a long-term offender under a long-term supervision order rather than to detain him indefinitely as a dangerous offender, courts sometimes seem concerned that medical personnel may not prescribe the anti-androgen drugs that the courts think are necessary to control the risk. For example, in *R. v. L.E.T*, the sentencing judge was concerned that there was no evidence that the drugs would work on L.E.T., and that there was no guarantee that the Parole Board would require him to take them if he withheld or withdrew his consent or if physicians thought there were harmful side effects in his case (*R. v. L.E.T.* 2003: para. 157, *R. v. L.E.T.* 2010: para. 32). This underscores the importance that an offender demonstrate willingness to attempt drug therapy at least, and preferably show that it is tolerated and effective in order to convince courts that a long-term supervision order will be appropriate. In *R. v. Evans*, the sentencing judge wrote:

> The evidence is clear that Mr. Evans cannot be compelled to take an anti-androgen against his will. Even if the National Parole Board made it a condition of a long-term supervision order that he take such medication, there is no way to force him to do so, as no physician will administer it against his wishes. Given his high risk of re-offence, it is no answer to suggest, as Dr. Gojer did, that a failure to take the medication could be dealt with as a breach of a supervision order. There is no evidence before me on behalf of the Parole Board or Corrections Canada that Mr. Evans would be re-incarcerated if, for example, he refused to take the medication because he could not or would not tolerate its side effects, as happened in the past. (*R. v. Evans* 2008: para. 120)

Evans suggests some judicial concern that the other parts of the system (medical and correctional) may not be able or willing to address risk satisfactorily through treatment. The sentencing judge declined to take the chance, and declared Evans to be a dangerous offender subject to indeterminate detention.

Where legally coerced consent to treatment occurs, the components of coercion and treatment are split between the judiciary and medical personnel. The judiciary supplies the pressure to consent to and subsequently comply with unspecified treatment through the threat of legal sanctions. Medical personnel recommend specific treatments, and provide them where the offender has given the consent. The significance of this splitting of the roles is addressed in the following section.

The Judicial and Medical Roles in Legally-coerced Consent to Treatment

The splitting of the judicial and medical roles in legally coerced rehabilitative treatment of criminal offenders has the consequence of making it possible for both judges and doctors to avoid conflicts with the social roles and ideologies that apply to them. It also poses certain risks. Judges will not be involved in assessing whether particular treatments might violate human rights laws, unless an offender returns to court to object. As for physicians, when they are not directly involved in the pressure being applied to offenders to consent, it is easier to accept an offender's consent at face value, and to ignore the ethical questions that ought to be raised about whether the ethical obligations of autonomy and beneficence are being met in each case. Other broader questions about the economic interests involved and the ideological commitments of the system are also obscured where there is no clear overarching responsibility for the entire system.

A. The Judicial Role

There are good reasons why judges should not include the specific treatments recommended by medical expert witnesses within their orders. Rehabilitative treatment involves an ongoing relationship in which various treatments may be tried, adjusted, or abandoned in light of their beneficial and harmful effects, the evolving needs of the offender, and progress in knowledge about treatment techniques. This kind of ongoing relationship cannot be captured in a one-off judicial order. Neither are courts equipped to exercise ongoing supervision and alteration of orders as treatment recommendations change over time (*R. v. Payne* 2001: para.131).

At the same time, the judicial distance from the treatments that will ultimately be imposed allows judges to avoid questions about whether particular treatments can legitimately be offered to offenders. Canadian law is quite clear that certain kinds of punishment are "cruel and unusual" and their imposition is a violation of constitutional human rights laws. The Supreme Court of Canada has stated that "[a]t a minimum, the infliction of corporal punishment, lobotomi[z]ation of dangerous offenders and the castration of sexual offenders will not be tolerated" (*Kindler v. Canada* 1991: 815).

It may be objected that the Court had in mind the forcible application of punishment rather than voluntary rehabilitative treatment. On this argument, we need not be concerned that courts do not have to consider the constitutionality of the treatments that may be recommended when they issue orders that offenders comply with whatever treatment is recommended to them later. However, the line between treatment and punishment can be blurry, as can the distinction between forced and consensual treatment. Surgical castration of sex offenders is an example of a procedure that has historically been used as punishment, and continues in some jurisdictions as a form of rehabilitative treatment (Council of Europe 2010a, 2010b, 2012a, 2012b). As for the question of voluntariness, the threat of indeterminate detention may induce offenders to seek surgical castration (*R. v. K.J.B.* 2003). Although some jurisdictions permit the voluntary physical castration of sex offenders as a condition of release (Scott and Holmberg 2003), others regard this practice as a violation of fundamental human rights. The Council of Europe recently criticized the Czech Republic for this practice, noting that most prisoners requesting surgical castration were at least partly motivated by the fear of long-term detention, and stating that the practice constituted "degrading treatment" contrary to European human rights laws (Council of Europe 2009, 2010a). The Supreme Court of South Carolina has also ruled that it was unconstitutional to suspend a sentence on the condition that an offender complete voluntary surgical castration (*State v. Brown* 1985). In the South Carolina case, the trial court initially suspended the 30-year sentences of three convicted offenders and then revoked the suspension. The offenders then applied to the Supreme Court to have the suspended sentences reinstated as they preferred castration. Given the blurring between punishment and rehabilitative treatment, and concern about voluntariness, it seems likely that legally coerced consent to certain treatments may violate the human right not to be subject to cruel and unusual punishment.

In sum, when judges issue "blank check" orders requiring offenders to comply with whatever treatments their treating physicians might recommend, they avoid the question of whether the specific treatments ultimately recommended and applied are constitutional. It is true that prisoners may return to the courts to contest the obligation to submit to particular treatments, although the extent to which they do this may be affected by the desire to appear cooperative (*Proctor v. Canada* 2002). Nevertheless, some offenders do return to the courts. In *Deacon*, the offender objected to the side effects of the anti-androgen drugs he'd been prescribed and he challenged the power of the Parole Board to require him to take medication as prescribed by a physician. The Federal Court of Appeal rejected his complaint, stating that this was not a matter of the forcible administration of medication, and "[if Deacon] does not want to take this medication, he may choose to refuse, but he thereby chooses also to face the consequences flowing from that decision, given his status as a long-term offender" (*Deacon* 2006: para 41, 74).

The Court did not rule on whether the specific treatment in Deacon's case was acceptable, stating that Deacon had not raised this matter. However, the Court left open the possibility that offenders could challenge the specific medication prescribed as well as the reasonableness or necessity of the medical treatment condition (*Deacon* 2006: para. 45).

B. The Medical Role

Forensic and correctional psychiatry exist between two major social institutions—medicine and law—and so encounter challenging ethical dilemmas flowing from the sometimes incommensurable objectives of those institutions (see Holmes and Murray 2011). In particular, psychiatrists practicing within the criminal justice system are at risk of dual agency problems. These arise where psychiatrists act as health care providers who are expected to act in a patient's best interests but may also have conflicting obligations to others, such as to the justice system as forensic evaluators or to the institutions (psychiatric hospitals or prisons) in which they work (Cervantes and Hanson 2013, Konrad and Vollm 2010, Verdun-Jones 2000, Robertson and Walters 2008). For this reason, it is generally accepted that a psychiatrist should not act as both forensic evaluator and therapist for the same patient—a clear separation of forensic and clinical roles (Cervantes and Hanson 2013). However, even when a correctional psychiatrist occupies a solely clinical role, challenging ethical problems arise with respect to the traditional medical-ethical principles of beneficence and respect for patient autonomy.

Beneficence

Physicians providing medical care to offenders are expected to adhere to the principles of medical ethics (Elger 2008, Robertson and Walters 2008, AMA 2013). The UN *Principles of Medical Ethics relevant to the Role of Health Personnel* states that physicians "charged with the medical care of prisoners and detainees have a duty to provide them with protection of their physical and mental health and treatment of disease of the same quality and standard as is afforded to those who are not imprisoned or detained" (UN General Assembly 1982: Principle 1). The American Medical Association Code of Ethics' opinion on "court-initiated medical treatments in criminal cases" states that physicians can ethically participate "only if the procedure being mandated is therapeutically efficacious and is therefore undoubtedly not a form of punishment or solely a mechanism of social control … " (AMA 1998).

However, it is not always clear what beneficence means in the case of rehabilitative treatment of prisoners, as is hinted at by the AMA's qualification that treatment not be "solely" a mechanism of social control. The implication is that treatment may ethically be partly a mechanism of social control. As Sen et al. (2006) put it, "it is often not clear whether "benefiting the patient" entails making the patient feel better or making the patient behave better. The clinician is often caught up in a web of divided loyalties, balancing the requirements of the State or the ward community with concern for the patient's welfare." Robertson and Walter (2008) make a similar point, suggesting that

> one view of the whole psychotherapeutic enterprise is that it represents a process of bringing the patient around to a world view consistent with his or her fellow citizens. Whether this is via dialectic behaviour therapy leading patients to experience their distress in less socially disruptive ways, or the radical reconstruction of the self into a more functional citizen, there is, perhaps, a tension between pseudosocial engineering and beneficence for the patient.

Our recent history of legally coerced "curative" treatment of homosexuality illustrates the dangers of assuming that behavioral modification that brings an offender into compliance with social norms is *ipso facto* beneficent (Pease 2012, Joyce 2009, King et al. 2004). It is clearly beneficial to the offender to avoid social condemnation and criminal punishment. We should not underestimate the value of avoiding "liberty-depriving 'total institutions' [such as prisons] … that sever ties to outside families, friends, jobs and communities" (Vrecko 2010). However, treatment—imposed paternalistically for an offender's own good—has also been criticized as dangerous since the ideology of beneficence and humaneness may distract practitioners from critical reflection about whether society is right in condemning the behavior in question in the way it does (see e.g. Lewis 1970). The conundrum for physicians is that regardless of their views of the legitimacy of the criminal law, they face a patient whom society has declared will be incarcerated unless he or she can be made to comply with behavioral norms. A physician who offers treatment participates in the system that declares and enforces those behavioral norms, but a physician who does not offer the treatment (having judged society's laws to be illegitimate and refusing to participate in coercive treatment) leaves the offender to face punishment. It is not clear what the ethical duty of beneficence entails in this case. Unfortunately, a retreat to the principle of autonomy—letting the offender decide—is not wholly satisfactory either, as discussed in the next section.

Autonomy

In addition to the medical-ethical principle of beneficence, respect for patient autonomy is a central principle of modern biomedical ethics (Beauchamp and Childress 2009). Evidently, legally coerced consent to rehabilitative treatment raises questions from the perspective of the ethical obligation to obtain voluntary consent.

Given that all of our decisions are made under a range of constraints and pressures, this fact on its own is not enough to invalidate consent. The issue of how much and what type of constraint or pressure is enough to invalidate consent is a thorny problem in biomedical ethics. There is debate, for example, on whether there is such a thing as a "coercive offer," the refusal of which leaves a person no worse off than before (Wertheimer and Miller 2008, McMillan 2010). Furthermore, coercion is not the only situation in which the validity of consent may be questioned. Undue inducement and exploitation are also recognized ethical problems (Beauchamp and Childress 2009, McMillan 2010). Finally, coercion is occasionally justified in medicine where competing interests outweigh a patient's autonomy, as with the involuntary treatment of virulent diseases.

For our purposes, it is worth noting that there are conflicting positions on legally coerced consent to rehabilitative treatment. Some take the position that if the conviction and sentence are justified, then there is no harm, coercion, or constitutional rights violation in offering a treatment alternative (Bailey and Greenberg 1998, *Deacon, R. v. V.M.*). The argument is that offenders may quite rationally prefer treatment to lengthy incarceration and, if this incarceration is legitimate, should they not be allowed to make this choice? The Czech government recently defended its practice of providing physical castration at the request of serious sex offenders against the criticisms of the Council of Europe (Council of Europe 2009, 2010a), noting that if other treatment options have been exhausted, "the only other alternatives are placement of the offender in a psychiatric hospital or in a detention facility" (Council of Europe 2010b). Some offenders also appreciate the relief from distracting and uncontrollable sexual drives (Harrison 2008, Gooren 2011, Grubin and Beech 2010). In fact, there may be an ethical and legal obligation to offer medically effective rehabilitative therapies including anti-androgen drugs to offenders facing indefinite preventive detention (Berlin 1989, Gooren 2011, Harrison 2008, citing US cases ordering correctional authorities to provide chemical castration to requesting offenders).

There are limits on how far one may take the argument that there is no ethical problem in offering a treatment alternative to incarceration. Presumably most people would agree that we cannot offer a lobotomy to reduce violent aggressiveness, even if a prisoner happens to prefer this to indefinite detention. As Appel (2012) points out, "some convicts might prefer having a hand lopped off to serving a long prison sentence for larceny, but this does not mean we as an ethical society should permit them that choice—and most reasonable people likely would agree that we should not." Thus the nature of the treatment offered will also affect whether it can ethically be offered. This point is recognized in ethical discussions of legally coerced treatment for drug addiction, where the commentary incorporates an obligation that the offender have a choice between treatments that are humane and effective (Stevens 2012, Hall and Gartner 2011, Porter et al. 1986).

Others are uncomfortable with legally coerced consent to rehabilitative treatment. They object that consent is not freely given when an offender is faced with a choice between two evils (Harrison and Rainey 2009). Gooren (2011) writes that "[i]f we genuinely believe in patient autonomy, we must be prepared to concede that there is indeed little freedom of choice when long-term detention is the only alternative to androgen deprivation." Although Grubin and Beech (2010) note the arguments in favor of sex offender treatments, and ask why an offender cannot make an informed choice even where the alternative to consent is imprisonment, they also clearly see the broader dangers to the therapeutic role. They warn of the risk that physicians who provide rehabilitative treatment to sex offenders may find that they have become "agents of social control," rather than physicians devoted to the best interests of their patients.

The challenge becomes even more acute where patients demand rehabilitative treatments that physicians feel are unethical and that judges cannot legally coerce—such as physical castration for sex offenders. It is not unprecedented for sex offenders to seek physical castration, even where anti-libidinal drugs are available (*R. v. K.J.B.* 2003, Alexander et al. 1993, Bailey and Greenberg 1998, *R. v. Racine* 1994). Physicians may thus encounter pressure to accede to patient requests for rehabilitative treatment that they may feel uncomfortable in providing. It is worth noting that judges, too, may find it difficult to respond where an offender succeeds in obtaining physical castration. The risk is that in granting a lighter sentence due to the offender's reduced risk of recidivism, it might encourage other offenders to seek the same treatment. The result is that the courts come indirectly to encourage a treatment that they could not encourage directly. This concern is reflected in the case described by Bailey and Greenberg (1998), who discuss an offender who sought physical castration and was granted permission to leave jail for this purpose. However, at the subsequent sentencing hearing, this did not appear to affect his sentence despite defense testimony that he was now unlikely to commit another crime. The judge remarked that "the trading of body parts for a lesser sentence" would set a "dangerous precedent." This is not an idle concern. In Canada, judges look at past cases to determine the appropriate sentences. The sentencing judge in *R. v. K.D.H.* (2012) considered the voluntary surgical castration case (*R. v. K.J.B.* 2003) as possible guidance, declining to follow it due to its "unusual facts, not the least that the offender underwent voluntary castration in an attempt to reduce the likelihood that he would reoffend"(para. 281, 420). The judge also noted that "I believe some special mitigating effect can be attributed to the very unusual step of voluntary castration that is reported in *R. v. K.J.B.*; it is difficult to argue that could be anything other than a sincere attempt to minimize the risk to reoffend" (*R. v. K.D.H.*, 2012, para. 420). It is not clear how much of an effect this had on the ultimate sentence for *K.D.H.* given that the cases differed in terms of crimes as well as in the fact of voluntary castration, but it was evidently in the judge's mind in comparing the two cases and deciding on a sentence. This case illustrates the mechanism by which the granting of lighter sentences risks "rewarding" voluntary surgical castration, and encouraging other offenders to seek it to avoid indefinite incarceration, even if neither physicians nor judges would themselves suggest or demand it of offenders.

The Significance of the Distance between the Judicial and Medical roles in Legally-coerced Consent to Treatment

Ultimately, the splitting of the roles between judicial and medical actors likely helps physicians to avoid confronting ethical problems related to patient autonomy. Where they have distance from the coercion, it is easier to avoid questions about the nature and legitimacy of the coercion, and to regard the coercion as a matter between the patient and the criminal justice system. It is up to the patient, in this view, to make his or her choice in light of whatever pressures and constraints may happen to exist, and it is not up to the physician to second-guess the voluntariness of the patient's decision. To be fair, physicians are caught in a system where they cannot win. Patient autonomy is in question if they accept legally coerced consent as valid. They also undermine the patient's constrained autonomy if they refuse to provide the treatment that the patient is requesting and leave the patient to face the greater evil of indefinite detention because of concerns about the validity of legally coerced consent.

The ethical comfort derived from the splitting of the roles can be observed in various discussions of the ethics of legally coerced rehabilitative treatment of offenders, which cite the ideas that "[t]he physician's aims are directed at the offender as a person in need of help and not primarily at the interests of the correctional system, which are legitimate but are not the physician's main professional responsibility" (Gooren 2011), or that "the psychiatrist herself is not coercing the sex offender; rather it is the state via the legal system that will continue to detain him" (McMillan 2013). The guidelines for the biological treatment of paraphilias promulgated by the World Federation of Societies of Biological Psychiatry (WFSBP) offers an analysis that clearly views consent as ethically required, but is quite comfortable with significant judicial pressure to "force" consent. For example, the WFSBP explains states that "in case of doubt of the validity of patient's consent … withdrawal of his consent or non-compliance with the treatment," the court "should … force the sex offender to comply with the treatment plan negotiated with the psychiatrist" (Thibaut et al. 2010: 607). These candid guidelines are consistent with the actual Canadian practice; however, they leave the impression that medical practitioners are "outsourcing" coercion to the judiciary rather than merely ignoring the existence of legal coercion.

There are potential risks in a system in which coercion and treatment are separated. First, both judges and physicians are enabled to distance themselves from those parts of legally coerced treatment that are inconsistent with ethico-legal constraints on their professional roles. Judges are entitled by the state to coerce, but not to practice medicine. State power to coerce is constrained by constitutional human rights guarantees, but in refraining from participating in the ultimate treatment decision judges avoid having to consider the constitutionality of specific treatments. As mentioned earlier, it is true that offenders (who are not afraid of the negative consequences of non-cooperativeness) may force them to consider the matter by launching a legal challenge. Physicians may provide beneficial treatment to consenting patients, but should not coerce them (with narrow exceptions). The split roles allow physicians to distance themselves from the coercion, such that they may approach the patient as a person who is consenting under constrained circumstances that are not the responsibility of the physician. In fact, beneficence even comes to mean providing the offender with the means to change himself to better conform to social demands.

Second, the role of the state in determining what treatment alternatives to indefinite incarceration will be available is also obscured. In its report on the use of surgical castration of sex offenders in the Czech Republic, the Council of Europe noted that the use of anti-androgen drugs may sometimes be constrained by financial limitations (Council of Europe 2009: 15). McMillan (2012) points out that "[n]ot being able to afford something is often a judgment about the opportunity cost, that is, what else can't be funded if this is. It's also relevant that not being able to fund something can be because an insufficient proportion of public funding has been allocated, a problem that might have a political solution." The state thus has a role in determining what alternatives to indefinite incarceration will be available, and the question of the allocation of resources is not a value-neutral proposition. An approach that regards the options as given, and the choice of whether to accept them as free and uncoerced, misses this dimension.

Third, coerced rehabilitative treatment as an answer to the problem of crime may be beguiling for society as the public purse may benefit. Sirotich (2006) notes that problem-solving courts were developed not just to help individual offenders by placing a healing or therapeutic function within the criminal justice system, but also to save money expended on trials and prison. Yet, a solely biological focus on crime encourages a therapeutic response that may miss other contributing causes. Holmes and Murray (2011) point out that treatments aimed at modifying the individual criminal ignore the "myriad socioeconomic, political and environmental factors … that have contributed to the patient being where he is today." Social and political reforms that might address these factors are likely more difficult and expensive than treating individual offenders, another possible reason why biological approaches are popular. There are thus underlying economic and ideological factors that are at work that are harder to see and address when the various actors in the overarching system of legally coerced treatment do not confront the system as a whole.

Conclusion

Legally-coerced consent to rehabilitative treatment should be understood as a component of a medico-legal apparatus that includes multiple actors, institutions, roles, and ideologies. A closer examination of how it actually operates reveals the importance of role fragmentation in allowing judges and physicians to play a part in a system while adhering to the limits prescribed for their respective roles. It also illustrates how power is distributed throughout an entire system of governing conduct, conscripting the governed individuals into the process and encouraging them to demand the very treatments that govern their behavior, even where the supposed agents of power (judges and physicians) might be reluctant for various reasons. The purpose here has not been to stake out a firm normative position on whether this system is right or wrong, but instead to inquire into how it functions and what might be its unintended consequences.

References

Alexander, M. 1993. Should a sexual offender be allowed castration? *British Medical Journal, 307*, 790.

AMA (American Medical Association). 1998. Opinion 2.065—Court-Initiated Medical Treatments in Criminal Cases. [Online] Available at: http://www.ama-assn.org/ama/pub/physician-resources/medical-ethics/code-medical-ethics/opinion2065.page?%3E. [Accessed: 19 May 2013].

AMA (Australian Medical Association). 2013. Medical Ethics in Custodial Settings—2013. [Online]. Available at: https://ama.com.au/position-statement/medical-ethics-custodial-settings-2013. [Accessed: 19 May 2013].

Amory Carr, W., Amrhein, C. and Dery, R. 2011. Research protections for diverted mentally ill individuals: Should they be considered prisoners? *Behavioral Sciences and the Law, 29*, 769–805.

Bailey, J.M. and Greenberg, A.S. 1998. The science and ethics of castration: Lessons from the Morse Case. *Northwestern University Law Review, 92*, 1225–1245.

BBC. 2012. Moldova introduces chemical castration for paedophiles. [Online: BBC News Europe]. Available at: http://www.bbc.co.uk/news/world-europe-17278225. [Accessed: 19 May 2013].

Beauchamp, T.L. and Childress, J.F. 2009. *Principles of Biomedical Ethics* 6th ed. New York: Oxford University Press.

Berlin, F.S. 1989. The Paraphilias and Depo-Provera: Some medical, ethical and legal considerations. *Bulletin of the American Academy of Psychiatry and Law, 17*, 233–239.

Canadian Psychiatric Association. 2009. Position Statement: The involvement of psychiatrists in coercive interrogation and torture. [Online] Available at: http://publications.cpa-apc.org/media.php?mid=863 [Accessed: 19 May 2013].

Candilis, P.J. 2009. The revolution in forensic ethics: Narrative, compassion, and a robust professionalism. *Psychiatric Clinics of North America, 32*, 423–435.

Cervantes, A.N. and Hanson, A. 2013. Dual agency and ethics conflicts in correctional practice: Sources and solutions. *Journal of the American Academy of Psychiatry and the Law, 41*, 72–78.

Cook, D.A.G. 1993. There is a place for surgical castration in the management of recidivist sex offenders. *British Medical Journal, 307*, 791.

Corrections and Conditional Release Act, S.C. 1992, c.20.

Council of Europe. 2009. Report to the Czech Government. CPT/Inf (2009) 8. [Online]. Available at: http://www.cpt.coe.int/documents/cze/2009-08-inf-eng.pdf. (Accessed: 19 May 2013).

Council of Europe. 2010a. Report to the Czech Government. CPT/Inf (2010) 22. [Online]. Available at: http://www.cpt.coe.int/documents/cze/2010-22-inf-eng.pdf. [Accessed: 19 May 2013].

Council of Europe. 2010b. Response of the Czech Government. CPT/Inf (2010) 23. [Online]. Available at: http://www.cpt.coe.int/documents/cze/2010-23-inf-eng.pdf. [Accessed: 19 May 2013].

Council of Europe. 2012a. Report to the German Government. CPT/Inf (2012) 6. [Online]. Available at: http://www.cpt.coe.int/documents/deu/2012-06-inf-eng.pdf. [Accessed: 19 May 2013].

Council of Europe. 2012b. Response of the German Government. CPT/Inf (2012) 7. [Online]. Available at: http://www.cpt.coe.int/documents/deu/2012-07-inf-eng.pdf. [Accessed: 19 May 2013].

Criminal Code of Canada, R.S.C. 1985, c. C-46.

Deacon v. Canada (Attorney General) 2006 FCA 265.

Elger, B. 2008. Medical ethics in correctional health care: An international comparison of guidelines. *Journal of Clinical Ethics*. 19(3):234–248.

Foucault, M. 1980. *Power/Knowledge: Selected Interview & Other Writings 1972–1977*. Edited by C. Gordon. New York: Vintage Books.

Foucault, M. 2003. The Subject and power. In P. Rabinow and N. Rose (Eds). *The Essential Foucault*. New York: The New Press, 126–144.

Gunn, J. 1993. Castration is not the answer. *British Medical Journal. 307*, 790–791.

Harrison, K. 2008. Legal and ethical issues when using antiandrogenic pharmacotherapy with sex offenders. *Sexual Offender Treatment. 3*(2).

Hall, W. and Gartner, C. 2011. Ethical and policy issues in using vaccines to treat and prevent cocaine and nicotine dependence. *Current Opinion in Psychiatry 24*, 191–196.

Holmes, D. and Murray, S.J. 2011. Civilizing the 'barbarian': A critical analysis of behaviour modification programmes in forensic psychiatry settings. *Journal of Nursing Management, 19*, 293–301.

Joyce, J. 2009. Gay injustice 'was widespread.' 12 September 2009. [Online: BBC News]. Available at: http://news.bbc.co.uk/2/hi/uk_news/8251033.stm. [Accessed: 19 May 2013].

Kindler v. Canada (Minister of Justice) [1991] 2 S.C.R. 779

King, M., Smith, G., and Bartlett, A. 2004. Treatments of homosexuality in Britain since the 1950s—an oral history: the experience of professionals. *British Medical Journal, 328*(7437), 427.

Klag, S., O'Callaghan, F., and Creed, P. 2005. The use of legal coercion in the treatment of substance abusers: An overview and critical analysis of thirty years of research. *Substance Use & Misuse, 40*, 1777–1795.

Konrad, N. and Vollm, B. 2010. Ethical issues in forensic and prison psychiatry. In H. Helmchen and N. Sartorius (Eds). *Ethics in Psychiatry*. International

Library of Ethics, Law and the New Medicine 45, DOI 10.1007/978-90-481-8721-8_22, 363–380.

Lewis, C.S. 1970. The humanitarian theory of punishment. Excerpt from Lewis, C.S. *God in the Dock*. C.S. Lewis Pte. Ltd. Reprinted in Tonry, M. ed. 2011. *Why Punish? How Much?* New York: Oxford Univ. Press, 91–96.

Miller, M. 2003. Chemical castration of sex offenders: Treatment or punishment. In B.J. Winick and J.Q. LaFond (Eds). *Protecting Society from Sexually Dangerous Offenders. Law, Justice and Therapy.* Washington DC: American Psychological Association.

Pease, R. 2012. Alan Turing: Inquest's suicide verdict 'not supportable' [Online: BBC News] Available at: http://www.bbc.co.uk/news/science-environment-18561092. [Accessed: 19 May 2013].

Peterson, A. 2003. Governmentality, critical scholarship and the medical humanities. *Journal of Medical Humanities*, *24*(3/4), 187–201.

Porter, L., Arif, A., and Curran, W.J. 1986. *The Law and Treatment of Drug and Alcohol Dependent Persons—A Comparative Study of Existing Legislation*, World Health Organization.

Proctor v. Canada (Attorney General) [2002] O.J. No. 350 (Ont. S.C.J.)

R. v Côté 2012 ONCJ 707.

R. v. Evans [2008] O.J. No. 3649; aff'd [2011] O.J. No. 1327 (C.A.)

R. v. Johnson [2003] 2 S.C.R. 357.

R. v. K.D.H. 2012 ABQB 471.

R. v. K.J.B. [2003] O.J. No. 4966 (Ont. S.C.J.)

R. v. K.O. 2013 ONSC 955.

R. v. K.W.B. 2013 BCPC 39.

R. v. L.E.T. 2003 BCSC 1154, aff'd B.C.J. No. 1797, aff'd 2010 BCCA 331.

R. v. M.B. [2000] O.J. No. 2135 (Ont. C.J.)

R. v. McDonald 2013 ONSC 1143.

R. v. Ominayak, 2012 ABCA 337.

R. v. Côté 2012 ONCJ 707.

R. v. Payne [2001] O.J. No. 146 (Ont. S.C.J.)

R. v. P.G. 2013 ONSC 589.

R. v. Racine [1994] O.J. No. 47 (Ont. Gen. Div.)

R. v. Ramgadoo 2012 ONCA 921.

R. v. R.B. 2011 ONCA 328.

R. v. Simmons 2010 ONSC 5894.

R. v. Taylor 2012 ONSC 1025.

R. v. V.M. [2003] O.J. No. 436 at para 130–136.

R. v. Weigel 2010 ONCJ 287.

Robertson, M.D. and Walter, G. 2008. Many faces of the dual-role dilemma in psychiatric ethics. *Australian and New Zealand Journal of Psychiatry*, *42*, 228–235.

Scott, C.L. and Holmberg, T. 2003. Castration of Sex Offenders: Prisoners' Rights Versus Public Safety. *Journal of the American Academy of Psychiatry and the Law*, *31*, 502–509.

Sen, P., Gordon, H., Adshead, G., and Irons, A. 2006. Ethical dilemmas in forensic psychiatry: two illustrative cases. *Journal of Medical Ethics*, *33*, 337–341.

Sirotich, F. 2006. Reconfiguring Crime Control and Criminal Justice: Governmentality and Problem-Solving Courts. *University of New Brunswick Law Journal*, *55*, 11–26.

State v. Brown 326 S.E.2d 410 (1985 S. Carolina Supreme Court)

Thibaut, F. et al. 2010. The World Federation of Societies of Biological Psychiatry (WFSBP) Guidelines for the biological treatment of paraphilias. *World Journal of Biological Psychiatry*, *11*, 604–655.

UN General Assembly. 1982. Principles of Medical Ethics relevant to the Role of Health Personnel, particularly Physicians, in the Protection of Prisoners and Detainees against Torture and Other Cruel, Inhuman or Degrading Treatment or Punishment. Resolution 37/194. 18 December 1992. [Online]. Available at: http://www.ohchr.org/EN/ProfessionalInterest/Pages/MedicalEthics.aspx. [Accessed: 19 May 2013].

Verdun-Jones, S.N. 2000. Forensic Psychiatry, Ethics and Protective Sentencing: What are the Limits of Psychiatric Participation in the Criminal Justice Process. *Acta Psychiatrica Scandinavica*, *101*, 77–82.

Vrecko, S. 2010. Therapeutic justice in drug courts: Crime, punishment and societies of control. *Science as Culture*, *18*(2), 217–232.

Wertheimer A, and Miller F. 2008. Payment for research participation: a coercive offer? *Journal of Medical Ethics*, *34*, 389–392.

Chapter 12
Psy Policing: The Borderlands of Psychiatry and Security

Rachel Jane Liebert

Introduction

In December 2012, Adam Lanza walked into Sandy Hook Elementary School in Newtown, Connecticut, and shot 27 people. Described on National Public Radio as "to schools like 9/11 was to airports," this shooting triggered another call for increased surveillance and security within schools in the United States (U.S.). Following a long (contested, and politically convenient) tradition of making individuals' psyches accountable for violence, psychiatric diagnoses and interventions have become central to these practices. The ghosts of Sandy Hook have materialized into the push of the Obama administration for a large-scale package of reforms to identify and intervene on young people "at-risk" of madness—an attention that resonates with the subsequent call by Dr. Oz on CNN's *Piers Morgan Tonight Show* that "We need a Homeland Security approach to mental illness."

In what follows, I critically explore these emergent borderlands of psychiatry and security, interested ultimately in how, and with what implications, psychiatric diagnoses circulate with/in the (bio)politics of terror that have come to dominate the post-9/11 U.S. context.

Psy Policing

Two years ago I attended an orientation for new faculty at a public university in New York City. The first presentation of the day was from representatives of the campus's Behavioral Intervention Team (BIT). These security personnel told us to be on the lookout for students showing "bizarre and unusual behavior" and to report any such thing for investigation and intervention. They directed us to their website, where I found a list of examples of what this behavior might look like as well as explicit assumptions that school-based violence emerges from "mental health issues," an emphasis on psychological or medical treatment, a focus on mitigating "risk" and facilitating "early" intervention, and an overarching discourse of "community" protection.

Randazzo and Cameron (2012) argue that it was the 2007 Virginia Tech shooting by Seung-Hui Cho that led to this kind of "intense focus" in campus security. Marking what they call a "critical turning point" in higher education, this event triggered the development and deployment of Threat Assessment (TA) practices, such as the BIT's, to identify, investigate, evaluate, and intervene on potentially threatening students in the name of violence prevention and school safety. While originating in a curious collaboration between the U.S. Secret Service and Department of Education following the Columbine High School shooting in 1999, and taken up then by a dozen or so schools, it was after the Virginia Tech shooting that TA spread to 80 percent of colleges and universities across the U.S. (Randazzo and Cameron 2012).

This widespread adoption of TA was pushed for by the 2007 *Report to the President on Issues Raise by the Virginia Tech Tragedy*, as co-authored by the then U.S. Attorney General, Alberto Gonzale, whose tenure included warrantless wiretapping and the authorization of torture. Indeed, as Reiss (2010) points out, this report "reads as a somewhat more chilling document when viewed in the context of national security more broadly" (p. 37). This context is also salient in the BIT practices I described above—several months after that initial orientation all faculty were sent an email (flagged with "high importance") reminding people to surveil students and deploying the well-known slogan from the U.S. Homeland Security campaign, "If you see something, say something."

Fast forward a year or so, and the Aspen Homeland Security Group is drawing upon the work of the 9/11 Commission to provide counsel on the Sandy Hook shooting to the U.S. Secretary of Homeland Security – advocating for the use of security measures, public education campaigns, and "validators" (including clergy members, celebrities, and grassroots organizations) to "broadcast … mental health indicators." And that same month, January 2013, Senator Al Franken of Minnesota introduces The Mental Health in Schools Act to train people who interact with children every day ("from bus drivers to principals") in the detection of "signs" of madness in order to prevent potential violence.

Despite this proliferation, TA remains remarkably unremarkable in academic literature; there is a loud absence of work documenting and questioning its broader logic and effects. The handful of pieces that do attend to these "invisible" security measures by-and-large focus on their evaluation and improvement—perhaps unpacking dilemmas around privacy and stigma, yet all-in-all taking TA's existence for granted. Even a critical review of campus security by Fox and Savage (2009)—while raising concerns about the "hyper-focus" on the Virginia Tech shooting and how this may lead to an exaggeration of risk, diversion of scarce resources, "counter-productive" and "knee-jerk" measures of questionable efficacy, and "needlessly sustaining the level of fear" (p. 1467)—depicts "educating faculty, staff, and students about recognizing and responding to signs of mental illness and potential threats" as simply "reasonable and practical" (p. 1468).

The contemporary classroom is thus, as Reiss (2010) argues, "in danger of becoming a barely acknowledged zone of quasi-psychiatric surveillance, risk assessment, and preventative intervention" (p. 27). One that, moreover, is proving fertile for a burgeoning industry. The BIT that I witnessed, for example, has its roots in the National Behavioral Intervention Team Association (NaBITA)—a U.S. association that provides support and professional development for BITs, with more than 800 active members and access to more than 180 model policies, training tools, templates, and other BIT-related materials. While proudly "independent and not-for-profit," it is of note that NaBITA's 3-day trainings cost $1500 a person; that their "partners"—including for-profit companies that provide administration software, training videos, assessment tools, and consultancy—have to pay a fee to be listed on their website and, in doing so, have the opportunity to receive the NaBITA "Endorsement of Excellence"; and that a standard campus NaBITA membership costs $639 per year (times 800 members, this means that the association brings in half a million dollars annually through dues alone).

In addition, NaBITA argues that the BIT model is distinguished from, and "more advanced" than, other forms of TA because of its focus on identifying and intervening on threats *before* they become manifest, as well as its emphasis on the heavily coordinated, long-term tracking of risky individuals (otherwise known as "red-flags"). This approach echoes with/in that of contemporary mental health more broadly—including in the substantial and increasing academic, clinical, public health, criminal justice, and corporate attention given to the risk of becoming psychotic. Such investment is despite "psychotic disorders" having a low prevalence in the general population; textbooks, policy documents, and social campaigns routinely cite (but do not reference) the figure of one percent. Advocates typically justify this disproportionate attention to the self-harm, suicide, violence, and criminality commonly associated with these diagnoses—problems that are thought to be especially high in "the early years" (e.g., Morgan et al. 2006) and to be exacerbated by delayed diagnosis (e.g., Muller et al. 2010). As Candilis (2003) therefore argues from nearly a decade ago, "the allure of early recognition and treatment is compelling. Indeed psychiatry has been committing significant attention to early psychosis research and its applications ... the movement to identify and treat early is building" (p. 75).

The epicenter for this "movement" is the Personal Assessment and Crisis Evaluation (PACE) clinic, which was originally established in 1994 in Melbourne, Australia (Yung 2003). Since that time, dozens of similar centers have emerged worldwide to produce knowledges on young people considered at-risk of psychosis, the vast majority of which are in the U.S. This transnational program of research has constructed a set of risk factors that can "distinguish" a population of "ultra high risk" (UHR) youth who are considered 500 to 1500 times more likely to develop a psychotic disorder within two years when compared to the general population (Carpenter and van Os 2011). In turn, these risk factors have been used to develop a number of *pre*-screening tools to arrest a person's potential psychosis—the most well-known of which is the Attenuated Psychosis Syndrome (APS). While moved to the Appendix at the last minute for further study, APS was released in the fifth edition of the Diagnostic and Statistical Manuals of Mental

Disorders (DSM-5) to identify people "at significantly increased risk of conversion to a full-blown psychotic disorder" (Psychotic Disorders Work Group 2012).

Importantly, the "treatment of choice" for this UHR population is anti-psychotic drugs (Thompson, Nelson, and Yung 2010)—an emphasis that reflects the involvement of the pharmaceutical industry in efforts to predict and prevent potential psychosis. The PACE center studies, for example, receive considerable funding from a number of drug companies—most especially Janssen Pharmaceuticals, Astra-Zeneca, Bristol-Meyers Squibb, and Eli Lilly—all of which have a vested interest in the creation and/or inflation of markets for their anti-psychotic products. In addition, 7 out the 11 Psychotic Disorders Workgroup members for the DSM-5 had financial ties to the pharmaceutical industry, and advocates for the APS diagnosis argue in part for its inclusion because it would facilitate large studies of pharmaceutical treatment and programs of pharmaceutical development (e.g., Woods, Walsh, Saks, and McGlashan 2010).

While a number of criticisms have been directed toward the APS in particular—many of which are from the UHR researchers and DSM Workgroup members themselves (e.g., Yung 2003, Carpenter and van Os 2011)—these are by-and-large more concerned with the inadequacy, and therefore improvement, of the UHR criteria's current predictive capabilities. Thus, like the advocates for TA, they are taking for granted the movement to capture the risk of becoming mad in the first place. Yet, "risk" is not a neutral term. As something malleable, dynamic, and contradictory, it can only be made intelligible when viewed in a "substantively political light" (Seddon 2010). Such illumination especially beckons, one might argue, in the context of attempts to capture potential psychosis given that these continue despite their low return after nearly two decades of investment and the skepticism of the people who "started it."

In addition what this movement does not reveal is that, while largely construed in the literature as a brain disease, psychotic disorders—like all "mental disorders"—are in fact "made possible by a contingent set of theoretical, social, and political phenomena" (Blackman 2001: 97). Indeed, although seemingly unquestioned in psy policing practices, diagnoses do not indicate an underlying objectively measurable entity; rather, they act as a situated, interpretive lens for people's experiences. For example, since the 1960's civil rights movement in the U.S., they have come to be affiliated with danger and to predominantly land on bodies that are young, brown, black, and/or alien (Metzl 2009). This is despite that these bodies have typically survived (as opposed to perpetrated) violence, which in fact typically emerges from maelstroms of rationality, whiteness, richness, and/or "America"—whether school shootings, police assault, gentrification, or neoliberal dispossession.

This ricochet of who or what constitutes a threat takes on additional significance in the context of U.S. schools given that it is also well established that "visible" security measures, such as metal detectors and "zero tolerance" disciplining, are largely implemented in those schools that serve predominantly Latina/o and African American communities—a dynamic that seems all the more amplified by abovementioned connections between the emergence of TA with the events of 9/11, which themselves perpetuated racist logics of "danger" and "nation." As Reiss (2010) suggests, "Cho's racial difference and foreign background may well have added to the chain of links between the national security apparatus and campus screening of the mentally ill" (p. 37).

These recurring silences and politics resonate with Katz's (2007) notion of "banal terrorism"—those "everyday, routinized, barely-noticed" reminders of terror, or the threat of terrorism, enacted through ("predictably ignorant, racist") material and social practices. Banal terrorism includes exhortations to report suspicious activity, people, and objects, diverse forms of screening, and anticipatory policing. While all three of these practices circulate within psy policing, it is the latter that Katz believes "puts the state and those it inculcates through the daily practices of banal terrorism on a slippery and dangerous slope"; "analogous to the U.S.'s unprecedented preemptive strike on Iraq … policing and security conducted in anticipation of certain people becoming criminals or terrorists is unacceptable, unwarranted and dangerously erosive to the boundaries of long-standing social and political-economic contracts and conventions" (p. 356). Perhaps, then, policing and security conducted in anticipation of certain people becoming "mentally ill" may warrant similar warnings.

Thus, in what follows, I critically examine the "common sense" of psy policing. Drawing on critical scholars of madness, security, and race, I trace the discursive and affective logic of the movement to capture the risk of becoming mad as it spirals through uneasy social imaginaries of "otherness" and "security." In doing so I consider how and with what implications psy policing circulates with/in post-9/11 (bio)politics, thus presenting the possibility that it moves as a form of banal terrorism.

(Bio)politics

Attempts to predict and prevent potential enact a peculiar form of Western governance that arose during the eighteenth century when, as Foucault (1978) famously writes, "the ancient right to take life or let live was replaced by a power to foster life or disallow it to the point of death" (p. 138). This new "biopower" was less concerned with "top down" sovereign decisions about whether people should live or die than it was with the "bottom up" unfolding and administration of life itself. It thus marks the emergence of a political condition in which our biology—our capacity to live—became drawn into governance.

These attempts include the deployment of regulatory mechanisms targeted at "man-as-species" in order to foster the capacity, and therefore ensure the sustainability, of a population. Such "biopolitics" relied upon the development of techniques for classifying, calculating, and comparing the biological capacities of individuals and the collective. In this way "society" as Hacking (1990) writes, "became statistical" (p. 1), and the "population" was foundational to this becoming. "Statistically organized and manipulated as groupings of characteristics, features, or parts" (Clough and Willse 2010: 51), the population is a biopolitical construct; "a postulated reality" defined by "abstract properties" (Hacking 1990)—risk factors—that effectively work to "dissolve" the subject (Castel 1991). This identification of risk factors directs pre-emptive interventions that target the at-risk population without regard to the specific present state or experiences of individuals. It is this weaving of pre-emption and dissolution, enabled by the construct of the population, that makes risk a biopolitical rationality: if disease can be identified and intervened upon in advance, "society" can continue undisrupted (Foucault 2009).

Thus, biopolitics works to both promote and protect "life" (Raman and Tutton 2010). In doing so it demands that the borders of citizenship be patrolled for threats, including those located in psyches (Liebert 2010). These security measures involve the "treatment of uncertainty" (via techniques that predict and prevent the unexpected) and the "management of contingency" (via techniques that identify and intervene on a calculated potential) (Foucault 2009). Hacking (1990) has called these statistical-cum-political moves the "taming of chance" and locates them in a nineteenth-century shift from notions of determinism to probability. Indeed, Press, Fishman, and Koenig (2000) argue that it is this "underlying cultural belief that probability statistics not only quantify but also tame uncertainty" that has produced the current-day "enthusiasm for risk knowledge" (p. 242).

Biopolitics, then, go hand-in-hand with risk, or what Rose (2007) describes as "a family of ways of thinking and acting that involve calculations about probable futures in the present followed by interventions into the present in order to control that potential future" (p. 70). This "family" has been reconfigured in contemporary times with the interweaving, intensifying ascendency of biomedicine and neoliberalism. Namely, the increased attention to risk comes with requisites for personal responsibility, surveillance, and intervention at the level of the individual (e.g. Rose 2007); requisites that allow the neoliberal State to retreat from its own accountability with regard to both the conditions and alleviation of dis-ease (Elliot 2002).

However, these biopolitical analyses typically link risk management to *self*-governance and as such appear to routinely assume the "choosing" middle-class subject, one that is further coded with whiteness and nation. These assumptions seem particularly limiting in the context of post-9/11 U.S. given Hier's (2008) contention that political events evoke "volatile and moralizing" discourses that invert everyday dialectics—including with regard to risk. Under these inverted conditions risk moves away from the self-governing (-responsible, -surveiling, -intervening) citizen and is instead transposed onto collectivizing discourses about defense from the "harm posed by "irresponsible" (i.e. dangerous, uncertain) others" (p. 175). In order to explore the post-9/11 (bio)politics of psy policing, then, I first turn to this construction of "otherness."

"Otherness"

As the guarantor of the integrity of the population, the State has an obligation to defend "the security of the whole from internal dangers" by driving out anything that biologically or politically threatens it (Foucault 2003: 249); maintaining the wellbeing of the population requires its "sanitation" through the "repelling" of contaminates (Bauman 2000). This "letting die" is what Foucault (2003) called "state racism," and what Clough (2008) has since developed into "population racism"—a phrase that (among other things) is more suited to the transnational circulation of biopolitics under contemporary geopolitical conditions.

Bauman (2000) argues that this racism is both product and tool of modernity, for "distinguished by its ambition to self-control and self-administration, racism declares a certain category of people endemically and hopelessly resistant to control and immune to all efforts at amelioration" (p. 215). This dynamic circulates in the story of how madness—most especially psychosis—came to be articulated and acted upon as a disease entity. In her critical analysis of "hearing voices," Blackman (2001) argues that U.K. governmental attention during the mid-nineteenth century to problems of "urban luxury and idle indifference" and "proletarian degeneracy and idle poverty" invoked a splitting of the sanities of the rich and the poor into the "morally mad" and the "heritably mad," respectively. The former had their reasoning "in error" and were curable through moral therapies that, premised on "self-prevention or auto-prophylaxis," educated people about "prior signs" of insanity, "warnings of danger," and "strengthening the self-will." The latter, however, congenitally lacked the capacity for reasoning, were more vulnerable to conditions that exacerbated madness, less able to be checked by "civilizing influences," and, thus, "simply uneducable."

By the early part of the twentieth century this "predisposition" of the poor was entrenched as an inherent, biological incapacity for reason, thereby naturalizing (ir)responsibility. It followed that that psy discourses and techniques could be used to "target those who were unable or incapable of practicing particular forms of individuality and sociality" (p. 122)—a targeting that moved in step with the concurrent politics of eugenics that constructed social problems of crime, poverty, and misery as problems of biological decay and deterioration.

Contemporary moves to predict and prevent potential madness can thus be understood as "citizenship projects," or "the ways that authorities thought [think] about (*some*) individuals as potential citizens, and the ways they tried [try] to act upon them in that context" (Rose 2007: 131, my emphases). The italics here are important: as suggested by Blackman's (2001) account above, rationalities and techniques of risk work to sort the "at-risk" from the "risky"—those potential citizens with the capacity to self-govern from those "anticitizens" or "intractable individuals unable to govern themselves according to the civilized norms of a liberal society of freedom" (Rose 2007: 249). O'Malley (2008) documents this sorting in his critical analysis of substance abuse in the Australian neoliberal context, where people are constructed as the "responsible drug user," or the "enslaved drug addict," or "drug abuser." These categories are in turn morally charged toward social inclusion and exclusion, respectively—the former is "like us" and thus a candidate for self-governance, the latter is "unlike us" and thus a candidate for more explicitly coercive governance.

The "unlike us" "anticitizen" has been explored by a number of scholars using the Foucauldian construct of "the monster." Through a critical analysis of the U.K. Dangerous and Severe Personality Disorder (DSPD) program advocating for the preventative detention of people diagnosed with certain "personality disorders," Seddon (2008), for example, argues that, despite how risk supposedly "dissolves" the subject, threat continues to land in some, specific bodies—"the dangerous individual." Or, those monstrous individuals who are implacably evil, different, or pathological—unhuman. Such excessive exceptionality is examined by Puar and Rai (2002) in their critical analysis of U.S. constructions of the terrorist psyche post-9/11, where the terrorist-monster is deemed ungovernable and thus distinguished from the "individual to be corrected" as the "incorrigible to be quarantined." These moral invocations work further to normalize citizenry; once quarantined the monster, "provides the occasion to demand and instill [a] certain discipline on the population … [that] aims to produce patriotic, docile subjects" (p. 130).

This dual function maps onto the historic twinning of madness and dangerous criminality, which itself worked to contain "the threatening" in insane asylums *and* to construct codes of conduct for "the non-mad" (Foucault 1988). Indeed, monstrosity seems especially relevant for contemporary constructions of madness given the hegemony of biomedical discourses that classify people's experiences as an abnormal, unreasonable, and chronic illness, and thus "the mad" as different, irresponsible and incurable. By identifying and intervening on potential monsters then, moves to capture the risk of becoming mad plausibly function to isolate those "individuals to be prevented"—sorting some for correction and some for quarantining—while normalizing the population as a whole through the pushing of a responsible, vigilant surveillance of self and others.

In addition, and especially relevant for psy policing, the monster routinely imbricates culture and race (Puar and Rai 2002). Critical race theorists have long documented how moves to locate and eradicate threat land in brown and black bodies, targeting "an evil they have inside of them" (Sartre 1962: li). "Over-determined from the outside" (Fanon 1951: 95), the "racialized person is seen as a threat, an infection, a symptom of social decline" (Bhaba 2004: xx). Moreover this threat is reliably biologized; as Fanon (1951) argues, "the black man is attacked in his corporeality … it is his actual being that is dangerous" (p. 142). Importantly however, this attack on raced bodies is done under the auspices of "a mother who constantly prevents her basically perverse child from committing suicide or giving free rein to it malevolent instincts. The colonial mother is protecting the child from itself, its ego, its physiology, its biology, and its ontological misfortune" (Fanon 1963: 149).

This notion of protection from an inherent, destructive potential of non-civility echoes with/in the history of madness, blackness, and illness in the U.S. For example, during slavery, "Negroes" were depicted as biologically unfit for freedom; if they escaped they were diagnosed with having a medical disorder—"drapetomania" (Cartwright 1851)—and "treated" with whipping, hard labor, and, in "extreme cases," toe amputation (Metzl 2009). These ideas continued to circulate through diagnostic categories for psychosis at the turn of the twentieth century. Resonating with the class analysis by Blackman (2001) above, Metzl (2009) suggests that accounts of psychosis as a biological entity ("dementia praecox") likewise landed on "the marginalized" when they crossed the Atlantic. However, not only did this American splitting reflect beliefs about class, it also met with the pre-existing dissociations between blackness and freedom as well as immanent anxieties about U.S. invasions by the "alien insane."

It was this assembling of raced representations, fears, and disease categories that marked the emergence of psy technologies to identify and intervene on potential madness—once again tied to broader projects of eugenics. Metzl (2009) for instance notes how at this time there were calls for laws that every steamship that landed in the U.S. would be met by a trained alienist who could screen people for dementia praecox using a test of 30 mental status questions—a score of less than 25 warranted deportation. And, Chief Justice Harry Olson urged national screening for insanity in adolescents, before they had "progressed so far as to commit murder or other serious crimes," by making young offenders of minor crimes "gaze for ten seconds at a drawing of a scroll and a box" and then draw these figures from memory. The "defective stock" could then be dealt with by "race betterment" strategies including prophylactic segregation and/or sterilization (p. 32).

Contemporary madness, then, is scarred with classed, raced, and nation-ed divisions between the at-risk and the risky, the nurtured and the natured, the vulnerable and the violent. Thus while the *intention* of today's (bio)politics may (at least explicitly) be less about cleansing the population of potential contaminants of the bloodlines, contemporary efforts to protect the population against potential threats may nonetheless enact similar, racist *effects* to these imperialist projects "of the past." One of which is deflection: According to Bauman (2000), racism not only enacts assumptions about people's capacity for modernity, but also functions to conceal the limitations of modernity by shifting their source into "a certain category of human beings" (p. 215). Such projection has been especially documented of late with regard to post-9/11 conditions; locating risk in some "fundamentally" unruly bodies deflects the insecurity of security measures. It is thus to this construction of "security" that I now turn.

"Security"

In his abovementioned analysis of the DSPD program of preventative detention, Seddon (2010) argues that these types of measures are emblematic of the twenty-first-century State's increasingly limited ability to assure the security of its citizens, leading to the resurgence of punitive, authoritative responses to perceived threats. Indeed, in contexts of uncertainty, interventions that might otherwise be considered intrusive, oppressive, discriminatory, or paternalistic, such as mass surveillance and screening, can be rationalized in the name of protecting, and thus benefiting, both the individual and society as a whole (Peterson 2011). While Rose (2010) agrees that risk-based approaches in mental health also echo a more generalized, contemporary demand for community protection and public defense, he adds further that such approaches simultaneously generate anxieties about the unpredictability and dangerousness of "the mentally ill" that help to justify the shift to, and maintenance of, these logics of regulation more broadly:

> The demand for risk management of those who have a psychiatric diagnosis is one more way of seeking to manage the insecurities that the fantasy of security itself generates and intensifies. Risk assessment, or the demand for it, has a significance which is more symbolic than instrumental—it answers not to the reality of dangers but to the politics of insecurity. (p. 87)

Similarly, Puar and Rai (2002) note that the psychologization of the terrorist is an attempt to know, predict, and prevent acts that we find incomprehensible and frightening. These analyses resonate with Massumi (2010), who contends that rather than evidence of a "clear and present" danger, it is fear that drives the repetitive practices and politics of security in post-9/11 U.S. as this "affective fact" legitimates and eternalizes threat vis-à-vis its invocation of pre-emptive practices that disallow the falsification of it's potential. It follows that measures to prevent the threatening not only feed off insecurities, but nourish them (see also DiProse et al. 2008, Salter and Mutlu 2012). Such currents are essential to the population racism of biopolitics—the circulation of "fear along with statistical profiles of populations ... [provides] neoliberalism with a rhetoric of motive" (Clough and Willse 2010: 51).

This affective twinning, or what Clough and Willse (2010) call "political branding," resonates with psy policing, as the profiles of those "at risk"—young, brown, black, and/or alien—come dripping with historical assumptions, and affective arousals, of inter/national threat. For example, the notion of "reason" that directed the abovementioned classifications of psychosis in the nineteenth century, also, according to Blackman (2001), separated "adult" from "child," "man" from "woman," "the civilized" from "the primitive"; the inability to reason was taken as a moral affront to that which "makes us human." Contemporary madness is therefore constructed as the antithesis to—thereby enabling it to become the scapegoat for—the (middle-aged, male, white, national) "rational actor" demanded under post/modern, Enlightened, imperialist pursuits, such as science (Bauman 2000), neo/liberalism (O'Malley 2002), and colonialism (Fanon 1951).

This projection of unwanted affects by the oppressors—in this case, their own inability to reason and control—into the oppressed, creates a "desiccated affectivity" in the former and a "hyperaffectivity" in the latter, thus further dividing the world into "the civilized" (those that have control over their emotions) and "the barbaric" (those that don't) (Oliver 2004). It follows that the very construction-cum-becoming of One as rational, superior, and in control, is dependent on the Other as irrational, inferior, and out of control—a dependence that haunts boundaries of "self" and "other" with fears and ambiguities that are themselves, as Oliver (2004) describes, also "disavowed to maintain the illusion of self-control" (p. xxiii).

Critical scholars have examined this dynamic using Kristeva's (1982) notion of "abjection." Based on "a type of dread that is always an anticipation of incoherence and dissolution," abjection ultimately enacts a self-protective bodily response to, offensive action toward, and political defense against, boundary threats (Hook 2012: 61). Perhaps then, as an in-between space of normal and pathological, citizen and monster, biopolitical life and death, being a *potential* threat may especially provoke such border anxiety and thus be especially subject to abjection. Importantly, however, the abject not only repulses but also "keys into prohibited modes of enjoyment" (Hook 2012: 70). With regard to madness, this desire may be about the very freedom that madness supposedly threatens; it is an experience of feeling, of acting "crazy," without social constraint—a longing that is *both* refused *and* encouraged under neoliberal demands for "the good citizen" to be both reasonable and autonomous. Perhaps, then, madness casts an unwelcome light on the paradoxical shadows of our current political regime. If so, this also lends explanation to the ferocity with which "we" seem to have grabbed on, and clung, to discourses of an inherited, diseased entity—it is a remarkably effective strategy for keeping Them from Us, and thus our own potential (and desire) for madness from Us, too.

These dynamics have been documented in Salter and Mutlu's (2012) critical examination of the persistence of "psychotic security measures" in the U.S. In a post-9/11 context of insecurity, Salter and Mutlu argue that such measures satisfy anxieties and reproduce desires that work to "shape the image of a safe United States" by enabling the regulation and exclusion of the Other alongside the assertion of the Self (p. 181). They are therefore "convinced" that "foreign policy constitutes national identity—and that we see in the construction of dangers, threats and traumas the construction of the self through the construction of the Other" (p. 182). Puar and Rai (2002) further argue that the aforementioned construct of the monster is drawn into nationalist discourses as an index of civilizational development and cultural adaptability— the monster signifies a "national deficit." In turn, the corollary may be that the absence, prevention, or correction of monsters signifies some sort of national surplus of civility, such that psy policing is perhaps also enacting "exceptionalism"—a narrative of "distinction and excellence" that claims the superior management of a people or population and is thus bound up with national identity (Puar 2007).

For example, in remarks given at the University of New Mexico in April 2002, then President George W. Bush launched the U.S. New Freedom Commission on Mental Health by invoking metaphorical "soldiers in the armies of compassion"—those "everyday people" committed to "fighting evil" to "make

America a welcoming place for people with disabilities"—as this "collective good ... will define the true value and character of our country." The subsequent Commission recommended TeenScreen, a program of "mental health check-ups," to identify and intervene on young people at risk of becoming suicidal. While recently withdrawn, TeenScreen was at the time soon implemented in primary care and high school settings across the U.S. If TeenScreen can prevent the emergence of young, burgeoning monsters, then the U.S. is marked as exceptionally civilized, progressive, secure, *and*, importantly, compassionate—a key discourse mobilized in the interests of twenty-first-century neoliberalism and the "war on terror" (Berlant 2004). Post-9/11 constructions of "the Baghdad mad," for instance, were used to depict Iraq as threatening, archaic, and lawless, and the U.S., vis-à-vis its imposition of mental health services, as benevolent, progressive, and promoting peace and safety (Howell 2010).

Lastly, the creation of an at-risk population is also the creation of a market for technologies of classification, surveillance, and intervention, as suggested by the involvement of industry in both the NaBITA and UHR examples given above. Importantly, in prevention efforts such as these, "what is treated ... is not disease but the almost infinitely expandable and malleable empire of risk" (Rose 2007: 87). This infinity is in part because, as mentioned above, pre-emptive practices mean that threat can never be falsified (Massumi 2010)—a profitability that is maximized if the "at-risk" population is considered not only treatable but also incurable. Herein lies another benefit of mobilizing discourses of psychosis as a chronic, biological illness: if people are forever potentially mad, then they must engage in life-long preventative intervention. This, then, is the "bio-value of risk" (Clough and Willse 2010) generated and circulated through the medico-security industrial complex of psy policing.

And so, psy policing circulates to make citizens, delineate monsters, expel threats, project anxieties, do nation, and push profits—all galvanized by the construction of "risk factors" that are soaked in (bio)politics, statistically spun into populations, thrown into bodies, and stuck down with fear. This raced process splits "the at-risk" from "the risky," propels people into life-long diagnoses and interventions, *and* ricochets accountability for violence away from other conditions of possibility; as a form of banal terrorism, psy policing incorporates us into particular regimes of seeing and not seeing, thereby doing the work, "of occluding, of repressing, of displacing the pain and price of the neoliberal security state" (Katz 2007: 354).

Imagination

In tracing the discursive and affective logic of psy policing, I hope to have made it intelligible within post-9/11 U.S. (bio)politics, thereby intervening on the "common sense" of these practices. An important companion to this logic, however, is how psy policing also moves to deny madness as a *dialogue* with social injustices.

Structures of domination mean that the "effects and affects of oppression" are "silenced" (Oliver 2004: 88); those "who are often devoid of a public voice, resort to dreaming, imagining, acting out, embedding the reactive vocabulary of violence and retributive justice in their bodies, their psyches" (Bhaba 2004: xx). Efforts to capture the risk of becoming mad threaten to imprison (sometimes literally) an embodied expertise that might otherwise offer a (nonetheless painful and at-times cryptic) source for social analysis and change.

For example, "day-dreaming" (Meyer, Finucane and Jordan 2011) and a belief that dreams "can come true" (Cylarova and Claridge 2005) have both been named as "pre-symptoms" of madness and thus targets for intervention. Yet both indicate a capacity for imagination—an awakening of which Watkins and Shulman (2008) argue as a central psychological task for the transformation and humanization of historically unjust, and pathologically repeating, social structures and relations. In addition, after the Virginia Tech shooting teachers were asked to surveil students' creativity as a means to predict and prevent violent madness—something that Reiss (2010) argues as representing, "a troubling call for the doubling of pedagogy and psychiatric scrutiny" (p. 30).

Reiss' critique joins an emerging body of work concerned more broadly with the transformation of U.S. higher education with/in a post-9/11 context. Giroux (2010), for example, argues that while higher education in the U.S. has long been a major site for the (re)production of neoliberalism, after 9/11 it has also become an intense site of militarization; both symbiotically mobilize an array of pedagogical practices to legitimate their related modes of governance and subject positions. Undermining the university's capacity for dissent, democracy, and critical and ethical thinking, these moves thus intersect with how governmental attempts to contain uncertainty, including through the prediction and prevention of threat, inhibit the imagination of alternative political futures and contestation of the status quo (Diprose et al. 2008).

These loopy dynamics demand more than a critique of the emergent borderlands of psychiatry and security, particularly one that simply re-instates the "objects" of psy policing as "objects." Instead, we need what Watkins and Shulman (2008) describe as "a new epistemology" that contains "possibilities for critical and utopian imagination that can continually rework and rethink experience in liberatory ways" (p. 26). O'Malley (2008), for instance, urges one to be on the lookout for "gaps" or "fault-lines" that would enable an experimentation with the "promise" of risk. Hook (2012) too contends, "[if] the negative reflection of the particular anxieties of a given culture [are] projected into another, then subtle shifts in cardinal anxieties and perceived societal lacks will be reflected in what is most angering, most menacing in today's other" (p. 145). It follows that it is to those very "risk factors" targeted by psy policing that we might turn for new ways of understanding insecurity, and therefore, perhaps, of doing security: Psy policing enacts not only a generalized fear of, but also an incapacity and desire for, imagination under contemporary (bio)politics of terror, including within psychiatry itself.

References

Bauman, Z. 2000. Modernity, racism, extermination. In L. Back and J. Solomos (eds). *Theories of Race and Racism*. London: Routledge.

Berlant, L. 2004. Compassion and withholding, in *Compassion: The Culture and Politics of an Emotion*, edited by L. Berlant. New York: Routledge.

Bhaba, H. 2004. Framing Fanon. Foreword to F. Fanon. *The Wretched of the Earth*, trans. Richard Philcox. New York: Grove Press.

Blackman, L. 2001. *Hearing Voices: Embodiment and Experience*. Free Association Press.

Candilis, P. 2003. Early intervention in schizophrenia: Three frameworks for guiding ethical inquiry. *Psychopharmacology*, *171*(1), 75–80.

Carpenter, W., van Os, W. and van Os, J. 2011. Should attenuated psychosis syndrome be a DSM-5 diagnosis? *The American Journal of Psychiatry*, *168*(5), 460–463.

Cartwright, S. 1851. Report on the diseases and peculiarities of the Negro race. In *De Bow's Review*, *Volume XI*. New Orleans.

Castel, R. 1991. From dangerousness to risk. In G. Burchell, C. Gordon, and P. Miller (Eds). *The Foucault Effect: Studies in Governmentality.* London: Harvester/Wheatsheaf, 281–298.

Clough, P. 2008. The affective turn: Political economy, biomedia, and bodies. *Theory, Culture and Society*, *25*(1), 1–22.

Clough, P. and Willse, C. 2010. Gendered security/national security: Political branding and population racism. *Social Text*, *28*(4), 45–63.

Cyhlarova, E. and Claridge, G. 2005. Development of a version of the Schizotypy Traits Questionnaire (STA) for screening children. *Schizophrenia Research*, *80*(2–3), 253–261.

Diprose, R., Stephenson, N., Mills, C., Race, K., and Hawkins, G. 2008. Governing the future: The paradigm of prudence in political technologies of risk management. *Security Dialogue*, 39, 267–288.

Elliot, A. 2002. Beck's sociology of risk: A critical assessment. *Sociology*, *36*, 293–315.

Fanon, F. 1951. *Black Skin, White Masks*. Paris: Editions du Seuil.

Fanon, F. 1963. *The Wretched of the Earth*. Présence Africaine.

Foucault, M. 1965. *Madness and Civilization: A History of Insanity in the Age of Reason*. New York: Random House.

Foucault, M. 1978. *The History of Sexuality, Vol. 1: An Introduction*. New York: Random House.

Foucault, M. 2003. *Society Must Be Defended: Lectures at the Collège de France, 1975–76*. New York: Picador.

Foucault, M. 2009. *Security, Territory, Population: Lectures at the College de France, 1977—1978*. New York: Picador.

Fox, J. and Savage, J. 2009. Mass murder goes to college: An examination of changes on college campuses following Virginia Tech. *American Behavioral Scientist*, *52*(10), 1465–1485.

Hacking, I. 1990. *The Taming of Chance*. Cambridge: Cambridge University Press.

Hier, S. 2008. Thinking beyond moral panic: Risk, responsibility, and the politics of moralization. *Theoretical Criminology*, *12*, 173–190.

Hook, D. 2012. *A Critical Psychology of the Postcolonial: The Mind of the Apartheid.* London and New York: Psychology Press.

Howell, A. 2010. Sovereignty, security, psychiatry: Liberation and the failure of mental health governance in Iraq. *Security Dialogue*, *41*, 347–367.

Katz, C. 2007. Banal terrorism: Spatial fetishism and everyday insecurity. In D. Gregory and A. Pred (Eds). *Violent Geography. Fear, Terror, and Political Violence*. New York: Routledge, 349–361.

Kuper, T. 2008. What to do with the survivors? Coping with the long-term effects of isolated confinement. *Criminal Justice and Behavior*, *35*, 1005–1016.

Kristeva, J. 1982. *Powers of Horror: An Essay on Abjection*. New York: Columbia University Press.

Liebert, R.J. 2010. Synaptic peace-keeping: Of bipolar and securitization. *Women's Studies Quarterly*, *38*, 325–342.

Massumi, B. 2010. The future birth of the affective fact: The political ontology of threat, in *The Affect Theory Reader*, edited by M. Gregg and G. Seigworth. Durham and London: Duke University Press.

Metzl, J. 2009. The Protest Psychosis: How Schizophrenia Became a Black Disease. Beacon Press.

Meyer, T., Finucane, L., and Jordan, G. 2011. Is risk for mania associated with increased daydreaming as a form of mental imagery? *Journal of Affective Disorders*, *135*(1–3), 380–383.

Morgan, C., Charalambides, Hutchinson, M., Murray, G., and Robin, M. 2010. Migration, ethnicity, and psychosis: Toward a sociodevelopmental model. *Schizophrenia Bulletin*, *36*(4), 655–664.

Müller, M., Buchli-Kammermann, S., Stieglitz, J., Stettbacher, R., and Riecher-Rössler, A. 2010. The self-screen-prodrome as a short screening tool for pre-psychotic states. *Schizophrenia Research*, *123*(2–3): 217–224.

Psychotic Disorders Work Group. 2012. Rationale: Attenuated psychosis syndrome (proposed for section III of the DSM-5). *DSM-5 Development*. American Psychiatric Association. [Online] Available at: dsm5.org/proposedRevisions/Pages/proposedrevision.aspx?rid=412#. [Accessed: August 21st, 2012].

Oliver, K. 2004. *The Colonization of Psychic Space: A Psychoanalytic Social Theory of Oppression*. Minneapolis, London: The University of Minnesota Press.

O'Malley, P. 2002. Globalizing risk?: Distinguishing styles of `neo-liberal' criminal justice in Australia and the USA. *Criminology and Criminal Justice*, *2*, 205–222.

O'Malley, P. 2008. Experiments in risk and criminal justice. *Theoretical Criminology*, *12*, 451–469.

Peterson, A. 2011. The 'long winding road' to adulthood: A risk-filled journey for young people in Stockholm's marginalized periphery. *Young*, *19*, 271–289.

Press, N., Fishman, J. and Koenig, B. 2000. Collective Fear, Individualized Risk: the social and cultural context of genetic testing for breast cancer. *Nursing Ethics*, *7*, 237–249.

Puar, J. 2007. *Terrorist Assemblages: Homonationalism in Queer Times.* Durham and London: Duke University Press.

Puar, J. and Rai, A. 2002. Monster, terrorist, fag: The war on terrorism and the production of docile patriots. *Social Text*, *20*(3), 117–148.

Raman, S. and Tutton, R. 2010. Life, Science, and Biopower. *Science, Technology & Human Values*, *35*, 711–734.

Randazzo, M. and Cameron, K. 2012. From presidential protection to campus security: A brief history of threat assessment in North American Schools and Colleges. *Journal of College Student Psychotherapy*, *26*, 277–290.

Reiss, B. 2010. Madness after Virginia Tech. *Social Text*, *28*(4), 25–44.

Rigakos, G. and Law, A. 2009. Risk, Realism and the Politics of Resistance. *Critical Sociology*, *35*, 79–103.

Rose, N. 2007. *The Politics of Life Itself: Biomedicine, Power, and Subjectivity in the Twenty-First Century*. Princeton, NJ: Princeton University Press.

Rose, N. 2010. Screen and intervene': Governing risky brains. *History of the Human Sciences*, *23*, 79–105.

Salter, M. and Mutlu, C. 2012. Psychoanalytic theory and border security. *European Journal of Social Theory*, *15*, 179–195.

Seddon, T. 2010. Dangerous liaisons: Personality disorder and the politics of risk. *Punishment & Society*, *10*, 301–317.

Thompson, A., Nelson, B., and Yung, A. 2010. Predictive validity of clinical variables in the 'at risk' for psychosis population: International comparison with results from the North American Prodrome Longitudinal Study. *Schizophrenia Research*, *126*(1–3), 51–57.

Watkins, M. and Shulman, H. 2008. *Toward Psychologies of Liberation.* New York: Palgrave MacMillan.

Whitaker, R. 2011. *Anatomy of an Epidemic: Magic Bullets, Psychiatric Drugs, and the Astonishing Rise of Mental Illness in America.* New York: Random House.

Woods, S., Walsh, B., Saksa, J., and McGlashan, T. 2010. The case for including attenuated psychotic symptoms syndrome in DSM-5 as a psychosis risk syndrome. *Schizophrenia Research*, *123*(2–3), 199–207.

Yung, A. 2003. Commentary: The Schizophrenia Prodrome: A High-Risk Concept. *Schizophrenia Bulletin*, *29*(4), 859–865.

PART III
Assistance

Chapter 13
Twenty-first-century "Snake Oil" Salesmanship: Contemporary Care of the Suicidal Person in Formal Mental Health Care

John R. Cutcliffe and Sanaz Riahi

Introduction

For those unfamiliar with North American historical colloquialisms, the original use of the phrase "Snake Oil" was to refer to fraudulent health products or unproven medicine(s). Picture a commonplace scene from a "Western" movie where the well-dressed salesman – most often complete with top hat and cane, is extolling the miracle virtues of his wonder product; the panacea for any and all ills, evils, and infirmity.

The unsuspecting (and often ill-informed) customer becomes convinced of the value and application of this wonder product as a result of the erudite sales pitch, the lack of any information that can refute the claims, and the use of accomplices in the audience who were able to provide compelling testimony as to the benefits of the preparation. And the reader could be forgiven for asking – "What does any of this have to do with twenty-first-century mental health provided to the suicidal person?" In response, the authors would point out that, for many, there is an almost automatic conflation of suicide with (or as a) mental health problem(s). Yet, if one looks closely at 'taken for granted 'truths' about suicide and commonplace "treatment" of suicidal people, then an argument can be constructed that posits much of contemporary mental health care for suicidal people as "Snake Oil" salesmanship.

Accordingly, this chapter focuses on several issues regarding care of the suicidal person, and in so doing, critiques the extant literature, such as it is.[1] This

1 Due to word limits, the authors have had to confine their critiques to specific issues and they are mindful that other related areas such as: the over-emphasis on risk (often at the expense of what follows risk assessment), insufficient use of interpersonal therapeutic communication skills, the lack of adequate and appropriate training for working with suicidal people, and major deficiencies in suicide risk assessment skills will have to be covered elsewhere.

critique shows that there is a disconcerting lack of empirical evidence to guide or support much of our contemporary care for suicidal people. It illustrates the often unquestioning adherence to antiquated, ill-thought-out ideas about how best to help suicidal people. Given that formal mental health care in the occidental world is purportedly operating in the epoch of "evidence-based" (or evidence-informed) care, and has embraced and endorsed "recovery-focused" national mental health policy positions (President's New Freedom Commission on Mental Health 2002, Canadian National Mental Health Strategy 2012), this chapter argues that it is disingenuous at best to camouflage containment-driven, defensive practices for "treating" suicidal people as either "recovery-focused" or "evidence-based" and that a radical re-think in our practice is long overdue.

Is Suicide Always the Result of Madness? Suicide, so-called Mental Illness and "Sleight of Hand"

Before we "take the plunge" and offer the substance of our arguments, we wish to preface this section by stating unequivocally that in no way are the authors suggesting that, or making the case for, practitioners adopting a cavalier, irresponsible approach to working with suicidal people. Indeed, quite the contrary; to continue to engage in care of the suicidal person without critiquing our practice (and the philosophical positions, theory, and evidence that underpins practice), would constitute the irresponsible position. Without such examination and deconstruction of practice during our past, perhaps Psychiatric/Mental Health practitioners would still be forcing clients into ice baths, providing so-called aversion "therapy" to "treat" homosexuals (see Barlow 1973), or God forbid, engaging in eugenics-driven forced sterilization of clients as occurred during World War II (Bonifazi 2004).

The general public's views of or attitudes towards suicide are not consistent overtime (Davis and Smith 1993, NORC 1983, 1985, Sawyer and Sobal 2001, Beautrais, Horwood, and Fergusson 2004, Hjelmeland and Knizek 2004); they can and do vary between different ethnic/culture groups (Xiao et al. 1999, Kamal and Lowenthal 2002, Fu and Li 2007, Yang and Li 2007, Oncu et al. 2008), and age groups and specific population groups (Domino et al. 1980, 1989, Domino and Perrone 1993, Zemaitiene and Zaborskis 2005). Furthermore, this body of work continues to illustrate how inaccurate or/and incomplete falsehoods about suicide can and do still prevail. For many "laymen", suicide is still synonymous with madness; it is seen as isomorphic with a dysfunctional brain and almost automatically associated with some so-called "mental illnesses", most commonly depression. Hjelmeland and Knizek's (2004) fascinating study, for example, found that within the Norwegian general population, common myths still prevail and that people in general mainly assign intrapersonal causes to suicide.

Yet personal experience of suicide and/or suicidal ideation appears to have a profound effect on attitudes towards suicide. Several studies undertaken with a variety of cultural population groups have repeatedly discovered that suicide ideation levels have the most impact on perceptions. Shearer (2003) and Renberg and Jacobsson (2004),for example, found that suicidal ideators were significantly more likely than non-ideators to view suicide attempters as more intelligent, and more justified in their actions. These findings signify that acceptance of suicidal behavior is positively correlated with one's own level of suicidal ideation (Shearer 2003, Renberg, and Jacobsson 2004).

An evenhanded examination of the literature in this area will show that a statistically positive correlation has been established between certain mental health diagnoses – most notably depression, and increased risk of suicide (see, for example, Barraclough et al. 1974, Stoff and Mann 1997, Powell et al. 2000, Arsenault-Lapierre et al. 2004). Some advance a more assertive case (see, for example, Isacsson and Rich 2008), claiming that suicide rarely occurs in the absence of depression and go on to posit a causal link between depression and suicide. While a comprehensive understanding of the literature in this area should acknowledge the statistical association between depression and suicide (methodological limitations notwithstanding), there are a number of problems with this association that cast significant doubt on any grandiose and premature claims of causality.

1. The vast majority of people diagnosed as suffering from depression, even so-called major depression, do not complete suicide; and it is reported that the majority never make as much as one suicide attempt (Goldsmith et al. 2002).

Numerous esteemed suicidologists contend that most people who complete suicide are sad, but they are not necessarily clinically depressed (see, for example, Maris et al. 2000, Tanney 2000, Shneidman 2001, van Praag 2004). Similarly, Van Heeringen (2001) draws on cross-sectional and longitudinal studies to illustrate that the occurrence of suicidal behaviour is not limited to the boundaries of psychiatric diagnoses. Furthermore, he highlights that although almost all so-called psychiatric disorders share a statistically increased risk with suicidal behaviour (when compared to the general population), there is no simple causal association between the two (van Heeringen 2001). Correspondingly, in their very well-argued rebuttal to Isacsson and Rich's claims, Jureidini and Raven (Isacsson et al. 2010) contend that the reasoning which posits a causal link between suicide and so-called mental illness (see Isacsson and Rich 2008) is flawed and that the state of the science in this substantive area indicates that it is premature to reach such a conclusion. They highlight how Isacsson and Rich privilege depression over the plethora of empirical evidence pertaining to more commonly found psychosocial factors and severe somatic disease (see also Zonda 2006). Without offering a robust or cogent case for so doing, Isacsson and Rich focus less attention on many other contributing factors to suicide, both proximal (e.g. alcohol intoxication, acute interpersonal conflict, access to lethal methods) and distal (e.g. poverty, unemployment) even when one of Isacsson and Rich's own studies found that only 36% of individuals had depression.

2. Conceptual and diagnostic limitations result in an inability to know for certain what a case of "real" depression is (and not an associated existential state, e.g. mourning) and what is a real case of suicide.

In order to make the case that there is a causal relationship between concepts, conceptual clarity is a pre-requisite. The question that should be asked is: How do we determine that we have a case of "depression" and suicide? Van Praag (2004) offers a persuasive argument for the existence of major imperfections in our systems/processes of diagnosis and classification of so-called mental illnesses. Focusing on depression, he draws attention to problems in distinguishing between "real"/clinical depression and sadness/distress/mourning. He states,

> The border then, between sadness/distress and depression is blurred … psychiatry, so far, has failed to study this issue systematically … that border, if such a zone exists at all, is *phenomenologically defined* [original emphasis] and poorly studied. Mourning, for instance, may, and often does, produce a mental state undistinguishable from major depression. (Van Praag 2004: 83)

Even the American Psychological Association acknowledges that the diagnostic categories contained in versions of the DSM are collections of expert opinion non-observable phenomena – clusters of signs and symptoms. Imperfections in diagnosing depression are also highlighted if one examines the process required in order to reach a valid medical diagnosis. Diagnosis requires: a) detecting any deviation from what is known to be normal, (be this anatomical, physiological, or psychological), b) identifying a complaint expressed by a patient/significant other, c) compiling a medical history, d) taking a physical examination and e) crucially, ordering various diagnostic tests. It is therefore important to note that no such biological markers, which constitute the necessary external validating criteria, exist for many mental health problems, including depression (Stevens 2007). No blood test, pathognomonic test, or specific anatomical lesion can be found for any major psychiatric disorder (see also Breggin 2000).

Diagnosis of so-called mental illness is more an art than a science (Zur and Nordmarken 2010). DSM-based research has repeatedly shown very poor reliability and, therefore, questionable validity. The DSM is more a political than scientific document (Zur and Nordmarken 2010). Decisions regarding inclusion or exclusion of disorders are made by majority vote rather than by indisputable scientific data (Caplan 1995, Caplan and Cosgrove 2004, Zur and Nordmarken 2010), with perhaps one of the most controversial examples being that of whether or not to include homosexuality in earlier editions. As Zur and Nordmarken (2010: 25) state,

> Homosexuality was listed as a mental disorder in the DSM until 1974, when gay activists demonstrated in front of the American Psychiatric Association Convention. The APA's 1974 vote showed 5,854 members supporting and 3,810 opposing the disorder's removal from the manual. At that time, the American

> Psychiatric Association made headlines by announcing that it had decided homosexuality was no longer a mental illness. Voting on what constitutes mental illness is truly bizarre and, needless to say, is political and unscientific.

Acknowledging the difficulties in diagnosing mental health issues is our conceptualization of suicide more robust? Regrettably, according to the literature, a parallel lack of conceptual clarity exists regarding suicide. Silverman (1997: 12), states that "after more than 25 years of discussion and debate, there does not exist a universally accepted set of definitions and classifications of suicidal behaviours for the reliable labelling, counting and study of individuals who are at risk for self-destructive injuries".

If one accepts then the difficulty in determining a genuine 'case' of depression, and similarly, recognizes the problems in defining what constitutes a genuine case of suicide, then it would be epistemologically imprudent to make the claim that depression is a necessary condition for suicide (Cutcliffe and Santos 2012). Arguably the most eminent suicidologist of his generation, Professor Ed Shneidman (2001) is equally critical of the automatic alleged isomorphic relationship between depression and suicide. He asserts (2001: 73) that converting suicide into depression is a kind of methodological sleight of hand. "The central fact about depression is that one can lead a long happy life with depression ... suicide and depression are not synonymous".

3. Health care systems classification and re-imbursement systems.

In many parts of the world, the health systems in which mental health care providers work require the recording of a formal psychiatric diagnosis in order for the client to receive treatment. Moreover, in the American insurance-driven health care system, a formal diagnosis is required in order for health care providers and institutions to receive reimbursement; the billing system for care provided is inextricably bound up with assigning a diagnosis. Tanney (2000) persuasively argues that such (systems-based) requirements lead to over-estimates in the numbers of people with psychiatric diagnoses who have also engaged in suicidal acts. Additionally, any comprehensive argument that seeks to identify causality between suicide and so-called mental illness should also be cognizant of the well-documented empirical data which shows that the majority of people who complete suicide never access or encounter formal mental health care services (Luoma et al. 2002). Their review of 40 studies for which there was information available on rates of health care contact indicated that only one-third of the suicide victims had contact with mental health services in the year prior to their suicide. These data led Tanney (2000: 314) to state that "in our efforts to establish associations to mental disorders, it is critical to realize that data about populations of persons who have performed suicidal acts are an incomplete sampling".

4. Recognized and documented methodological limitations of psychological autopsies.

The argument that suicide rarely occurs in the absence of depression is strongly supported by studies utilizing the psychological autopsy methodology. However, psychological autopsies consist of a number of methodological short-comings. These studies are almost exclusively researched under the paradigmatic auspices of medicine (Pouliot and De Loe 2006). This biomedical approach permits only a restricted lens on a multifaceted phenomenon. It is also common for those interviewed to seek relatively socially acceptable explanations and they may consciously or unconsciously omit revealing certain problems due to shame or embarrassment (Isacsson et al. 2010).

Defensive and Custodial Practices: The Efficacy of Close or "Special" Observation

Defensive practices in the care of suicidal persons include, or more accurately, are epitomized by, "close observation".[2] The first point to note is that the authors could not locate any randomized control trial which attempted to compare the effects on rates of suicide in psychiatric units that use close observation with those that do not. Neither could they find any empirical study which examined the effect that being observed might have on a person's inclination to try suicide. The second point to note is that because of the limited literature in this area, only tentative rather than firm conclusions can be drawn. Nevertheless, the literature is consistent in showing that close observation as a means to ensure inpatients' physical safety fails 18% to 48% of clients, depending upon which study one refers to (see Table 13.1).

While a range of 18–48% may not seem statistically or clinically significant, especially given the relatively small numbers of people, the authors would beg to differ[3] and wonder: How many people are going to complete suicide while "under" observation before we replace this archaic and often ineffective "intervention"? And if the empirical evidence indicates that the use of observation has only limited efficacy as a means of preventing suicide, maybe the qualitative (and/or anecdotal) evidence offers a more compelling case for using it? Alas, this is also not the case. The qualitative literature has focused on the experiences of being "under" observation and while lacking uniformity, the findings tend to suggest that the experience is often less than therapeutic and in some cases counter-productive

2 Different vernacular terms for "close observation" are used in different countries, e.g. specialing, 'one-to-one', arms-length observations and to a lesser extent, constant observation can also be carried out in seclusion rooms, or by the use of physical restraints and closed-circuit TV monitoring

3 For example, the authors wonder how many people would ever board an aircraft if the chances of surviving the flight were 52–72%?

Table 13.1 Findings regarding inpatient suicides and levels of observations

Study/Reference	Year	% completed suicides while under observations
United Kingdom Dept. of Health	2001	18% of those who died on the ward were under observation
National Suicide Prevention Strategy for England (National Institute for Mental Health in England	2007	22% and 48% of those who died on the ward were under close/special observation
The National Confidential Inquiry into Suicide and Homicide by People with Mental Illness Annual Report	2012	2009–2012, almost twice as many suicides occurred under crisis resolution/home treatment services.
Powell et al.	2000	26% of completed inpatient suicides were 'under' or 'on' observation, and two were under constant/ close/special observations at the time
Busch et al.	2003	20% of completed inpatient suicides were monitored every 30 minutes or seen by staff within 30 minutes of suicide, 9 were checked every 15 minutes or observed at least 15 minutes before the event, and 4 were continuously observed
Meehan et al.	2006	8% of patients ended their lives after absconding while on medium- or high-level observation.

(see for example Horsfall and Cleary 2000, Dodds and Bowles 2001, Bowles et al. 2003). Being under observation has been associated with both therapeutic and non-therapeutic perspectives. The described therapeutic aspects included observer intentions, optimism, acknowledgement, distraction, emotional support, and protection; those described as non-therapeutic aspects included lack of empathy, lack of acknowledgement, lack of information, lack of privacy, invasion of personal space, and confinement (Cutcliffe and Stevenson 2008). In summary and while acknowledging the limited scope and extent of the literature in this area, it is clear that:

a) Close or special observation clearly does not ensure the physical safety of all those individuals placed "under" observation.
b) Close or special observation is often experienced as less than therapeutic and in some cases, actually counter-productive.
c) Little empirical evidence "speaks" to whether or not being under observation adversely affects a person's psychache, inclination to suicide, or sense of hope.

As a result, it would be disingenuous at best to make the case that close or special observation as an intervention for suicidal people is "evidence-based" or "evidence-informed".

Suicide, Anti-depressants and Pharmacocentrism: More Smoke and Mirrors?

In the Western world, the bio-medical view of health and health care is the dominant discourse. Perhaps not surprisingly, this has led to situations where the principal intervention for "treating" suicidal people is pharmacological. In a previous section, we highlighted how, for the many who champion a bio-medical view, suicide is conflated with depression (Anderson and Jenkins 2006, Isacsson and Rich 2010). This conflation makes space for (some would say "encourages") pharmacological responses and the most common treatment for depression is an anti-depressant in the form of a selective serotonin reuptake inhibitor (SSRI), according to the NIMH (recovered 2013) –Indeed, such is the influence of the dominant discourse that has so successfully transmuted suicide "into" depression, that often the only "treatment" or help that suicidal people receive is pharmacologically based (Maris et al. 2000, Campbell 2005).

Compelling evidence indicates that prescriptions for SSRIs have increased dramatically during the last two decades or so. In Ireland, the number of prescriptions more than doubled from 13.3 million in 1995, to 27.7 million in 2005. In the United Kingdom the number of prescriptions more than doubled from 8.2 million in 1999, to 18.5 million in 2005 (MIND 2008). In Canada, between the years 1981 and 2000, total prescriptions for antidepressants increased by 353% from 3.2 to 14.5 million (Hemels, Koren, and Einarson 2002). In the USA, the number of people taking anti-depressants (most commonly SSRIs) has doubled in the last decade (ref) (Tracy 2013 – recovered may 2013)) In Iceland, since the introduction of the SSRIs in the early 1990s a sharp increase in the prescription and sales of anti-depressants has also been recorded (Helgason et al. 2004).

Various explanations have been advanced to try and explain these remarkable increases in prescriptions of anti-depressant drugs, most especially the SSRIs. They include such factors as assertions that the (so-called) disorder is "growing" in successive generations; an increased awareness of and comfort in diagnosing depression among physicians' (especially general practitioners') ; and a growing population of better informed, more demanding consumers.

These assertions warrant exploration. Not only is it the case that these theories lack convincing empirical support, alternative evidence and explanations exist. Munoz-Arroyo, Sutton, and Morrison (2006), for example, analysed data from the Information and Statistics Division in Scotland, including psychosocial morbidity culled from the Scottish Health Surveys of 1995 and 1998, and the general practitioner consultations from the continuous morbidity recording (CMR) dataset. They examined antidepressant prescribing trends for all Scottish practices and 54 stable CMR practices (175 955 patients). They concluded that "there is no evidence of an increase in incidence, prevalence, care-seeking behaviour or identification of depression during the period of a sharp increase in anti-depressant prescribing. Further work is required to explain the increase" (p. 427).

If the chain of reasoning advanced by Isacsson and Rich (1997) and others – that depression is a necessary condition for suicide – or/and the hypothesis that suicide rarely occurs without depression, is accurate, then given the well-documented increase in prescriptions of SSRIs to treat depression (and suicide), one would logically expect to see corresponding reductions in the rate of suicide within the population. Stated frankly, the facts simply do not support this hypothesis; there has been no such corresponding and proportionate drop in suicide rates. In most countries the suicide rates remain fairly stable; in some cases it has increased and in other places, there have been modest reductions (see Table 13.2).

Table 13.2 Suicides

Country	National Suicide Rate (per 100,000) for 1995	National Suicide Rate (per 100,000) 2008/9*	Increase in SSRI prescriptions
Ireland	Males – 17.9 Females – 4.6	Males – 19.0 Females – 4.7	13.3 million in 1995, to 27.7 million in 2005.
United Kingdom	Males – 11.7 Females – 3.2	Males – 11.7 Females – 3.2	8.2 million in 1999, to 18.5 million in 2005
Canada	Males – 21.5 Females – 5.4	Males – 10.9 Females – 3.0	3.2 million in 1981 and 14.5 million in
Iceland	Males – 16.4 Females – 3.8	Males – 16.5 Females – 7.0	Reported "sharp increases"
United States of America	Males – 19.8 Females – 4.4	Males – 17.7 Females – 4.5	Doubled in last decade

* It is also noteworthy that these data do not include any effects that the 2008/9 economic crisis had on national rates of suicide. It is important to acknowledge this given that the emerging evidence for both Europe and USA clearly indicates profound and more significant effects on national rates than previous economic "downturns" (Reeves et al. 2012). As a result, the alleged effectiveness of anti-depressants to treat depression and thus reduce rates of suicide may be further undermined by these latest data.

Van Praag (2004), the former chief psychiatrist of New York State and interestingly a pioneer of the biological basis for mental health problems concludes that

> Over the past decades the rate of completed suicide has remained quite stable, and that of suicide attempts seems to have increased. These are puzzling observations, since (it is often purported) that depression is the major precursor of suicide and antidepressants have been used increasingly in the treatment of

> depression. These observations have not attracted sufficient attention, possibly because they do not accord with consensus opinions about depression treatment in psychiatry today. (van Praag 2005: 254)

As an attempt to make sense of these puzzling observations, the authors extend the following tentative (untested) statements:

1. The apparent limited effectiveness for SSRIs in reducing suicide rates might be explained by the issue of the questionable efficacy of SSRIs (and antidepressants per se). Far be it for the authors of this article to attempt to resolve the question of whether or not SSRIs are effective, as such a resolution falls outside of the scope of this article. However, the questionable efficacy is well-documented.[4,5,6,7,8,9]
2. If the prescribed SSRIs and other anti-depressants are effective at treating any underlying depression, then it is theoretically possible that they have

4 1.The Medicines Regulation Board of the Netherlands reported the results of their systematic review of 77 studies, between 1983–1997, each focusing on treatment of major depression (Storosum, van Zwieten, van den Brink, Gersons and Broekmans 2001). The report concluded that suicide attempt rates did not differ significantly between placebo and experimental groups (those taking antidepressants).

5 Kahn et al. (2000, 2001) reviewed 19,639 and 23,201 cases from the FDA database and found that attempted suicide rates did not differ significantly in depressed patients treated with either placebo or antidepressants. Annual rates for attempted suicide were 0.4% and 2.7% on placebo, compared to 0.7% and 2.8% with antidepressants.

6 Kirsch et al. (2008) found that antidepressants were no better than placebo in treating anything but the most severe depression and then differences were negligible (Kirsch, Deacon, Huedo-Medina et al. 2008). Interestingly, this lack of effectiveness in clinical trials has been documented over many years. Antonuccio, Burns and Danton (2002) point out that similar negligible effect sizes in favour of antidepressants have been found repeatedly in individual trials for more the thirty years. For example, in Moncrieff, Wessely, and Hardy's 1998 meta-analysis of trials comparing antidepressants with active placebo, it was found that in only 2 out of 9 trials was there any significant effect in favour of antidepressants. Moncrieff and Kirsh (2006: 156) concluded that SSRIs have no clinically meaningful advantage over placebo and claims that antidepressants are more effective in more severe conditions have little evidence to support them.

7 Moncrieff and Kirsh (2006: 156) concluded that SSRIs have no clinically meaningful advantage over placebo and claims that antidepressants are more effective in more severe conditions have little evidence to support them.

8 Moncrieff et al. (1998) meta-analysis of trials comparing antidepressants with active placebo found that in only 2 out of 9 trials was there any significant effect in favour of antidepressants.

9 Antonuccio, Burns and Danton (2002) point out that similar negligible effect sizes in favour of antidepressants have been found repeatedly in individual trials for more than thirty years.

treated the depression but not the desire for suicide. This would therefore further refute the theory that suicide rarely occurs without depression.

In summary, an even-handed review of the relevant evidence seems to suggest that large increases in prescriptions of SSRIs have not brought about a corresponding drop in suicide rates. Yet the orthodox view of contemporary psychiatry (or as van Praag, 2004 states – consensus opinion) continues to uphold pharmacological responses to suicide as sacrosanct; even to the extent that dissenting opinions are actively discouraged and psychiatrists who advance an alternative discourse are reprimanded (James 2006). For instance, James (2006) reports how a psychiatrist who was disinclined to diagnose schizophrenia in a patient hearing abusive voices and to prescribe anti-psychotic drugs[10] was told that his practice was a clinical risk and he was advised to undergo retraining in "organic psychiatry".

Conclusion

Epidemiological data indicate, limitations notwithstanding, that the trend line for the global rate of suicide has been on the rise since the 1950s. All of our well-meaning efforts at studying, understanding, predicting, and ultimately preventing suicide then do not appear to have produced overwhelmingly positive results; there is little evidence that shows how these efforts have led to (and maintained) significant reductions in global suicide rates.[11] Indeed, the principal "treatments" or approaches most commonly encountered in twenty-first-century mental health care for suicidal people actually have inconclusive and in some cases – damning evidence – to 'support' their continued use; yet their use continues unabated.

First, this chapter has presented evidence which casts doubt on, if not actually refutes, the notion that suicide is a mental health disorder or rarely occurs without the presence and influence of a so-called mental illness. While it is abundantly clear that there is a relationship between suicide and mental health problems, it is also abundantly clear that it is epistemologically premature to convert suicide into depression.

Second, the continued use of close or special observation as the *modus operandi* for "treating" suicidal people is, at best, an ill-informed measure that has a very weak supporting evidence-base and is, at best, an antiquated defensive practice that arguably speaks, indirectly, to the discomfort some mental health care services have in providing "care" to suicidal people. It is very difficult to reconcile such impersonal practices, practices that erect and maintain "emotional-distance" between clients and those caring for them with other literature that demonstrates recovery is inextricably linked to clients having close, supportive, interpersonal

10 Instead, he might try to help that person understand what the voices represent and work out how to control them – à la Voice Hearing network)

11 It could be argued that rates might be even higher were it not for our scholastic efforts.

relationships. As Deegan (2006) reminds us, "Service systems that have given up hope attempt to cope with despair and hopelessness by distancing and isolating the very people they are supposed to be serving".

Thirdly, the pendulum of pharmacocentrism in psychiatry has swung so far in recent decades despite the fact that massive increases in rates of SSRI prescriptions have not produced corresponding reductions in the global rate of suicide – yet this (for some) uncomfortable truth is ignored and those who champion an alternative discourse to biologically-driven psychiatry are pilloried, reprimanded, and warned. In this epoch of evidence-based or evidence-informed practice, should we not be mindful of what the evidence actually says? Should we not abandon or alter a practice when it is not shown to be efficacious? While the reader may reach a different conclusion, this counter-intuitive situation speaks, for the authors of this paper, to the influence and power that big pharmaceutical companies have over contemporary mental health care. For us, the continued championing of SSRIs to "cure" depression and thus "cure" suicide (as some authors advocate) can be thought of as a modern-day version of "Snake oil Salesmanship".

References

Anderson, M. and Jenkins, R. 2006. The national suicide prevention strategy for England: The reality of a national strategy for the nursing. *Profession Journal of Psychiatric and Mental Health Nursing, 13*(6), 641–650.

Antonuccio, D.O., Burns, D.D. and Danton, W.G. 2002. Antidepressants: A triumph of marketing over science? *Prevention & Treatment*. [Article 25] 5(1). Available at: http://www.journals.apa.org/prevention/volume5/pre0050025c.html [accessed 2013)].

Arsenault-Lapierre, G., Kim, C. and Turecki, G. 2004. Psychiatric diagnoses in 3275 suicides: a meta-analysis. *BMC Psychiatry, 4*, 4–37.

Barraclough, B., Bunch, J., Nelson, P. and Sainsbury, P. 1974. A hundred cases of suicide: Clinical aspects. *British Journal of Psychiatry, 125*, 355–373.

Barrkman, H. 2013. The Prozac Revolution. [Online]. Available at: http://www.wej.com.au/newmoon/features/prozac/prozac.html [accessed 2013].

Barlow, D.H. 1973. Increasing heterosexual responsiveness in the treatment of sexual deviation: A review of the clinical and experimental evidence. *Behavior Therapy, 4*, 655–671.

Beautrais, A.L., Horwood, L.J. and Fergusson, D.M. 2004. Knowledge and attitudes about suicide in 25-year-old. *Australian and New Zealand Journal of Psychiatry, 38*, 260–265.

Bonifazi, W.L. 2004. Cruelty and courage: Nurses in the Nazi era. [Online]. Available at: http://www.nurseweek.com/news/Features/04–10/ThirdReich.asp.

Bowles, N., Dodds, P., Hackney, D., Sunderland, C., Thomas, P. 2002. Formal observations and engagement: A discussion paper. *Journal of Psychiatric and Mental Health Nursing, 9*(3), 255–260.

Breggin, P.R. 2000. *Reclaiming our Children.* Cambridge MA: Perseus Books.

Busch KA, Fawcett J, Jacobs DG. 2003. Clinical correlates of inpatient suicide. *Journal of Clinical Psychiatry. 64*(1), 14–19.

Campbell, P. 2005. Book Review: Coming off psychiatric drugs: Successful – withdrawal from neuroleptics, antidepressants, lithium, carbamazepine and tranquilizers. *Mental Health Practice, 8*(7), 33.

Caplan, P.J. (1995). *They Say You're Crazy: How the world's most powerful psychiatrists decide who's normal.* Reading, MA: Addison Wesley.

Caplan, P.J. and Cosgrove, L. (Eds). 2004. *Bias in Psychiatric Diagnosis.* New York: Jason Aronson.

Conbs, H. and Romm, S. 2007. Psychiatric inpatient suicide: A literature review. *Primary Psychiatry, 14*(12), 67–74.

Cutcliffe, J.R. and Santos, J.C. 2012. *Suicide and Self-Harm: An Evidence-informed Approach.* London: Quay Books.

Davis, J.A. and Smith, T.W. 1993. *General Social Survey, 1972–1993.* Chicago: National Opinion Research Center.

Deegan, P. 2013. *Recovery and the Conspiracy of Hope Presented at: "There's a Person In Here": The Sixth Annual Mental Health Services Conference of Australia and New Zealand. Brisbane, Australia Date: September 16, 1996.* [Online]. Available at: https://www.patdeegan.com/pat-deegan/lectures/conspiracy-of-hope [accessed 2013].

Department of Health. 2001. *Safety First – Five Year Report of the National Confidential Inquiry into suicides and homicides by people with mental health problems.* London: HMSO.

Department of Health. 2005. *National Suicide Prevention Strategy for England (2nd) Annual Report on progress.* London: HMSO.

Dodds, P. and Bowles, N. 2001. Dismantling formal observation and refocusing nursing activity in acute inpatient psychiatry: A case study. *Journal of Psychiatric and Mental Health Nursing, 8*,173–188.

Domino, G., Gibson, L., Poling, S., Westlake, L. 1980. Students' attitudes towards suicide. *Social Psychiatry and Psychiatric Epidemiology, 15*,127–130.

Domino, G., MacGregor, J.C., Hannan, M.T. 1989. Collegiate attitudes towards suicide: New Zealand and United States. *Omega: Journal of Death and Dying, 19*, 351–364.

Domino, G. and Perrone, L. 1993. Attitudes toward suicide: Italian and United States physicians. *Omega: Journal of Death and Dying, 27*, 195–206.

Fu, X.H. and Li, L.P. 2007. A study on suicide attitude and depression of university students. *Clinical Journal of Health Psychology, 15*, 42–45.

Goldsmith, S.K., Pellmar, T. ., Kleinman, A.M. and Bunney, W.E. 2002. *Reducing Suicide: A national imperative.* Washington, DC: The National Academies Press.

Hemels M., Koren G. and Einarson, T. 2002. Increased use of antidepressants in Canada: 1981–2000. *The Annals of Pharmacotherapy, 36*, 1375–1379.

Hjelmeland, H. and Knizek, B.L. 2004. The general public's views on suicide and suicide prevention, and their perception of participating in a study on attitudes towards suicide. *Archives Suicide Research*, *8*(4), 345–59.

Horsfall, J. and Cleary,M. 2000. Discourse analysis of an 'observation levels' nursing policy. *Journal of Advanced Nursing*, *32*(5), 1291–1297.

IMS Canada (retrieved 2013) Retail Prescriptions Grow at Record Level in 2003. [Online]. Available at: http://www.imshealthcanada.com/vgn/images/portal/cit_40000873/0/37/78325962retail_prescriptions_grow_record_level.pdf [accessed 2013].

Isacsson, G. and Rich, C.L. 2008. Antidepressant medication prevents suicide – a review of ecological studies. *European Psychiatric Review*, *1*, 24–26.

Isacsson, G., Bergman, U. and Rich, C.L. 1994. Antidepressants, depression, and suicide: An analysis of the San Diego Study. *Journal of Affective Disorders*, *32*, 277–286.

Isacsson, G., Rich, C.L., Jureidini, J. and Raven, M. 2010. The increased use of antidepressants has contributed to the worldwide reduction in suicide rates. *The British Journal of Psychiatry*, *196*, 429–433.

James, A. 2006. *'My tutor said to me, this talk is dangerous' from Times Higher Education.* [Online]. Available at: http://www.timeshighereducation.co.uk/202721.article.

Kahn, A., Warner, H.A. and Brown, W.A. 2000. Symptom reduction and suicide risk in patients treated with placebo in anti-depressant drug trials: An analysis of the Food and Administration Database. *Archives of General Psychiatry*, *57*, 311–317.

Kahn, A., Kahn, S.R., Leventhal, R.M. and Brown, W.A. 2001. Symptom reduction and suicide risk in patients treated with placebo in antidepressant clinical trials: An analysis of the food and Drug Administration Database. *International Journal of Neuropsychopharmacology*, *4*, 113–118.

Kamal, Z. and Lowenthal, K.M. 2002. Suicide beliefs and behavior among Muslims and Hindus in the UK. *Mental Health, Religion & Culture*, *5*, 111–118.

Kirsch, I., Moore, T.J., Scoboria, A. and Nicholls, S.S. 2002. *The emperor's new drugs: An analysis of antidepressant medication data submitted to the U.S. Food and Drug Administration.* [Prev Treat 5 article 23]. Available at: http://www.journals.apa.org/prevention/volume5/pre0050023a.html [accessed 2013].

Kirsch, I., Deacon, B.J., Huedo-Medina, T.B., Scoboria, A., Moore, T.J. and Johnson, B.T. 2008. Initial Severity and Antidepressant Benefits: A Meta-Analysis of Data Submitted to the Food and Drug Administration. *PLoS Medicine*, 5(2), e45 doi:10.1371/journal.pmed.0050045.

Luoma, J.B. and Pearson, J. 2002. Suicide and Marital Status in the United States, 1991–1996: Is Widowhood a Risk Factor? *American Journal of Public Health*, *92*(9), 1518–1522.

Luoma, J.B., Martin, C.E. and Pearson, J. 2002. Contact with mental health and primary care providers before suicide: A review of the evidence. *American Journal of Psychiatry*, *159*, 909–916.

Maris, R.W., Berman, A.L. and Silverman, M.M. 2000. *Comprehensive Textbook of Suicidology.* New York: Guilford Press.

Meehan, J., Kapur, N., Hunt, I.M., et al. 2006. Suicide in mental health inpatients and within 3 months of discharge. National clinical survey. *British Journal Psychiatry, 188*, 129–134.

Mental Health Commission of Canada. 2012. *Changing Directions, Changing Lives: The Mental Health Strategy for Canada*, MHCofC, Ottawa.

MIND (retrieved 2013) MIND News, Policy and Campaigns – MIND releases latest drugs report Coping with Coming off. [Online]. Available at: http://www.mind.org.uk/News+policy+and+campaigns/Press+archive/CWCO0905.htm [accessed 2013].

Moncrieff, J. and Kirsch, I. 2006. Efficacy of antidepressants in adults. *British Medical Journal*, 331, 155–157.

Moncrieff, J., Wessely, S. and Hardy, R. 1998. Meta-analysis of trials comparing antidepressants with active placebos. *British.Journal of Psychiatry, 172*, 227–231.

Moncrieff J, Hopker S. and Thomas P. 2005. Psychiatry and the pharmaceutical industry: who pays the piper? *Psychiatric Bulletin, 29*, 84–85.

Munoz-Arroyo, R., Sutton, M. and Morrison, J. 2006. Exploring potential explanations for the increase in antidepressant prescribing in Scotland using secondary analyses of routine data. *British Journal of General Practice, 56*(527), 423–428.

National Institute of Mental Health (recovered 2013) How is depression diagnosed and treated? [Online]. Available at: http://www.nimh.nih.gov/health/publications/depression/how-is-depression-diagnosed-and-treated.shtml [accessed on 2013].

National Opinion Research Center (NORC). 1983. *General Social Survey: 1972–1983, Cumulative Codebook.* Chicago: NORC.

National Opinion Research Center (NORC). 1985. *Cumulative Codebook, General Social Survey: 1972–1985.* Chicago: NORC.

Oncu, B., Soyka, C., Ihan, I.O. and Sayil, I. 2008. Attitudes of medical students, general practitioners, teachers and police officers towards suicide in a Turkish sample. *Crisis, 29*, 173–17.

Pouliot, L. and De Leo, D. 2006. Critical issues in psychological autopsy studies. *Suicide and Life-Threatening Behavior, 36*(5), 491–510.

Powell, J., Geddes, J. and Hawton, K. 2000. Suicide in psychiatric hospital in-patients. *The British Journal of Psychiatry, 176*(3), 266–27.

President's New Freedom Commission on Mental Health. 2003. Achieving the Promise: Transforming Mental Health Care in America. [Final Report]. Available at: www.mentalhealthcommission.gov/reports/FinalReport/FullReport.htm.

Reeves, A., Stuckler, D., McKee,M., Gunnell, D., Chang, S. and Basu, S. 2012. Increase in state suicide rates in the USA during economic recession. *The Lancet, 380*, 1813–1814.

Renberg, E.S. and Jacobsson, L. 2003. Development of a questionnaire on attitudes towards suicide (ATTS) and its application in a Swedish population. *Suicide and Life-Threatening Behavior, 33*, 52–64.

Sawyer, D. and Sobal, J. 2001. Public attitudes towards suicide-demographic and ideological correlates. *Public Opinion Quarterly, 51*, 92–101.

Shearer, K. 2003. A survey examining the attitudes in a college population toward suicide attempters. *Suicide and Life-Threatening Behavior, 33*(1), 52–64.

Shneidman, E.S. 2001. *Comprehending Suicide: Landmarks in 20th-Century Suicidology.* Washington: American Psychological Association.

Silverman, M.M. 1997. Current controversies in suicidology. In R.W. Maris, M.M. Silverman and S.S. Canetto (Eds). *Review of Suicidology 1997.* New York: Guilford Press, 1–21.

Silverman, M.M., Berman, A.L., Sandadal, N., O'Carrol, P.W. and Joiner, T. 2007. Rebuilding the tower of Babel: A revised nomenclature for the study of suicide and suicidal behaviors – Part 2: Suicide-related ideations, communications, and behaviors. *Suicide and Life-Threatening Behaviors 37*(3), 264–277.

Stoff, D.M. and Mann, J.L. (Eds). 1997. *The Neurobiology of Suicide: From the Bench to the Clinic.* New York: The New York Academy of Sciences.

Storosum, J.G., Van Zwieten, B.J., Van den Brink, W., Gersons, B.P.P. and Broekmans, A.W. 2001. Suicide risk in placebo-controlled studies of major depression. *American Journal of Psychiatry, 158*, 1271–1275.

Tanney, B.L. 2000. Psychiatric diagnoses and suicidal acts. In R.W. Maris, A.L. Berman and M.M. Silverman (Eds). *Comprehensive Textbook of Suicidology.* New York: Guilford Press, 311–340.

Van Heeringen, C. 2001. Suicide, serotonin, and the brain. *Crisis, 22*(2), 66–70.

Van Praag, H.M. 2004. Stress and suicide: Are we well-equipped to study this issue? *Crisis, 25*(2), 80–85.

Van Praag, H.M. 2005. Why haven't antidepressants reduced suicide rates? In *Prevention and Treatment of Suicidal Behaviour: From Science to Practice.* K. Hawton (Ed.) Oxford: Oxford University Press, 239–260.

Yang, L. and Li, L.L. 2007. Undergraduates' attitude to suicide and its correlative factors. *Chinese Journal of Social Medicine, 24*,126–131.

Xiao, S., Yang, H., Dong, Q. and Yang, D. 1999. The development, reliability and validity of suicide attitude inventory. *Chinese Mental Health Journal, 13*, 250–251.

Zemaitiene, N. and Zaborskis, A. Suicidal tendencies and attitude towards freedom to choose suicide among Lithuanian schoolchildren: Results from three cross-sectional studies in 1994, 1998, and 2002. *BMC Public Health, 5*, 83.

Zonda T. 2006. One-hundred cases of suicide in Budapest: a case-controlled psychological autopsy study. *Crisis, 27*, 125–9.

Zur, O. and Nordmarken, N. 2010. DSM: Diagnosing for Money and Power. Summary of the Critique of the DSM. [Online]. Available at: http://www.zurinstitute.com/dsmcritique.html.

Chapter 14
Sex Offender Therapy: Collusion, Confession and Game-Playing

Dave Mercer

Introduction

This chapter draws on discursive and ethnographic data from a research project (Mercer 2010) that explored the language of mental health nurses and detained patients in relation to "talk" about the treatment of sexual offenders in one forensic hospital. In contrast to a body of literature that understands the fashionable status of relapse prevention in terms of risk management, and assessment as a pseudo-scientific enterprise and measurement tool, it adopts a critical analysis of collusive relations that defined patient-professional interactions at the subterranean level of a high-security hospital. Drawing on the intellectual contribution of philosophers like Goffman, Szasz, and Foucault, attention is given to micro-power relations, struggles, and resistance strategies characteristic of everyday relations within carceral institutions–settings where the inmate is "hostage to therapy" (Pilgrim 1988a, 1988b). The functions of sex offender treatment programmes [SOTP] are discussed as a symbolic ritual in the process of gaining self-knowledge and presenting versions of the self through contrition and confession. Here, engagement is as much a part of the disciplinary and institutional apparatus of detention as high-walls, barred windows, and locked doors, where treatment is a "game" and adherence is the "rule". Forensic nurses adopted an evangelical role in promoting and policing patient attendance at therapy sessions, but shared a dismissive discourse about maintaining control and manufacturing a marketable commodity for less secure services.

The design of the study that generated the data discussed in the chapter has been reported in detail elsewhere (Mercer 2013a). Here, it is enough to note that the broad focus was to critically explore the socially constructive nature of language (Potter and Wetherell 1987) and discursive-practices (Holmes 2002, Perron et al. 2005) in one UK forensic hospital. Alongside observations, interviews were undertaken with 18 mental health nurses [13 men and 5 women] and 9 male sexual offenders with a diagnosis of personality disorder. The chief topic of co-constructed accounts (Kvale 1996) was around managing sexually explicit media in secure settings. Given, though, that "fantasy" is accorded a central role in talk about offending and risk-management, attention was also devoted to accounts of sex offender treatment [SOT] in the context of nursing care. The setting of the study was one of the former English "special hospitals". Though these institutions have, latterly, been incorporated into National Health Service [NHS] provision, their roots date back to the "criminal lunatic asylums" of the mid-nineteenth century – isolated and insular communities managed centrally alongside the penal system (Cohen 1981). This, in part, explains their unique cultural formation (Pilgrim 2007, Quinsey 1999), much troubled history (e.g., Blom-Cooper et al. 1992), and calls for closure (Bluglass 1992, Fallon et al. 1999). Early work into the hybrid role of nurses who worked in such secure environments was dominated by the "therapeutic custody" debate (e.g., Burrow 1991).

Despite reorganization, restructuring, and the adoption of an overt therapeutic discourse, these institutions characterize the last vestige of the "total institution" (Goffman 1961) in psychiatric care. They contain long-stay populations comprising those deemed to be both disordered and dangerous – men detained, often without limit of time, for treatment rather than punishment. Foucault (1978) interrogated the "will to power" of the forensic psychiatric apparatus, and offered an insightful "history of the present" as it relates to the borderline between law and medicine and struggle for the soul of the deviant individual. His article begins with an exchange that took place in 1975 in the Paris criminal courts between the presiding judge and a man accused of rape. The defendant is asked to "reflect" on his crimes and "analyse" himself, but a refusal to speak results in the gears of criminal justice machinery grinding to a standstill. For Foucault, the silence of the accused denied the "modern tribunal" an essential answer, "Who are you?" As he noted: "Beyond admission, there must be confession, self-examination, explanation of oneself, revelation of what one is. The penal machine can no longer function simply with a law, a violation and a responsible party; it needs something else, a supplementary material" (Foucault 1978: 2).

The early origins of therapeutic sentencing (e.g., Brookes 2010) and psi-discipline interventions like SOTP can be traced back to the historical collaboration between law and psychiatry and the "psychiatrization of criminal danger" (Foucault 1988), which introduced "new techniques of management focusing on the instincts, motivations, and will of individuals needing to be transformed" (McCallum 1997: 70). In the UK, sex offender treatment programmes operate across a range of mental health settings, probation services (Mandeville-Norden et al. 2008), and the prison system (Wakeling et al. 2013). Typically, these adopt a cognitive-behavioral approach ("relapse prevention"), premised on breaking down "denial", challenging "distorted thinking", identifying "offence-cycles" and "triggers", and developing empathic attitudes toward victims (Marques et al. 2005, Marshall et al. 2005). This, though, is dependent on "disclosure" and acceptance of a "sexual offender" identity. "Talk" is central to the therapeutic process, but clinicians pay little attention to the political and ideological functions of language in producing, and reproducing, oppressive power relations (Fairclough 1992, 1989). Current critical scholarship has explored the role of discourse in constructing masculinities (Cowburn and Pringle 2000), and has analysed discourse in prison sex-offender groups (Auburn 2005) where cognitive distortion is understood as "social resource" rather than "pathological mental entity".

The sections below utilize extracts of nurse and patient data to reconstruct everyday relations in one forensic unit. This individual "talk" is organized in relation to the discursive repertoires, or shared ways of speaking, that characterized a typically taken-for-granted world. Attention is given to the nursing role with a specific client group of men defined in terms of disorder and dangerousness – a "pathology of the monstrous" (Foucault 1978) revisited. The centrality of talk that is part of SOT and promoting engagement is identified in constructing a psychiatric subject but is focused on long-term control and surveillance. Though sceptical about the value of therapy, each group of respondents adopted dramaturgical roles (Goffman 1963, 1961) to satisfy the needs of the institutional apparatus. Finally, consideration is given to the way male nurses distanced themselves from the sex offender as "other", by opting out of therapeutic relations and protecting the "sexual self".

Talking about Treatment: The "Sexual Offender" and the "Serious Offender"

When nurses talked about their role they clearly identified the physical and human impact of security, but a counterpart philosophy of treatment was less clearly articulated. Concepts such as "treatment", "therapy", and "nursing care" were used uncritically and interchangeably. This suggested an ill-defined professional persona for nursing, and represented part of a larger semantic conflation about interventive work with medicalized offenders (Pilgrim 2007). Only three nursing respondents had direct experience of facilitating groups as part of the SOTP, and this hinted at an institutional division of labour. Typically, a routine distinction was made between the generic practice of forensic nursing [done on the wards] and the expertise of offence-focused work [done off the wards]:

> as someone's ICC [individual care co-ordinator] you wouldn't discuss their offending but you'd tend … from a personal point of view … and I think for most people … you tend not to get too deeply involved … just on the one-to-one basis [pause] it's mostly preferred if it's … done off the ward where you might [coughs] psychologists may well be involved in it … but they tend to frown on sex … certainly sexual index offence work on like a one-to-one basis … it's geared up towards the group work. (male nurse 15)

> I don't feel trained enough to open basically a bag of worms [break] obviously you do have to talk about his offence … during interviews and sessions … but with regards to the more specific nature of it … it's not worth having SOTP groups to me … and then we do the work on the ward … but obviously these people are trained in some way to facilitate groups … and they understand how to interpret responses. (male nurse 5)

Nurses described a key part of their professional role in terms of "treatment", but this was often a superficial statement that lacked substance or evidence. Frequent references to SOTP provided a convenient pigeonhole to evade talking about the therapeutic input of ward-based staff, and constructed a potentially effective strategy for a group of patients typically seen as resistant to any form of intervention. But, it was a therapeutic approach which needed to be promoted through hard-sell techniques. If it could not guarantee a "cure", there was symbolic value in "something" being better than "nothing", And this was an opportunity that was embraced with zeal:

> it's on two levels ... it's something that might stop people sexually offending and it's something that might treat people that you previously thought were untreatable [pause] so I think there is that evangelical side to it [break] it's not going to be a cure-all but I think it's something ... we've spent so many years with nothing [pause] I think people do see it in that evangelical way. (male nurse 6)

> I think you've got to hope you can do something otherwise you're wasting your time [pause] and I mean in the past it was [pause] I don't think anyone knew ... what we were doing ... I think we're still learning about dealing with sex offenders ... and we are still learning ... but there is treatment and you've got the opportunity that you can do something ... otherwise you might as well just incarcerate people. (male nurse 10)

Despite the discursive dominance of talk about SOT at an institutional level, it was reported that a shortage of available places relative to need meant rhetoric differed from lived-experience. It was suggested that commodification of treatment, as package and product, had created an internal market subject to laws of supply and demand:

> but we haven't really got the treatments ... we acknowledge that most of them need to do SOTP ... if not now they need to do ETS [enhanced thinking skills] or other work to prepare them to do SOTP but we haven't had the SOTP courses being run 'cos we haven't had the facilitators ... so they've been identified needs for most of the patients ... but unmet ... because of the service. (female nurse 11)

Nurses commonly portrayed therapy as unwanted and enforced, the principle of choice being usurped by involuntary and indeterminate containment. Patient participation in treatment programmes was, in this sense, interpreted as an instrumental and grudging gesture, motivated by *self-interest* rather than *self-help*:

> the only reason ... the majority of them [pause] attend any of the therapy ... or take on any of the therapy that's offered to them is because it's the only bloody way they'll get out [pause] they know that ... and I hope we know that ... really [pause] so it's not a sort of ... it's not a freedom of choice thing is it? ... It's

> [pause] "you're here … and unless you do something to improve your chances of not offending you'll be here for a very long time". (male nurse 6)

These sentiments formed a part of most nursing accounts, where it was suggested therapy was undertaken only because it earned merit for the patient when being considered for transfer to less secure settings. Staff and patients each talked about attendance at SOT groups as clinical currency that overtly signalled an internal desire to change. Cynicism, though, was not universal and there was shared recognition of institutional impediments to the uptake of offence-specific interventive work, not least the fear of exposure and threat of visibility:

> I'll tell you exactly what the problem with the group work is [pause] sex offenders do not want to go on sex offender treatment programmes because they don't want to be seen to go on the movement … to a group … and to get criticised by others … or seen by others [pause] their fear of a group … work is … hard work to get them to even attend. (female nurse 12)

> You're always in the open … you're open y'know … on movement they go to SOTP they go "Oh he's a nonce … he's a nonce … he's a nonce" [pause] then people start slagging them off … that's what … they're scared … I think a lot of them are scared of going. (patient 9)

Commenting on the admission of sexual offenders for treatment, other nurses echoed the idea of an atypical group of offenders defined by political imperative rather than clinical criteria or diagnostic need. Here, conviction for sexual offences was secondary to indeterminate detention under the Mental Health Act (DoH 1983, 2007). If patient motivation and engagement to participate in SOTP type interventions represented the focus of clinical-management, a legislative expedient of public safety was prioritised in secure-hospital "disposal":

> when people come here legally they're deemed to be having a mental disorder … whether or not … you or me agree with a particular person having that disorder … because there's probably quite a few people in gaol who should be here and vice versa [pause] I think a lot of it's political as well [pause] if someone's … like a recidivist [pause] this is the best place for them legally because it keeps them off the streets indefinitely … because the Mental Health Act's quite a powerful piece of legislation. (male nurse 8)

> and part of the [admission] criteria is that people have to opt in … wanting to come [pause] and of course … that gets trumped when you get a court decision to a hospital … that's regardless of whether they even want it or not. (female nurse 13)

Discussion about the role of the ward-based nurse in relation to specific treatment needs of sexual offenders was riven with tensions around the nature of interventions and relations between nursing and therapy. A composite profile set the men in the unit apart from other offenders convicted of sexual crime. The hospital was described as a facility for atypical individuals marked out from other criminal groups by the degree of deviance that accompanied offences: excessive violence, abuse of the very young and elderly, and gratification through the infliction of pain:

> the extent of the violence … the extent of the stranger violence is markedly different to some other offenders … the multiple … victim groups … multiple age range … the indiscriminate level of the violence … the use of violence before during and after offences [pause] the level of sadism I would say was different … or the level of sexual deviancy would be marked. (female nurse 13)

Patients, likewise, talked about tensions between legal and psychological definitions of sexual-crime expressed in a distinction between sexual *offence* and sexual *motivation*. The aetiology of crime took precedence over offence category in an argument reminiscent of feminist debate about gendered language in criminal justice (Allen 1987) and the concept of "femicide" (Russell and Radford 1992), where sexual murder of women is concealed by the terms "manslaughter" and "homicide". It was proposed that a large number of detained men had avoided confronting their offending behaviour and were under little pressure from clinical teams to engage in treatment. The suggestion that, in the acronym SOT, *sexual offender* should be replaced by *serious offender*, promoted an awareness of sexual violence in terms of culture, language, and power inequities:

> Some people do sadistic torture and sadistic … say murder or taking someone else's life [pause] whether they get … sexually sadistically off on it … makes them a sex offender really [pause] but it's hard to prove whether they've committed … actually … a sexual act … is another thing [break] there's no way that they're trying to push them into dealing with their behaviour and say you need to do SOTP [pause] 'cos they'll say "I never raped anybody … y'know I just slaughtered and tortured somebody" [pause] but … maybe it's a case of they should change SOTP … instead of being sex offenders treatment programme … to serious offenders treatment programme. (patient 9)

Talking about Therapy: A New Way of Speaking, or a New Way of Being?

Though nurses had minimal involvement in delivering SOT, they readily adopted a propagandist and policing function. Commenting on the cost of failure to engage with the treatment ethic, they noted, in stark terms, how the patient was hostage to therapy (Mason and Jennings 1997, Pilgrim 1988a, 1988b). Reminiscent of the search for the soul of the "criminal man" (Sapsford 1981, Foucault 1977), the patient had to do more than fulfil the criteria of a modularized programme, such as demonstrating empathy or identifying risk factors. He had to know himself and share this self-knowledge with others. The reduction of future recidivism required understanding the *archaeology* of offending, accessible through dialogue with the perpetrator; to be heard was to be helped. This message represented induction into secure services – treatment as the "game", adherence as the "rule":

> [Staff from a Regional Secure Unit ask what treatment has been done] and if that's nothing then it's goodbye … we'll come back in five years and have a look at them [pause] and patients know that because obviously we … that's what we instil in them … you're gonna have to look at your offence … you're gonna have to look at who you are. (male nurse 5)

> People need to know what they've come into … but they also need to know the rules of the game to actually get out … and that is one of the rules of the game … to be involved in treatment. (female nurse 13)

Group therapy interactions were described as a double-edged dialogue, where information imparted to the patient was conditional upon confession. Risk-reduction strategies initiated in treatment, it was posited, would continue to be transacted by successive therapeutic agents as their "moral career" (Goffman 1961) continued. Respondents talked about SOT as one component of ongoing intervention that defined a group of men for whom treatment had no end-point. Completing the programme offered a gateway to future movement out of high-secure care, but progress was contingent upon continued surveillance. Unlike physical treatments, completing therapy was not judged in terms of success or failure. Rather, it signalled the engagement of a receptive subject with a wider network of agencies that would orchestrate, scrutinize, and monitor the life of the "dangerous individual" (Foucault 1978). With no date for eligibility to leave the forensic system, and no final destination for the treatment journey, these people, as Menzies (1987) noted, become ensnared within the "gravitational field of the transcarceral network". While there was considerable variance in the extent to which staff invested in the idea that risk factors could be calculated with any degree of actuarial confidence, risk remained an innate quality that defined the being of the disordered offender:

> a ninety odd session programme just … really gets to the point where somebody's comfortable talking about their sexual deviance … that's all it does … after that … and you get a lot of information … and patients get a lot of information … but really … for me the work starts there … after that point. (female nurse 13)

> 'cos that's what we do … I hope so [pause] I hope it [treatment] makes a bit of a difference [pause] and if it doesn't make a difference to the person … it gives us … it gives the nurses … it gives us a clearer picture of what's going on. (male nurse 2)

Talking about the size and complexity of the forensic enterprise, akin to a "web of power" (Thiele 1986, Foucault 1973), one nurse reflected on SOT in absolutist terms. "Risk" was replaced by "chance", and long-term incarceration represented a more realistic option than the "pretence" of rehabilitation. Combining concepts of "quality care" and "life imprisonment" permitted envisaging a form of containment where limited *freedoms* could be granted, without the individual ever being *free*. Other colleagues shared this pessimism in relation to the therapeutic management of sexual offenders:

> well I think it's containment … I don't know if we manage them … or we keep them away from doing those dangerous things again … we risk assess them on the basis that we don't let them do things that might be a danger to a particular target group [break] I think probably if there's a chance of them … of offending it's probably best that they go into some long-term institution that is not about treatment … is not about pretending to treat … but is really about giving them a quality of life [pause] and what I mean by that is lots of freedom … within a perimeter … lots of chances to do things escorted [pause] but with no pretension that there was any chance of them not being a risk to other people. (male nurse 1)

> there's no easy answer to it [pause] I mean there really isn't … I mean build a [pause] if you were to build another ten [name of hospital] to cater for those people that I've just identified it would mean probably locking them up for thirty years … so where do you begin and end with that? I really don't know. (male nurse 17)

For inhabitants of the high-secure hospital system, "community" ceased to exist at all, and a taxonomic ordering of clinical risk was matched by graded tiers of secure provision. It was commonly reported that ambitions to manage people within the lowest level of security deemed appropriate had been sacrificed to a political agenda that prioritised public safety. Comparing detained patients with a prisoner population sentenced for similar offences, one nurse located debate within a human-rights agenda. Admission into a secure hospital represented a miscarriage of justice, masked by diagnostic disposal and medical management:

> it seems to me that there are endless numbers of people who are in prison who escape [name of hospital] and go back out into the community having served their prison sentence and reoffend … and how the authorities cope with that I've really no idea because it's … they end up locking people up here under the guise of treatment for endless numbers of years [break] to some degree I think the people who are here are the unfortunate ones [pause] somewhere along the line the system has decreed that they require treatment at [name of hospital] and the others have managed to get away with it … basically. (male nurse 17)

Commenting on the constant scrutiny and subjective interpretation of inmate behaviour by nurses, one patient discussed the centrality of therapeutic talk in evaluations of risk, with treatment interventions and surveillance mechanisms inextricably linked to notions of *cure* and *control*, and where honesty carried little incentive. The dilemma of truth-telling in therapy suggested a collusive and ritual enactment between nurse and patient, where attendance had greater import than meaningful participation. It implied a Goffmanesque game (e.g., Maynard 1991, Swedberg 2001) was being played, for which there were formal and informal rules, and fair play had a high cost. Within the bureaucratic structure of the hospital, "therapy" represented an administrative exercise that transformed the patient into a commodity. The therapeutic process as change-agent, like feigned patient participation, was dismissed as superficial and fraudulent:

> I've said to them … look I'm struggling with this SOTP … I'm being really honest … I'm telling people that I still get these fantasies [pause] and yet I sit there and I hear other people say 'I don't get that anymore' … and I know they're lying [pause] not everyone might be lying … but a good proportion of them are [my nurse said] it doesn't matter whether you've changed at the end of it [pause] as long as you can tick that box we can then sell you to an RSU [pause] and I really think that is wrong [pause] I do because [pause] I think it's wrong that the system is set up that way. (patient 7)

Compliance with treatment placed a symbolic distance between those colloquially referred to as "treated" and "untreated" sex offenders. The SOT programme emerged as a benchmark of progress. Treatment was about becoming a better person, a living embodiment of the therapeutic being. The rewards of engagement, it was assumed, would encourage others to appreciate the value and tangible benefits of taking part. The process was likened to a spiritual experience – an awakening, to see the light and crawl from the shadows. The metaphor of salvation emerged during interviews, where a changed attitude toward treatment was equated with changed personae. This was nicely illustrated in the description of a patient, who, in his denial and rejection, was characterised as macho, spirited, and rebellious. The entry of this recalcitrant man into treatment, described as part maturation and part mystical, signalled more than compliance. It constructed a transformative and cathartic experience, of being re-birthed in the baptismal font of therapy, precipitating a journey from ignorance to self-awareness and knowledge:

> well I'm working with somebody at the moment that for many years went through [name of hospital] as … denying … I mean he is a sex offender he's raped two women and for many years he sort of denied this … denied that he had any problems within that area … wouldn't get involved in any therapy … tended to be a bit of a jack the lad and being with the patients round the hospital who are perhaps a little bit notorious [break] maybe suddenly one day they're ready for treatment … he agreed to do the sex offender treatment programme … did it … and did absolutely fantastic on it and is now [pause] ready to go out … and is a changed lad [pause] totally changed … matured … quite aware of his

> problems … why he committed offences … what triggers could affect him in the future. (male nurse 3)

Success was measured in terms of the ability to articulate an offender identity and the "triggers" to future risk. Other respondents, though, would proffer a more cynical interpretation of such performance rituals. If life inside without faith in therapy was bleak, it could also be long, and another nurse punctuated this interpretation with anecdotal evidence that was salutary and sad:

> and so they slowly but surely come out of the woodwork and start to attend the groups … but there's some that adamantly will not … in fact I know one sex offender here who spent thirty years here because he was not going to address his offending behaviour [pause] and thirty years later … eventually [pause] attended the group … and has moved on. (female nurse 12)

Self-report as a component of risk assessment was deemed unreliable owing to the possibility that patients learned a *new way of speaking* rather than a *new way of being*. The therapeutic process here resembled an organisational charade, or "no-win" situation, where the game was rigged. Adherence to the rules (accepting therapy) confirmed the diagnostic symptomatology of devious and untrustworthy "psychopaths", while rejection of the rules (declining therapy) invited other forms of negative attribution, conjuring up the image of service-*losers* rather than service-*users*:

> they play the therapeutic game … it's not the content [pause] it's the "I've done this therapy now … so I move on now" … and we have patients on this ward who have done that … and they're involved in the therapeutic jargon [pause] rather than "well I've learned from it" … it's "I have done that … so I can move on now" [pause] yeah and that's … they're playing the therapeutic game. (male nurse 10)

> they're told they're psychopathic [pause] if they play the game … engage in therapy they're said to be manipulative [pause] if they don't engage and take therapy they're said to be deviant [pause] and that's of course if there's any therapy available … because we're told we're excellent at providing therapy … but if I was a patient here I'd be completely pissed off. (male nurse 1)

Talking about the "thrill" of sexual offending that persisted long after the offence, one patient recalled the experience of undertaking SOT "fantasy work", with programme integrity premised on the disclosure of thought patterns seen to promote sexually abusive behaviours. He questioned, though, claims by other group members that they had actually exorcised high-risk cognitions. Similarly, a nurse noted that "fantasy" existed only as a part of the offender-patient's internal world, and modification of the imaginary was dismissed as unthinkable, unworkable, and fundamentally flawed:

> they sit there and they say "don't fantasise about anything like that anymore" [pause] I sit there and I think you lying bastard [laughs] I do … I never say it … because it would be controversial and it would be against the group ethics [pause] but I do sit there … and I think you lying fucker … you're trying to pull the wool over people's eyes. (patient 7)

> you can't measure it … it's self-reported and who in their right minds … if they know they're never going to get out the front gate if they're still having the fantasy about rape [pause] "I'm still having that fantasy" … they're going to come up and go "well I've sorted that … it worked … thank you". (male nurse 6)

It was not unusual for patients to retell stories from the perspective of another person by using reported speech. Critically attacking SOT, one man augmented personal reservations about therapy with alleged experiences of a fellow inmate. He suggested those undergoing treatment mobilized different discourses according to context. Though keen to stress no therapeutic boundaries had been violated, "disclosure" appeared to have an equivalent, unofficial version, with offence-specific details being shared amongst patients on the wards. One unnamed individual emerged as a skilled and intelligent performer, graduating the programme with merit. At the same time as winning support and approval from facilitators, it was intimated he had outsmarted them:

> he went on the SOTP [pause] now he's kept the confidence of the group … he hasn't told me about the group … but what he's told me is about himself [pause] I've read his papers so I know his history … I know all his rapes … all the gory details [pause] this guy … is so fuckin' angry … he's clever too … he went in there … he became at the end of the SOTP the star patient [pause] "look what we've done for him … look how well he's done" [pause] he said to me "I could go out tomorrow cut their fuckin throats and hack the fuckin' heads off these motherfuckers … who've tortured my fuckin' mind with this sick fuckin' … rape therapy thing" [pause] he said "I've learned more over there about fuckin' sexual offending than I even knew before I went in". (patient 3)

Nurses identified therapeutic talk as an important way of demonstrating reduced risk, but this account indicted the process as dangerous farce – a game played, and a role adopted to project appropriate responses. Veneers of transformation masked a rehabilitative success story, with the hostile rebuke of "rape therapy" as "torture". Rather than equip offenders with knowledge or skills to prevent recidivism, it was suggested the experience refined offence techniques; new or novel acts of abuse were shared among group members. This reported discussion might never have happened, or represent a selective re-telling of events, but the emergent discourse evidenced a casual, aggressive language to communicate aspects of offending behaviour:

> I said "tell me" [pause] so he did … he was giving me a few scenarios … tie up's and whatever … and he'd not thought of that [pause] I said "you're kidding?" he said "oh no … that's the trouble … they're fuckin' gross" he said "really gross" he said "and I wouldn't mind trying it out" [pause] I said "you're kidding me?" he said "well" he said "put it this way … I don't want to" he said "but now it's in me head I'm not so sure I can handle it". (patient 3)

Talking About the Sexual Self: "Normal Men" and "Dangerous Others"

If the physical act of attending a treatment group could be stress provoking, the spectacle of therapy and the ritual performance of disclosure amplified the level of potential risk for patients, where there could be no hiding place from the clinical gaze. One nurse described the experience of facilitating SOT in terms of the demands it placed on group members; each word was discussed and dissected under the technological lens of camera conditions; the patient was stripped of defences and revealed before their peers; every utterance and gesture was recorded, and replayed, as the property of the group. It was contended that there was a powerful incentive to conceal aspects of the self that could attract shame and stigma, particularly as sexual offenders rated low in the institutional pecking order of inmate status:

> and to do that under camera conditions in a very tight environment … where people are going to be talking about it … where other people are going to hear … other patients are going to hear … it's a very difficult thing to ask people to do [pause] and I guess patients may not be able to articulate that … but they'd certainly understand it [pause] and there are consequences for them being … labelled as a sex offender … 'cos it's still pejorative … as a nonce and so on. (female nurse 13)

Fear and emotional cost were less common themes that related to male nurses distancing themselves from SOT work. First was a concern about the inescapable emotional penalty of prolonged exposure to the *offensive* details of *offending* behaviour:

> Right but can they cope with the information they're getting? 'Cos it's hard isn't it? I've watched … as I say I've probably seen a bit more SOTP than I like to let on being honest and I've … the hot chair etc. … and lads … and all that … and I think if you're facilitating that day in, day out and reflecting on it … feedback … you take it home … don't care what anyone says … you take the job home … can they handle that? (male nurse 16)

This nurse also questioned the motivation to undertake the SOTP, locating discussion in hypothetical qualities of a *normal individual* with a *normal job.*

Contact with an unpopular and outcast group was described as shameful and contaminating in comparison with honest labour, the implication being that those who elected to engage were themselves of dubious character:

> Do they feel like they can help? Or do they enjoy it? 'Cos what average man … there's a stereotype bloke isn't there? Works on a building site … does whatever … talks to you in a pub and you say "What do you do for a job?" "Building site" … whatever … you say "Oh I work with sex offenders" [pause] A normal man's instinct … I say "normal" loosely … a normal man's instinct … wouldn't it? It'd be "Why the fuck do you work with them?" (male nurse 16)

The account paralleled that of a patient who suggested that, beyond monetary payment for the job, some nursing staff derived prurient pleasure from the opportunity to spend time with incarcerated offenders:

> these people [nurses] I've come to learn … actually enjoy people killing because if I hadn't killed they would not be in a fucking job for Christ's sake [pause] they almost come off on it … some of them … talking to them [pause] and it makes me sick. (patient 3)

Reflections on the relationship between sexual-self and offence-focused therapy embroiled the personal and professional lives of male nurses in a way that generated threat and fear, making it equally challenging for facilitators and patients alike. The patient could not be, or was reluctant to be, honest in his disclosures because this could result in prolonged detention. Likewise, the honesty of staff about feelings or fantasy could be compromised in an institutional setting where suspicions of blurred boundaries could be perceived as an error of clinical/custodial judgement. Given that the format of treatment was premised on an ideological difference between two sets of men, representing the "normal" and the "deviant", there could be no overt recognition that their respective sexualities (women were excluded) might overlap (Mercer 2013b):

> I'm not going to go into my sexual fantasies … but I'd like to think they're fairly normal … I mean this is one of the things I noticed about [pause] sex offender therapy is talking with … certainly [pause] again it's like the sort of demonising normal behaviour [pause] if you're involved in it [pause] from a sort of staff point of view [pause] nobody is going to admit in public … as a member of staff … . that "I had the same fantasy the other night as he's just described … 'cos he's an offender" [pause] if I was sat there … as a patient was describing some sexual fantasy about a young girl … we're not gonna go "Oh I've had the odd one like that … I was fantasising about this fourteen-year-old". (male nurse 6)

Another nurse explained his refusal to engage in SOT in terms of fear, exposure, and the danger of self-knowledge. Types of offending defined deviant categories, such as "paedophile", constructed the "other" as an outsider and threat. For these nurses, the cultural iconography of a sexually precocious child-woman (Kincaid 1998, 1994) became problematic only to the extent that it invited a connection between the average man and the convicted sexual predator:

> I am sometimes scared that you might see something in other offences that … now I don't mean obviously … about kids … young y'know and that … but sometimes I've been over to them [therapy group] like and a fella's talking about like older schoolgirls like [pause] I'm a man … you go past a school sometimes … so there's a bit of that as well … I don't want … I don't like … I wouldn't like to [pause] see something. (male nurse 16)

Concluding Remarks

The findings and ideas reported in this chapter represent an alternative account of sex-offender treatment to the dominant discourse of forensic psychiatry and much behavioural science research. Clinicians clearly recognize the merit of qualitative inquiry in this sphere of practice (e.g., Clarke et al. 2013), but the focus is driven by a need to evaluate service provision and support organizational goals. The approach adopted in the previous discussion is about more than interviewing patients regarding their experiences of therapy. It has attempted to situate language in the cultural context where therapy is transacted, and understand talk as collective, constructive, and functional. Patients and nurses spend the greater part of their time together, and their interactional speech textures a shared social space. Typically, their voices are unheard by the wider professional academic community and, in this sense, critical research is not only illuminating but potentially empowering.

References

Allen, H. 1987. *Justice Unbalanced: Gender, Psychiatry and Judicial Decisions*. Milton Keynes: Open University Press.

Auburn, T. 2005. Narrative reflexivity as a repair device for discounting 'cognitive distortions' in sex offender treatment. *Discourse and Society*, *16*(5), 697–718.

Blom-Cooper, L., Brown, M., Dolan, R., and Murphy, E. 1992. *Report of the Committee of Inquiry into Complaints about Ashworth Hospital*. Cm 2028. London: HMSO.

Bluglass, R. 1992. The special hospitals should be closed. *British Medical Journal*, *305*, 323–324.

Brookes, M. 2010. Supporting uniformed officers delivering therapy within a prison therapeutic community for sexual offenders. *Mental Health Review Journal*, *15*(4), 40–45.

Burrow, S. 1991. The special hospital nurse and the dilemma of therapeutic custody. *Journal of Advances in Health and Nursing Care, 1*(3), 21–38.

Clarke, C., Tapp, J., Lord, A., and Moore, E. 2013. Group-work for offender patients on sex offending in a high security hospital: Investigating aspects of impact via qualitative analysis. *The Journal of Sexual Aggression*, *19*(1), 50–65.

Cohen, D. 1981. *Broadmoor*. London: Psychology News Press.

Cowburn, M. and Pringle, K. 2000. *Pornography and men's practices*. The Journal of Sexual Aggression, *6*(1/2), 52–66.

Department of Health. 2007. *The Mental Health Act*. London: DoH.

Fairclough, N. 1992. *Discourse and social change*. Cambridge: Polity Press.

Fairclough, N. 1989. *Language and power*, 2nd edition. London: Longman.

Fallon, P., Bluglass, R., Edwards, B. and Daniels, G. 1999. *Report of the Committee of Inquiry into the Personality Disorder Unit, Ashworth Special Hospital* . Cm 4194. London: HMSO.

Foucault, M. 1973. *The Birth of the Clinic: An Archaeology of Medical Perception*. London: Tavistock.

Foucault, M. 1977. *Discipline and Punish*. London: Penguin.

Foucault, M. 1978. About the concept of the 'dangerous individual' in nineteenth century legal psychiatry. *International Journal of Law and Psychiatry*, *1*, 1–18.

Foucault, M. 1988. The dangerous individual. In L.D. Kritzman (Ed.). *Michel Foucault: Policy, Philosophy, Culture*. New York: Routledge.

Goffman, E. 1963. *Stigma: Notes on the Management of the Spoiled Identity*. Harmondsworth: Penguin.

Goffman, E. 1961. *Asylums: Essays on the Social Situation of Mental Patients and other Inmates*. Harmondsworth: Penguin.

Holmes, D. 2002. Police and pastoral power: Governmentality and correctional forensic psychiatric nursing. *Nursing Inquiry*, *9*, 84–92.

Kincaid, J.R. 1998. *Erotic Innocence: The Culture of Child Molesting*. London: Duke.

Kincaid, J.R. 1994. *Child Loving: The Erotic Child and Victorian Culture*. London: Routledge.

Kvale, S. 1996. *Inter-views: An Introduction to Qualitative Research Interviewing*. London: Sage.

Mandeville-Norden, R., Beech, A. and Hayes, E. 2008. Examining the effectiveness of a UK community- based sexual offender treatment programme for child abusers. *Psychology, Crime and Law*, *14*(6), 498–512.

Marques, J.K., Wiederanders, M., Day, D.M., Nelson, C. and van Ommeren, A. 2005. Effects of a relapse prevention program on sexual recidivism: Final results from California's Sex Offender Treatment and Evaluation Project (SOTEP). *Sexual Abuse: A Journal of Research and Treatment*, *17*(1), 79–107.

Marshall, W.L., Ward, T., Mann, R.E., Moulden, H., Fernandez, Y.M., Serran, G. and Marshall, L.E. 2005. Working positively with sexual offenders: Maximising the effectiveness of treatment. *Journal of Interpersonal Violence*, *20*(9), 1096–1114.

Mason, T. and Jennings, L. 1997. The Mental Health Act and professional hostage taking. *Journal of Medicine, Science and the Law*, *37*(1), 58–68.

Maynard, D.W. 1991. Goffman, Garfinkel and games. *Sociological theory*, *9*(2), 277–279.

McCallum, D. Mental health, criminality and the human sciences. In A. Peterson and R. Bunton (Eds). *Foucault, Health and Medicine*. London: Routledge.

Menzies, R. 1987. Cycles of control: The transcarceral careers of forensic patients. *International Journal of Law and Psychiatry*, *19*(3), 233–249.

Mercer, D. 2010. *A discourse analysis of staff and patient accounts of pornography in a high-security hospital*. University of Liverpool [unpublished PhD thesis].

Mercer, D. 2013a. Girly mags and girly jobs: Pornography and gendered inequality in forensic practice. *International Journal of Mental Health Nursing*, *22*, 15–23.

Mercer, D. 2013b. Theorising sexual media and sexual violence in a forensic setting: Men's talk about pornography and offending. *The International Journal of Law and Psychiatry* [in press].

Perron, A., Fluet, C., and Holmes, D. 2005. Agents of care and agents of the state: Bio-power and nursing practice. *Journal of Advanced Nursing*, *50*(5), 536–544.

Pilgrim, D. 1988a. Psychotherapy in British special hospitals: A case of failure to thrive. *Free Associations*, *11*, 58–72.

Pilgrim, D. 1988b. Hospitals-cum-prisons: British special hospitals. In S. Ramon and G. Giannichedda (Eds). *Psychiatry in Transition: The British and Italian Experiences*. London: Pluto Press.

Pilgrim, D. (ed.) 2007. *Inside Ashworth: Professional Reflections of Institutional Life*. Oxford: Radcliffe.

Potter, J. and Wetherell, M. 1987. *Discourse and Social Psychology: Beyond Attitudes and Behaviour*. London: Sage.

Radford, J. and Russell, D.E.H. 1992. *Femicide: The politics of Woman Killing*. Milton Keynes: Open University Press.

Sapsford, R.J. 1981. Individual deviance: The search for the criminal personality. In: In M., Fitzgerald, G., McLennan and J., Pawson (Eds). *Crime and Society: Readings in History and Theory*. London: Routledge & Kegan Paul.

Swedberg, R. 2001. Sociology and game theory: Contemporary and historical perspectives. *Theory and Society*, *30*(3), 301–335.

Thiele, L.P. 1986. Foucault's triple murder and the modern development of power. *Canadian Journal of Political Science*, *19*(2), 243–260.

Quinsey, V.L. 1999. Report of the committee of inquiry into the personality disorder unit, Ashworth special hospital, Vol. 1, *The Journal of Forensic Psychiatry*, *10*(3), 635–648.

Wakeling, H., Beech, A.R., and Freemantle, N. 2013. Investigating treatment change and its relationship to recidivism in a sample of 3773 sex offenders in the UK. *Psychology, Crime and Law*, *19*(3), 233–252.

Chapter 15

Shock Therapies as Intensification of the War against Madness in Hamburg, Germany: 1930–1943[1]

Thomas Foth

Introduction

In May 1937, the international conference of the Swiss Psychiatric Association in Münsingen was devoted to *The Treatment of Schizophrenia: Insulin Shock, Cardiazol, Sleep Treatment*. The founder of the hypoglycemic insulin convulsant therapy of schizophrenia, Manfred Sakel, described the interplay between epileptic seizures and hypoglycemic coma. "The epileptic attack is the artillery [and] the hypoglycemia is the infantry in the battle against the disease. According to military theory, the artillery never conquers and occupies hostile territory. It can only open the way for the infantry." As he continued,

> the artillery might be able to create a breach in the walls of the city. However, at this stage, the battle is not finished. The city must still be occupied and pacified. The besieging troops must penetrate the city and must establish an intelligent and coordinated system of occupation that assures the return to the normal. The restoration of normality needs very subtle means able to reach the damaged parts and the finest mental processes in order to restore larger clarity in the mental and emotional spheres. (Sakel 1938: 25)

The military vocabulary used by the Jewish Austrian-born Sakel was a precise description of the rationale behind the deployment of shock treatments in psychiatry. As I argue below, shock therapies incorporated the strategic power field of psychiatric practice and were used as an effective tool to implement the will of psychiatrists and nurses deep into the core of the patient. In an attempt to decipher this rationale, I use the notes of psychiatrists, and particularly of nurses, that were kept on Anna Maria Buller, who was admitted to both the Langenhorn and Friedrichsberg asylums in Germany between 1931 and 1943. This one specific patient record, used as a kind of "microstorie [sic]," highlights the fact that shock therapies were used more or less randomly by asylum staff as a means

1 First published in the *Canadian Bulletin of Medical History*. Used with permission.

of disciplining this patient's behavior (for the use of "microstorie" for a history of psychiatry and more specifically for a history of psychiatric nursing, see for example: Huisman 2005: 405–423).

In an attempt to contextualize German psychiatric practices, this chapter will also touch on international discussions among psychiatrists that took place during the 1930s and 40s on how these therapies were presumed to operate. Although Buller was in these asylums over the period of the Nazi regime, and without denying or downplaying cruelties committed during the Nazi era, I contend, along with some historians writing currently in the field, that German psychiatric practice demonstrates more continuity than discontinuity from the First World War into the post-Second World War era. Conventionally, historians writing after the Second World War have subdivided the history of German psychiatry into three fairly distinct stages, paralleling German political history (regarding the periodization of German psychiatry: Roelcke 2002). Written for the most part by psychiatrists themselves, this traditional historiography was an attempt to create a respectable self-image by distancing themselves from their past and presenting the Nazi era as exceptional and German psychiatry as the victim of political circumstances. The first decades after 1900 were characterized by the development of an academic psychiatric discipline and the development of nosology, classification, and neuropathology based on the work of Emil Kraepelin or Alois Alzheimer. The advent of Nazi rule marked the beginning of the second phase, which lasted from 1933 to 1945, when psychiatrists were purportedly forced to adhere to Nazi racial ideologies. The third stage that began after the Second World War was characterized "by a slow but more or less successful 'normalization' of German psychiatry," (Roelcke 2005: 162) and German psychiatrists adjusted to international developments in psychiatry.

This compartmentalization of the German history of psychiatry began to be contradicted by historian Klaus Dörner as early as the 1970s when he points to the continuities in mental health care, and particularly the treatment of chronic patients, since the 1920s (Dörner 1967, 1984). Historian Heinz Faulstich's work points out that psychiatric patients had been killed both before and after the Nazi regime (Faulstich 1998). Newer research on the history of military psychiatry in Germany highlights that the treatment of "war neurotics" arose during and after the First World War (Kaufmann 1999), and heralded the era of "heroic therapies," where psychiatrists began to search for therapeutic success regardless of the risk that these treatments posed for patients or how much they exposed them to pain or fear (Quinkert, Rauh, and Winkler 2010, Allard 2012). And preliminary results from my research at a Toronto Hospital (Canada) suggest that shock treatments and other chemical and physical measures employed there in the 1930s and 1940s were not that different from those given in German psychiatric asylums. Some nursing practices at the Toronto hospital, and especially the way that nurses perceived their patients, also appear to be comparable to German nursing practices of the same time period.

While my research perspective is much more aligned with that of this new generation of historians of German psychiatry, I assert, nevertheless, that even these newer approaches are not far reaching enough. Although historian Volker Roelcke, for example, suggests that the interests of the profession drove the development of German psychiatry, his focus remains on reasons exterior to psychiatric practice and to psychiatric knowledge as such. In contrast, this chapter is based on Michel Foucault's work, which argues that psychiatry at its very core is a discriminatory practice, and that the Nazi exclusionary practices were extreme variants of scientific, social, and political exclusionary practices that were already in place (Foucault 1973, 1999). German psychiatrists, whether before or after the extremes of the Nazi era, were following a rationality that was part and parcel of psychiatric practice (termed a practice by Foucault and not a discourse because the asylum cannot be understood by scientific discourses alone). As Foucault notes, these exclusionary practices are necessarily bound to symbolic and physical violence, which begins with the differentiation between those considered "normal" and those defined as abnormal, and the definition of madness as the absolute 'other' of reason (Foucault 1999). Once these distinctions were in place, lunatics could easily be identified without any doubts by psychiatric experts because of their difference, even if the causes of their lunacy could not always be determined. When the theory of degeneration allowed psychiatrists to link deviant behavior with theory, and when the idea that the degenerated person was abnormal became the foundation of biological psychiatry, psychiatry was able to extend its power beyond its traditional focus on curing (Foucault 1997). The idea of incurability had formerly represented a kind of psychiatric horizon, since it defined the effective limits of treatment for diseases that had been perceived as essentially curable. However, from this moment on, madness appeared to be more the technology of the abnormal, and when that status of abnormality was fixed by heredity onto the individual, the project of curing no longer made any sense. Foucault also argued that as the pathological content of the psychiatric domain disappeared, so too did the therapeutic dimension of psychiatry (Foucault 1999). The German psychiatrist Kankeleit made this correlation visible in 1925 when he argued that, although it would be easier and less expensive to "re-integrate the inferiors as viable members into society," the power of psychiatry was insufficient to achieve this goal: "however successful the care, it can only reform but it can never transform inferiors into normal humans" (Kankeleit 1925: 25).

If the insane could not be cured but only influenced by the rationality of psychiatry, then, Foucault argues, psychiatric practices could best be described as disciplinary, aiming to influence the conduct of the patient and based on a power structure that hierarchically placed the psychiatrist at the top. Admission to the asylum was a demonstration of the medical power that ruled the asylum, conveying to patients that they had entered a specific space where the distribution of power had nothing in common with the "ordinary world" (Foucault 2003). Using a Foucauldian discourse analysis approach to history thus enables one to analyze this very specific distribution of power and the way psychiatrists conceptualized their interventions, in this case, shock treatments. The underlying question is to analyze how humans govern themselves and others through the production of a specific truth (Foucault 2007). This kind of historical analysis can help to decipher the ways in which certain practices are justified as well as the intentions and evidences of these practices.

Psychiatric Practice

To analyze the strategic power field of psychiatric practice means grasping the intricate connections between a myriad of "technologies of power" that are directed onto the bodies of patients and are aimed at profoundly transforming them. Technology approaches the forces of the body and the aptitudes and capabilities of individuals in order to shape their behavior (Dean 1996). It is invested with a strategic rationality that seeks to subsume the patient's conduct to the requirements of psychiatry, to introduce the will of the psychiatrist into the patient's core.

The asylum can thus be perceived as a kind of machine and psychiatric practice as a complex interplay between discourses, technologies, architecture, and institutions—in other words, a *dispositif* (Deleuze 1989). German psychiatrist, Carl Schneider, best described it in the 1930s as, to "biologically influence sick persons" a strategic interplay of different psychiatric interventions is necessary. Work therapy is only one component and must be combined with other biological treatments such as shock treatments. Schneider emphasized that these different interventions were mechanisms aimed to "make the sick persons realize the superiority of the healthy [i.e psychiatrists and nurses], [their] greater quick-wittedness, greater flexibility and [their] greater cautiousness." In order to achieve this goal, Schneider emphasized that it was necessary to

> carefully block every possibility to withdraw. Partly as a matter of fact (by locking the doors of sick persons who want to get out of their rooms), and partly through figurative indications or through orders to the personal to shut down possibilities that would enable the sick person to draw back into his symptoms. If necessary everything the sick person does or how he behaves must be regulated through the constraint of being always observed, accompanied and being subjected to the healthy. (Schneider 1939. This book was considered ground breaking and influenced psychiatric theory even after the end of the Nazi regime.)

Schneider called this strategy a "psychological pair of tongs" and emphasized that "many persons are needed in order to regularly affect the sick person." These persons [psychiatrists and nurses] must pursue the same goal: "to fight against a symptom, to achieve certain indoctrination, or to force the sick person to make a specific decision" (Schneider 1939: 160).

The psychiatrist attempted to transform all parts of the asylum into a therapeutic apparatus solely through his presence; he made rounds through all departments every morning in order to transform discipline into therapy, to control all the small wheels of the system, to inspect all disciplinary mechanisms. According to Eugen Bleuler, an influential Swiss psychiatrist who introduced the concept of schizophrenia at the beginning of the twentieth century, the physical appearance of the psychiatrist alone should be sufficient to convince the patient that any resistance to the asylum was futile. As he stated: "One cannot forget that it is very rare to persuade the sick person to back down through logic itself, but rather through the appearance of the one who applies the logic" (Bleuler 1923: 163, 1943).

Since the asylum itself could be understood metaphorically as the body of the psychiatrist, with every part of the asylum and everyone working within the asylum functioning as an extension or part of his body (Foucault 2003), the "logic" of the asylum writ large was physically imposed on the patient, hinting at the rationale behind psychiatric practice. Psychiatric practice was never founded on scientific discourses but was based more on the play of this disciplinary power, what historian Jean-Noël Missa calls the "therapeutic empiricism" of psychiatry (Missa 2006). The psychiatrist can only take on the role of doctor if the patient demonstrates symptoms of a recognized illness, and only transforms from jailer to physician when the patient plays out the symptoms of a mental illness. This aspect was a crucial part of the admission ritual that aimed to provoke a situation in which patients could not avoid acknowledging their madness. Admitting madness meant that patients also admitted that they were actually ill, in need of a physician and of being interned, and that they were the kind of patients for whom psychiatric asylums were built. Foucault calls this moment the "double enthronement" (*double intronisation*), when the interned individual was "enthroned" as a sick person, while the interning individual was "enthroned" as psychiatrist and physician. This is also the reason why psychiatrists regularly carried out interviews with patients to interrogate them about events recorded in their medical chart. Only if patients were able to recognize themselves in the written case history of the record was there a chance of being released and being considered "cured" or in "remission." The desire to find a way out of madness implied acknowledging this medical power as all powerful, renouncing the omnipotence of madness, and accepting the documentary-biographical identity.

This strategic power imbalance erected one kind of a reality within the asylum, but caused an endless battle with patients because it had nothing in common with their reality. The insurmountable, disciplinary power of psychiatry confronted the "absolute" power of the insane—absolute because patients tried to force their own reality onto their surroundings by, for example, claiming that "somebody is talking to me." By imposing their own "rules," patients attempted to oppose the "reality of the asylum." Bleuler described the negativistic logic of the "sick person":

> When the sick persons ought to get up, they want to stay in bed; if they ought to stay in bed, they want to get up. They neither want to dress nor do they want to undress, whether or not they are complying with an order or doing this according to the asylum's rules. They either refuse to come to eat, or else refuse to leave the table; if they can do all these actions beyond the desired time or if they can somehow do it against the will of those surrounding them, they will do it. They

> will not use the toilet spontaneously if they are accompanied there, they withhold their excrement in order later to soil their beds or their clothes. They eat soup with a fork or with a dessert spoon, the dessert with a tablespoon. Many resist with might and main (*Leibeskräften*) against any influences, often with agitated insulting and swiping … It can develop into a real harassment (*Chicanose*), into an active desire to always in a provocative manner annoy those surrounding them. (Bleuler 1923: 312)

The only possibility of influencing madness was through "purposeful education," especially for people considered to be chronic who were "for the most part to be trained to normal behavior and work." Nurses had a specific part to play in this education. As the delegated representatives of the psychiatrist's power, nurses were strategically positioned "beneath" the patient, because only from this position was it possible for them to understand the patient in every detail and to influence his or her behavior in depth. German psychiatric nurse Heinrich Becker specified that the function of nursing was "to find out in all patients how they are best to be influenced." But in order to be able to do so, the nurse had to "try to infiltrate the trains of thoughts or peculiarities of the sick persons, and when he succeeds, to act out of this knowledge" (Becker 1936: 117). The following analysis highlights the strategic interplay between different actors and the specific rationale behind the use of shock treatments in the case of Anna Maria Buller.

Anna Maria Buller

Eighteen-year-old Anna Maria Buller was first admitted to the psychiatric hospital in Friedrichberg, Germany, in 1931. Although originally admitted to the general hospital on a suspected diagnosis of influenza, she was transferred to Friedrichsberg within the first week because her behavior was classified as "abnormal." Apart from short stays in her parental home, she spent the rest of her life, until 1943, between Friedrichsberg and the other nearby asylum of Langenhorn. Her diagnosis during her admissions swung among schizophrenia, amentia, dementia praecox, and feeblemindness. Any and every available medication and shock therapy was tested on her Cardiazol, Insulin, Eugenozym (an unlicensed medication) combined with Digitalis, Morphium-Scopolamine, and Paraldehyde, and she endured continuous baths, isolation, and forced bed rest, among other "treatments." She was sent on 25 June 1943 to Hadamar. Although Hadamar had been a gassing facility for so-called euthanasia killings between 1940 and 1941, patients admitted after those years continued to die there through starvation, medication, and neglect. Anna Maria died there eleven days after she was admitted.

Buller's medical record comprises more than 200 pages of primarily nursing and physician notes. Her record was chosen because she had a very long "asylum biography" that started before the Nazi regime and ended in the gas chamber at Hadamar, covering more than ten years (1931–1943). This record therefore enables me to compare the nurses' notes from before the time the Nazis came to power with the notes taken during World War Two, and to determine similarities and differences in the nurses' and psychiatrists' perception of Anna Maria Buller. This kind of micro-research allows for a kind of "debunking" because it challenges the "history of ideas and institutions," and is "an important correction to the 'Big Picture' history of psychiatry" (Huisman 2005: 411).

The notes in Buller's record document an escalating fight over the course of her admissions between the professional staff and her madness. The nurses' notes appeared to detail Buller's "education," because every time she behaved in a way deemed illegitimate, the nurses intervened with a whole range of disciplinary measures that became more and more severe. On her first admission in 1931, nurses focused on detailed descriptions of Buller's behavior that they attempted to "correct" through forced bed rest and the application of the sedative Paraldehyde. Her behavior, however, became more unpredictable. On 13 April 1931, one nurse wrote:

> 13.4.: Pat. jumped out of bed at 1.00 a.m., ran to the door noisily and screamed. When pat. was taken back to bed she insulted the nurse saying: "bitch with the red cross, you Satan." Pat. spat at the nurse, scratched her and tried to bite her. Pat. was very resistant. After the injection, the patient got up again, went to the bathroom, said then, "Oh I feel so sick to my stomach." Lay down flat on the floor, was persuaded to get up, went to the dormitory and lay down in patient Kuscher's bed, propped herself up with both feet against the bed, so that it was very difficult to get her out. At 2:00 a.m. patient fell asleep again. This disruption woke up all the other patients (Wa.). (PR, FMR, PN)

The nurses' reactions to this unpredictability and perceived dangerousness escalated over the following years, and they began to administer continuous baths (often over periods of whole days), inject her with Morphine-Scopolamine, confine her to an isolation cell, apply cold wet sheet packs, and administer shock treatments. The record reads like a continuous struggle in the "war against madness" and with every admission to the psychiatric hospital the range of disciplinary means used on Buller was gradually broadened. Nurses had a decisive function in this war, because not only did they command most of these disciplinary means but their descriptions of Anna Maria Buller in her medical record also determined how she was perceived and how her prognosis would evolve.

Before her death in 1941, however, her therapy had taken a radical twist. To begin with, her diagnoses changed dramatically from schizophrenia, which carried hope for amelioration, to "dementia praecox," which implied an escalating process of stupefaction with no possible cure, through to "schizophrenic final state." The record contains the medication plan kept by the nurses in order to record the multiple Morphine-Scopolamine injections and the Paraldehyde that she was receiving. However, on her final admission in 1940, she started receiving a new drug, Cardiazol (or Metrazol), that she had never received before. Furthermore, the Cardiazol treatment was combined with an "Insulin deep coma" therapy.

According to procedures in the asylum in Friedrichsberg, Cardiazol treatment, which was meant to induce seizures in patients, was to follow a precise scheme of two shocks per week at intervals of two to three days (Widenmeyer 1937). Buller's Cardiazol injections started on 26 April 1940 with the usual dose for women, but the psychiatrists considered this treatment ineffective and the injections were repeated one day later with a slightly larger amount, eventually leading to a seizure. From then on, the nurses reported only from time to time on Buller's Cardiazol injections, and the psychiatrist did not mention them again until 12 June, more than two months after they began. In Buller's case, however, the medication plan shows that no regular schedule was employed. She received these injections on an irregular basis; in June, for example, she was given seven while in July, she received none. The Cardiazol injections were combined with insulin injections from 6 May to 16 May 1940. Nowhere in the record were the Cardiazol injections defined as a "therapy," whereas the insulin injections explicitly were.

Comparing the medication plan with the nurses' notes and the descriptions of Anna Maria Buller's behavior, it is clear that the Cardiazol injections were used as a disciplinary measure against what the nurses (and through them, the physicians) deemed bad behavior. On 29 October 1940, the nurses wrote:

29.10.	Pat. [patient] is very inhibited, stands around and must be urged to eat. Nurse Olga
	Pat. was very blocked. In the evening beat another patient with her slipper. Cried a little. Got Paral [dehyde].
Night	Restless, often out of bed, disturbs other sick persons, pinched them. (Inj.) [Morphine Scopolamine]
31.10.	Pat. was restless in the morning, ran around crying, got Cardiazol +, became quiet afterwards. [Nurse Olga (PR, FMR, PN)]

Between 24 and 28 November, Buller received both Paraldehyde and Cardiazol at least once and was also strapped to the bed several times for her restlessness. The entry on the afternoon of 28 November demonstrated well the aim of "treatment" and the type of behavior that the nurses desired. During the periods that Anna Maria seemed to "behave well," according to the nurses' perceptions, she received no Cardiazol injections. Cardiazol was only applied when nurses and psychiatrists estimated her behavior to be disruptive.

Night	
25.11.	Pat. [patient] stood always in front of the window, slept after she received Paral [Paraldehyd]. Pat. ran around sobbing, came into the belt. Nurse Olga
26.11.	Pat. got Cardiazol. Was very restless, always out of the bed, talked quietly to herself.
Aftern.	The same
27.11.	Pat. was very restless, was put into the belt.

Aftern.	Pat. was very excited during visiting hours, transferred to ward #13. Nurse Lotte
28.11.	Pat. got Cardiazol, very restless.
Aftern.	The same Nurse Senta
Aftern.	Pat. nice and orderly, [did] housework, [laughed] and [answered] questions. Nurse Senta
Morn:	Pat. helps with sewing.
30.11.	Pat. was nice and friendly. [Nurse Senta (PR, FMR, PN)]

By January 1941, Buller had received Cardiazol injections, however irregularly, for nearly one year. Within a psychiatric dispositive, even medications that were initially prescribed according to a certain conception of the etiology of mental illness or its organic correlations were re-utilized in a directive system. As one psychiatrist reported, a "young schizophrenic male patient" had been "threatened by his physician [that he would] get [Cardiazol], the 'shaking treatment,' (accompanied by a demonstration of it), if he [did] not soon wake up, get peppier and work faster and with more interest. Immediately he [began to defend himself against [Cardiazol]], worked with more zest, looked brighter, and when he saw his doctor approaching he busied himself where he could not be overlooked" (Kerschbaumer 1943: 394).

Shock Treatments and Psychiatric Practice

Although Cardiazol was not used until the end in Anna Maria's case, it was part of what Bleuler called "the active therapy" that complemented the "educational therapy of schizophrenia" (Bleuler 1943), or what was known as "psychotherapy" at the time (Schneider 1939). Cardiazol shock therapy—intravenous injections of pentamethylentetrazol, a camphor-like substance used to provoke an epileptic seizure—was introduced by neuropathologist and neurologist Lazlo (Ladislaus) Meduna in 1934, and from June 1936 on, insulin and Cardiazol shock therapies were carried out at Friedrichsberg. In the US, Metrazol/Cardiazol therapy was introduced in 1937 (Colomb and Wadsworth 1941), and in Canada, at the Ontario hospital in Hamilton, in September 1938 (Cummins 1944). Meduna's theory was that genuine epilepsy rarely occurred in combination with schizophrenia, creating what he called a "biological antagonism" between these two diseases. Because the two diseases were mutually exclusive, he contended that synthetically provoking artificial epileptic seizures should positively influence schizophrenia. However, this theory was immediately challenged. As an international debate highlights, practitioners like military psychiatrist Hirsch Gordon identified 50 different shock therapy theories (Gordon 1948). Psychiatric journals published an overwhelming number of studies that tried to discover the exact mode of action and the impact of different shock therapies on patients' behavior, but they were less interested in finding theoretical underpinnings for the causes for schizophrenia and how shock therapies influenced them.

American psychiatrist Louis H. Cohen emphasized that the Cardiazol procedure was relatively simple, economical, and did not involve restraint. Whereas all conventional forms of treatment, such as continuous baths, packs, seclusion and chemical sedation, were effective only during the immediate period that they were applied, shock therapies appeared to last longer over time. Cohen stated that even after shock treatment was discontinued "most patients remain[ed.] quiet and cooperative" and many of them "for the first time in years, [were] capable of doing productive work." Cardiazol therefore was considered one solution for administrative problems concerning the handling of "chronically disturbed patients" (Cohen 1938a: 228). Another American psychiatrist summarized that the duration of the illness was shortened and that "some of the others [patients who could not be discharged] became better hospital citizens" (Colomb and Wadsworth 1941: 58). Even if patients remained unchanged, most of them improved regarding their over-activity, aggressiveness, and destructiveness. "Necessary sedation has been diminished to practically nil" (Cohen 1938a: 332).

These considerations were also sometimes closely related to eugenic arguments. For example, Professor H. Mouttet at the Swiss Psychiatric Association meeting in 1937 mentioned at the beginning of this article, that "we officers of the state who are concerned with prosperity, the health and the well-being of our fellow citizens expect from you the transformation of useless human beings into individuals useful to society" (Mouttet 1938: 3). Leading psychiatrists like Carl Schneider in Germany emphasized on the one hand the necessity "to furnish the new times with new humans" and underlined, on the other hand, the connection between curing and devastation (see for example: Schneider 1939). "Psychiatric patients should receive intensive "biological" therapy, but if they were incurable and could not be integrated into society, they lost their reason for existence in the biological sense as well" (Rotzoll and Hohendorff 2012: 317).

No consensus among psychiatrists existed as to exactly how the therapy should be carried out or for how long. Higher doses of the drug were to be administered within a couple of minutes if any seizure occurred, but if no seizure could be provoked, further injections were to be held off until the following day. According to Bleuler, who followed Meduna's recommendations, patients would ideally receive two shocks per week—15 to 20 in all (Bleuler 1943). But a look at the international literature shows that the suggestions regarding the duration of the course and the frequency of injections were quite arbitrary (Cohen 1938b: 1004). Sometimes the injections were given daily (Cohen 1938a), sometimes every second day (Ziskind 1941).

Psychiatrists usually gave the intravenous injections. Because patients often vomited following the injection, they were fasting and placed in bed with a piece of rubber hose inserted between their teeth to prevent them biting their tongues (Widenmeyer 1937). As was the case with epileptic seizures in general, induced seizures also left patients unconscious, although they often suffered dislocations of joints, bone fractures, and other surgical complications. Ten to 15 seconds after the injection, a so-called pre-paroxysmal phase occurred that was characterized by a short interval of coughing, which watchers stated was "followed by [an interval] usually lasting not more than ten seconds during which the patient [made] thrashing movements and [flailed] his arms and legs about, his facial expression closely resembling terror" (Cohen 1938b: 1004). The assistant physician at the Illenau asylum in Achern, Germany explained that "most sick persons oppose the Cardiazol treatment; because in the short interval that lasts only several seconds ... [they] experience a displeasing feeling, especially in the cardiac region, that can bring on a mortal fear. Nevertheless, it is just a misperception that is not based on a real specific danger" (Widenmeyer 1937: 163).

This "misperception" is worth analyzing in more detail. Psychiatrists generally agreed on the fact that the fear provoked in patients during the therapies (especially in the case of Cardiazol shock therapy) had an impact on the outcome of the treatments. They disagreed only to what extent. From 1937 to 1939, a large number of studies carried out in US asylums tried to determine the impact of fear in shock therapies, for example, by artificially provoking prolonged sequences of fear that sometimes lasted up to three hours. Cohen described the fear experienced by patients as a "threat to the self which arises out of the experiences of impending catastrophe" (Cohen 1939). Humbert and Friedemann described this feeling as a "falling into non-existence" which invoked in the patient "the primitive complex of the association of life-death ... that appeared to have cumulative effects" (Humbert and Friedemann 1938: 180).

Psychiatrists who studied the impact of fear agreed on the fact that the "animal-like expression of fear" was a sign of a kind of fear articulated at a lower biological level, and they differentiated this kind of fear from that consciously expressed by patients, which often led them to resist treatment. As two researchers asserted, a patient "suddenly and in the course of a few seconds after the injection of [Cardiazol] receives a terrific assault upon his entire economy including [his] consciousness and his instinct of self-preservation. He almost dies but does not" (Clark and Norbury 1941: 197). Schilder described this condition as a "threat of annihilation and death and indeed during the epileptic fit and the following coma the patient comes very near to death" (Schilder 1939: 142). The patient is "dead for a minute or so in an average attack. He goes through a terrifying experience of which he is aware, in active consciousness or in a subconscious state, only for a short time." The fear of impending death is "probably more real than that of the angina patient" (Clark and Norbury 1941: 197). This profound fear on a "lower biological level" was only experienced if it was followed by seizures. However, it was possible to produce a less profound kind of fear by provoking "abortive seizures," which occurred if the dose of Cardiazol was too low or if it was injected too slowly. Patients clearly remembered the fear brought on by these abortive seizures, leading to the speculation that the injection of lower levels of the drug or injecting it too slowly had the potential to be used deliberately. Cohen regarded shock therapies as "the twentieth-century variety of shock treatments of the past, in which fear [was] instilled [for a] therapeutic purpose" (Cohen 1939: 1349).

This suspicion is pertinent in Anna Maria Buller's case, because the medication plan clearly indicates that, in the course of her treatment, "single shot injections" became more frequent. For some of these injections, she successfully experienced a seizure (in these cases, a + sign is marked beside the entry) but some injections obviously not did not provoke seizures. According to standard procedures, in these cases the injections had to be repeated until a seizure occurred (or the injections had to be resumed on the next day), but in Buller's case, this did not happen. It seems as if the rationale behind these single injections was to discipline specific behavior that the nurses reported in order to obtain permission from the psychiatrist for another injection.

Shock therapies were enthusiastically received in Germany and abroad. An overwhelming number of case studies were published that demonstrated astonishing results for patients who had successfully recovered from schizophrenia. It must be emphasized that psychiatrists referred only to "remissions" of patients, not to cures. Bleuler believed that heredity or "congenital disposition [was] of critical importance" and considered schizophrenia to be a "heredodegeneration," even though he admitted that no medically sound idea existed for its causes (Bleuler 1923: 326–7). The term heredodegeneration, a combination of "heredity" and "degeneration," implied that the cause was to be found in the patient's family history, and that it was possible to locate the reason for the illness in former events that had induced a degeneration of a family member and was later passed on. The inability to find an organic cause of illness could be balanced by a kind of "virtual body," the "body of the family." Through heredity, it was possible to re-introduce a pathological "material substratum" and give the illness certain physicality.

From this perspective, the course of the illness could be influenced only through psychotherapy, meaning that patients could be educated, but not really cured. Psychiatrists internationally thus tried to define the success of therapies through classification of patient behavior. The psychiatrists L.v. Angyal and K. Gyárfás distinguished four forms of "remission": "complete (A), good (B), social (C), and none (0)." People with complete remission, it was thought, had gained complete insight into their illness, were able to work, and were thought to have attained a complete cure by those close to them. In the everyday life of the asylum, patients were judged according to how they were able to adjust to the regulations of the institution (Angyal and Gyárfás 1937: 2).

To reduce the purpose of shock therapies to produce only more manageable patients, however, is too simplistic. As the quote from Angyal and Gyárfás highlights, patients who were considered in complete remission were said to have complete insight into their illness. Solomon et al. described in his case study how patients who were "hostile to questioning" about their mental illness before shock treatment exhibited "a cooperative cordial attitude towards" the psychiatrist after they recovered (Solomon, Darrow and Blaurock 1939: 125). They were able to give an "objective outlook and an apparently adequate rationalization" of their problems (Colomb and Wadsworth 1941: 57–58). The authors defined "psychologic resistance" as a "hostile, angry, disputing attitude towards the examiner" (Solomon, Darrow and Blaurock 1939: 120). Psychiatrist Hamlin A. Starks carried out interviews on the subjective experiences of patients receiving insulin and Metrazol therapy. As one patient stated, "Before the treatment, I was in a little world by myself, having bad feelings. After I got the treatment, I felt rather the reality [became more aware of his surrounding]. Another patient admitted that he had been mentally ill, that he had "imagined things that didn't exist in reality." After the treatment "my mind began to look at things realistically again. It made me very reasonable, very rational, and [able to] think clearly" (Starks 1938: 703). In contrast, a patient who did not "change" through the treatment "admitted only what she wished to admit, often answering one question by asking another. The patient made no attempt to use the interview to gain insight into her problems" (Solomon, Darrow and Blaurock 1939: 131). From this perspective, shock therapy became a means to achieve these confessions, and could be defined as introducing the psychiatrist's will into the body of the patient. What happened in these moments was Foucault's "double enthronement," when patients acknowledged both the reality of the asylum and their own biography in their case histories as preserved in their patient records. But shock therapies had an even more far-reaching effect because they let patients acknowledge the all-embracing power of psychiatrists and nurses.

Psychiatrists acknowledged that the effects of Cardiazol and insulin were "deeper than the effects of what we call psychic influence. The treatment is an organic treatment reflected in psychological attitudes." The psychosis was not forgotten, "but the individual changed his emotional attitude" (Schilder 1939: 143). This was especially true in cases of "degenerative schizophrenia" (classical dementia praecox) in which the "psychotherapeutic influence is forcibly limited to superficial re-education." These cases that were considered as hopeless appeared to be "responsive to shock treatment either by insulin or by Cardiazol" (Bleuler 1943). Here we find the idea that Sakel developed through his use of military vocabulary, that shock therapies somehow overcame a blockage in patients in order to open them up to the possibilities of "re-socialization" through education.

Shock therapies in general thus had a very specific effect on patients, because they not only changed the way they communicated verbally but also how they acted in front of psychiatrists and nurses. Kerschbaumer described these changes as "a positive transference" leading to a "close patient-physician relationship," where, for example, "some male patients [saw] in the woman-psychiatrist a sweetheart, wife, beloved sister or mother-substitute." This "close patient-physician relationship" seemed to be a consequence of extreme fear because patients appeared to almost cling to their rescuers (Kerschbaumer 1943: 390). Schilder noted that after a fit, a patient "experiences … a slow revival of his interest in the world and an enormous feeling of relief in which he grasps for any contact offered to him"(Schilder 1939: 142). In this final stage of shock treatment the patient perceived psychiatrists and nurses as rescuers and tried to establish close contact with them.

Perceiving the psychiatrist as "rescuer" resembles the description of what Foucault called the "foundational scene" of psychiatry (Foucault 2003). In what has become a famous scene, Pinel, at the beginning of the nineteenth century in Bicêtre, liberated the furious lunatics from their chains. They had been kept in chains because, it was feared, they would become a danger to all. But, merely by recognizing Pinel as their rescuer and by expressing their gratitude to him, they entered the path to a cure. Similarly, the recovery of patients from their seizures was often accompanied by a kind of "infantile regression in their verbal expressions and gestures, beginning with the most primitive ones like thumb-sucking and calling frequently for "mamma" (even when hostile maternal complexes were present), then reaching out for support and behaving as if struggling for life, both in the state of torpidity and in the awakening" (Humbert and Friedemann 1938: 177). As theoretical considerations developed at the beginning of this article suggest, this part of shock treatment could be interpreted as a sign of an inevitable submission to psychiatric power.

Furthermore, as was the case for Anna Maria B., Cardiazol therapy was often combined with insulin shock therapy. The addition of insulin, which had been developed by Manfred Sakel in the 1930s, was based on the theory that insulin antagonized the neuronal effects of products of the adrenal system that were considered the physiological cause of the patient's illness. Insulin shock therapy was employed on a grand scale in Hamburg and elsewhere. The former medical director of Friedrichsberg, Prof. Dr. Hans Bürger-Prinz, stated after the end of the Second World War, that a quarter of the patient beds had been reserved for insulin shock treatments, or 80 beds out of 320 (Ebbinghaus 1984: 141).

"Deep insulin coma therapy" was extremely rigorous. It was administered in a separate unit, with the patients staying together with the same doctors and nurses throughout the therapy.

Comas were induced on five or six mornings a week. Typically, the "therapy" began with an initial dose of 10–15 units of insulin with a daily increase of 5–10 units until the patient showed a severe hypoglycemia. Treatment continued until there was a satisfactory psychiatric response or until 50–60 comas had been induced. In Anna Maria B's case, the "therapy" started with 30 units and with a daily increase of 10 units, reaching up to 100 units on the ninth day.

Experienced therapists in Great Britain let patients spend up to 15 minutes in "deep coma" (Jones 2000). Bleuler believed that one could leave a patient in deep coma for up to an hour with hypotonia and absent corneal and pupillary reflexes (Bleuler 1943). Hypoglycemia made patients extremely restless and susceptible to major convulsions. Comas were terminated by administration of glucose via a nasal tube or through intravenous injection. Patients required continuous nursing supervision for the rest of the day since they were liable to experience hypoglycemic "after-shocks" and a doctor had to be immediately available.

Bürger-Prinz pointed out that patients experienced these periods of "forced unconsciousness in slow motion," which caused "panicky anxiety states in them" (Bürger-Prinz as cited in: Ebbinghaus 1984: 141). Cardiazol shock provoked a profound fear of death in the patient, but insulin coma therapy was literally a death threat. Although American psychiatrist Smith Elly Jellife believed that innumerable forms of death threats existed, with varying degrees of significance for patients, he asserted that the hypoglycemic death threat was unique. "Genetically considered it may be thought of as a very primordial, primitive and massive type of threat which strikes at the very initial stages of life" since "carbohydrates were among the first energy transforming substances creating life." Insulin coma therapy produced, similarly to Cardiazol shock therapy, a reaction on a deep and profound level but the actual mechanisms differed. Insulin has a specific impact because of carbohydrates' long phyletic history. Hence, "the death threat is a much more vital one coming from this direction than from almost any other." The death threat experienced by the "withdrawal of glycogen forces a definite withdrawal of libido from the aggressive, hostile anal, oral and other negativistic behavior patterns" because it strikes at the initial stages of life. It is as if the patient is catapulted into a coma that is comparable to an "intrauterine bath of primary narcissistic omnipotence" (Jelliffe 1937: 577).

The insulin units were mostly the sole responsibility of nurses (Missa 2006), who administered not only the insulin but also the glucose via a nasal tube (Enge 1941). Nurses thus conducted patients systematically into a "twilight state" between life and death. However, as the example below suggests, they were also very concerned in recording patient behavior, as they did for Anna Maria Buller.

> 15.5. Afternoon: Pat. got Insulin. Pat. walked around nude. Was drowsy. Must be urged to eat. Ate well then. (Nurse H.)
> Night: Slept. (Nurse M.)
> 16.5. Pat. got Insulin. Is always out of the bed. (Nurse M.)
> Afternoon: Pat. removed her shirt, walked around.
> Night: Slept till morning. (Nurse K.)
> 17.5. Got Cardiazol (+ ['seizure']) afterwards unchanged. (Nurse L.)
> Night: unchanged
> 18.5. Pat. got Cardiazol. Afterwards quiet. Vomited a bit. (Nurse M.)
> Afternoon: Pat. was quiet. [Nurse O. (PR, FMR, PN)]

The patients not only imagined the possibility of death through these shock therapies, but fatalities were very real, as was reported in all the medical literature of that time. Historian Angelika Ebbinghaus presumes that the increase in the mortality rate in Friedrichsberg before the Nazi regime was due partly to the new "active" therapies. According to her research, patients were already dying from these shock therapies long before the beginning of the planned and systematic assassination of patients. (See Table 15.1) While the table indicates that the number of admitted patients did not double between 1936 and 1941, the number of deaths more than tripled in the same period of time.

The example of Anna Maria Buller highlights the fact that shock therapy was a technique that embodied the whole rationale of psychiatric practice, that

Table 15.1 Number of treated patients and number of patients who died in Eilbektal, the asylum at the University of Hamburg (Ebbinghaus 1984: 143)

Year	Number of patients treated in the asylum of the University of Hamburg	Number of deaths in the asylum of the University of Hamburg
1936	1333	85
1937	1990	142
1938	2196	154
1939	2516	188
1940	2113	235
1941	2391	290

of forcing the reality of the asylum onto the individual. In Buller's case, for example, Cardiazol and insulin coma therapy was combined with the usual Morphine-Scopolamine injections, with Paraldehyde, often given via enema in order to increase the sedative effects, and with a whole array of other disciplinary interventions. All these interventions were aimed at correcting her behavior, and the nurses' notes only focused on potential changes in her behavior.

As the nurses' notes pointed out, Buller was considered a chronic case. The nurses saw her as increasingly disoriented: "Sitting around and does not know what to do," or "Pat. sits at one place with her head down for hours." On 20 February1941, the psychiatrist noted that "she was completely unchanged and negativistic in character." Buller remained alternately stuporous and excited, out of touch with her surroundings, and "must be strapped down." As a consequence, B. was diagnosed as "schizophrenic final state." This state might also have been due partly to the extensive use of Cardiazol and other medications, since Ziskind reported on memory defects in patients who had received this drug: "Persistent amnesia resulting from metrazol therapy resembles the memory impairment noted in organic psychoses" and the more "pronounced forms present in Korsakoff syndrome" (Ziskind 1941: 230). These findings coincide with the findings of Platner and Müller who reported Korsakoff syndrome, a brain disorder usually associated with heavy alcohol consumption, as a complication of shock therapy of both insulin coma and Cardiazol shock therapies. Other abnormalities in severely affected patients included "impaired sensorium, silliness, and neglect of personal appearance, mental retardation, emotional lability, decreased self-preservation and feelings of familiarity."(Plattner 1938, Müller 1938) Ziskind argued that these symptoms were significant because "they are readily recognized as being due to the treatment and not part of the original disease." He further emphasized that shock therapy augmented memory defects in patients depending on the duration of treatment and the spacing of convulsions (Ziskind 1941: 230).

The psychiatrists and nurses knew very well what they were doing when they employed shock therapies. Bürger-Prinz's assistant, psychiatrist Fred Kögler, stated that "Insulin shock therapy and especially Cardiazol shock therapy are very brutal somatic interventions." Patients become helpless and feeble, "which clears the way for psychotherapeutic guidance … The shock itself might perhaps function like a concussion to the core of the personality due to the deep impact on vegetative and other cerebral functions and thereby influences the mysterious biological events of schizophrenia" (Kögler 1939: 111).

The notes on Buller in her record described her as "mentally dead," a term coined by psychiatrist Alfred Hoche. Hoche contended that it was not difficult for physicians, especially alienists and neurologists, to identify mentally dead persons, because these people had no clear imagination, no feelings, wishes, or determination. They had no possibility of developing a "world view" (*Weltbild*), no relationship to their environment, and most importantly, they lacked self-consciousness or the possibility of becoming conscious of their own existence. They had no subjective claim to life because they had only simple, elemental feelings such as are found in lower animals. A mentally dead person, therefore, was not able "to raise a subjective claim to life nor [was] he able to perform any kind of mental process" (Binding and Hoche 2006). Seen against the backdrop of these findings, it does not seem to be an exaggeration to assume that psychiatrists and nurses actively contributed to the "final state" of Anna Maria Buller.

Conclusion

These kinds of perspectives refuse to assume the idea of progress in psychiatry. The article began with a brief theoretical outline of psychiatric practice to argue that the asylum was organized around the absolute power of the psychiatrist, which created an insurmountable reality to be forced onto the patient. Shock therapies must be analyzed within this frame of reference, since they incorporated the entire rationale of psychiatric practice and can be seen as technologies that were able to reach the inner core of patients. While the supporting evidence for this theoretical perspective was drawn from a patient record that spanned the era of Nazi Germany, I attempt to demonstrate that German psychiatrists were part of an international network whose members viewed the integration of shock therapies into psychiatric practice in similar ways.

But psychiatry and its practices cannot be analyzed through scientific discourses alone. The patient record as historical evidence is useful, on a "microlevel," to demonstrate the perceptions of patients held by the professional medical staff and to better understand, in a concrete fashion, how they tried to "force their reality" onto their patients. Nurses were profoundly implicated in these practices, since they played a strategic role in influencing the behavior of their patients through a multitude of disciplinary interventions, including shock therapies. Even if they did not always administer the injections, they were required to report on patients' behavior, maintain surveillance over them, and decide whether or not patients "treated" with shock therapies had improved. This analysis thus not only highlights the fact that nurses were powerful, if seen from the perspective of patients, but also complicates the perception of nursing as a benevolent vocation.

References

Allard, G. 2012. *Névrose et folie dans le corps expéditionnaire Canadien (1914–1918). Le cas Québécois*. Outremont, Québec: Athéna.

Angyal, L. v., Gyárfás, K. 1937. Über die Cardiazol-Krampfbehandlung der Schizophrenie. *Archiv für Psychiatrie*, *106*, 1–12.

Becker, H. 1936. Der Umgang mit widerstrebenden Kranken. *Geisteskrankenpflege. Monatsschrift für Geisteskranken- und Krankenpflege*, *40*(8), 116–118.

Binding, K. and Hoche, A. 2006. *Die Freigabe der Vernichtung lebensunwerten Lebens. Ihr Maß und ihre Form (1920)*. Berlin: Berliner Wissenschaftsverlag.

Bleuler, E. 1923. *Lehrbuch der Psychiatrie*. Berlin: Springer.

Bleuler, E. 1943. In Bleuler M., Berze J. (Eds), *Lehrbuch der Psychiatrie*. Berlin: Springer-Verlag.

Clark, S.N. and Norbury, F.G. 1941. A possible role of the element of fear in Metrazol therapy. *Diseases of the Nervous System*, *2*(6), 196–198.

Cohen, L.H. 1938a. The early effects of Metrazol therapy in chronic psychotic over-activity. *American Journal of Psychiatry*, *95*, 327–333.

Cohen, L.H. 1938b. Observations on the convulsant treatment of schizophrenia with Metrazol. The *New England Journal of Medicine*, *218*(24), 1002–1007.

Cohen, L.H. 1939. The therapeutic significance of fear in the Metrazol treatment of schizophrenia. *American Journal of Psychiatry*, *95*, 1349–1357.

Colomb, H.O. and Wadsworth, G.L. 1941. An analysis of results in the Metrazol shock therapy of schizophrenia. *Journal of Nervous and Mental Disease*, *93*(1), 53–62.

Cummins, J.A. 1944. Metrazol shock therapy administered in the general hospital. *Canadian Medical Association Journal*, *50*, 420–421.

Dean, M. 1996. Putting the technological into government. *History of the Human Sciences*, *9*(3), 47–68.

Deleuze, G. 1989. Qu'est-ce qu'un dispositif? *Michel Foucault philosophe. Rencontre internationale* Paris, *9,10,11 Janvier 1988*. Paris: Éditions du Seuil.

Dörner, K. 1967. Nationalsozialismus und Lebensvernichtung. In K. Dörner, C. Haerlin, R. Schernus and A. Schwendy (Eds). *Der Krieg gegen die psychisch Kranken. Nach "Holocaust": Erkennen—Trauern—Begegnen*. Rehburg-Loccum: Psychiatrie Verlag, 74–111.

Dörner, K. 1984. *Bürger und Irre. Zur Sozialgeschichte und Wissenschaftssoziologie der Psychiatrie*. Frankfurt a.M.: Europäische Verlagsanstalt.

Ebbinghaus, A. 1984. Kostensenkung, "Aktive Therapie" und Vernichtung. Konsequenzen für das Anstaltswesen. In A. Ebbinghaus, H. Kaupen-Haas and K.H. Roth (Eds), *Heilen und Vernichten im Mustergau Hamburg. Bevölkerungs- und Gesundheitspolitik im Dritten Reich.* Hamburg: Konkret Literatur Verlag, 136–146.

Enge, D. 1941. Aufgaben des Pflegepersonals bei der Insulinschock- und der Cardiazol- bzw. Azomankrampf-Behandlung. *Geisteskrankenpflege. Monatsschrift für Geisteskranken- und Krankenpflege, 44*(11), 134–136.

Faulstich, H. 1998. *Hungersterben in der Psychiatrie 1914–1949. Mit einer Topographie der NS-Psychiatrie*. Freiburg im Breisgau: Lambertus.

Foucault, M. 1973. *Madness and Civilization: A History of Insanity in the Age of Reason* (R. Howard Trans.). New York: Vintage Books.

Foucault, M. 1997. *Il faut défendre la société. Cours au Collège de France. 1976.* France: Gallimard/Seuil.

Foucault, M. 1999. *Les Anormaux. Cours au Collège de France. 1974–1975.* Paris: Seuil/Gallimard.

Foucault, M. 2003. *Le pouvoir psychiatrique. Cours au collège de France. 1973–1974* (Hautes études ed.). France: Seuil/Gallimard.

Foucault, M. 2007. *Les mots et les choses. Une archéologie des sciences humaines.* France: Gallimard.

Gordon, H.L. 1948. Fifty shock therapy theories. *The Military Surgeon, 103*(5), 397–401.

Huisman, F. 2005. From exploration to synthesis. Making new sense of psychiatry and mental health care in the twentieth century. In M. Gijswijt-Hofstra, H. Oosterhuis, J. Vijselaar, and H. Freeman (Eds). *Psychiatric Cultures Compared: Psychiatry and Mental Health Care in the Twentieth Century.* Amsterdam: Amsterdam University Press, 405–423.

Humbert, F. and Friedemann, A. 1938. Critique and indications of treatments in schizophrenia. *American Journal of Psychiatry, 94*(2), 174–183.

Jelliffe, S.E. 1937. Discussion paper presented at the section of neurology and psychiatry, New York, academy of medicine, and the New York neurological society. Joint meeting, January 12, 1937. *Journal of Nervous and Mental Disease, 85*(5), 575–578.

Jones, K. 2000. Insulin coma therapy in schizophrenia. *Journal of the Royal Society of Medicine, 93*, 147–149.

Kankeleit, D. 1925. Was kosten die Minderwertigen den Staat? *Hamburger Anzeiger*, (21. 12.1925), 10.

Kaufmann, D. 1999. Widerstandsfähige Gehirne und kampfesunlustige Seelen. Zur Mentalitäts- und Wissenschaftsgeschichte des Ersten Weltkrieges. In M. Hagner (Ed.), *Ecce Cortex! Beiträge zur Geschichte des modernen Gehirns.* Göttingen: Wallstein, 206–233.

Kerschbaumer, L. 1943. Spontaneous reactions to Metrazol therapy. *Journal of Nervous and Mental Disease, 98*, 390–395.

Kögler, F. 1939. Beitrag über das Ergebnis der Insulinschockbehandlung der Schizophrenie. *Allgemeine Zeitschrift für Psychiatrie und ihre Grenzgebiete, 110*, 111–117.

Missa, J. 2006. *Naissance de la psychiatrie biologique: Histoire des traitements des maladies mentales au XX. siècle*. Paris: Presses universitaires de France.

Mouttet, H. 1938. The treatment of schizophrenia Insulin shock, Cardiazol, sleep treatment. *American Journal of Psychiatry*, *94*(suppl.), 1–5.

Müller, M. 1938. Insulin therapy of schizophrenia. *American Journal of Psychiatry*, *94*(supl.), 5–15.

Plattner, P. 1938. Amnestisches Syndrom nach Insulin-Cardiazolbehandlung. *Zeitschrift Für Die Gesamte Neurologie Und Psychiatrie*, *162*, 728–735.

Quinkert, B., Rauh, P. and Winkler, U. (Eds). 2010. *Krieg und Psychiatrie 1914–1950*. Göttingen: Wallstein.

Roelcke, V. 2002. Die Entwicklung der Psychiatrie zwischen 1880 und 1932: Theoriebildung, Institutionen, Interaktionen mit zeitgenössischer Wissenschafts- und Sozialpolitik. In R. v. Bruch, and B. Kaderas (Eds). *Wissenschaften und Wissenschaftspolitik: Bestandsaufnahmen zu Formationen, Brüchen und Kontinuitäten im Deutschland des 20. Jahrhunderts*. Stuttgart: Franz Steiner, 109–124.

Roelcke, V. 2005. Continuities or ruptures? Concepts, institutions and contexts of twentieth-century German psychiatry and mental health care. In M. Gijswijt-Hofstra, H. Oosterhuis, J. Vijselaar, and H. Freeman (Eds). *Psychiatric Cultures Compared. Psychiatry and Mental Health Care in the Twentieth Century: Comparisons and Approaches*. Amsterdam: Amsterdam University Press, 162–182.

Rotzoll, M. and Hohendorff, G. 2012. Krankenmord im Dienst des Fortschritts? Der Heidelberger Psychiater Carl Schneider als Gehirnforscher und "therapeutischer Idealist." *Der Nervenarzt*, *83*(3), 311–320.

Sakel, M. 1938. The nature and origin of hypoglycemic treatment of psychosis. *The American Journal of Psychiatry*, *94*(suppl.), 24–40.

Schilder, P. 1939. Notes on the psychology of Metrazol treatment of schizophrenia. *The Journal of Nervous and Mental Disease*, *89*(2), 133–144.

Schneider, C. 1939. *Behandlung und Verhütung der Geisteskrankehiten. Allgemeine Erfahrungen, Grundsätze Technik Biologie*. Berlin: Julius Springer.

Solomon, A.P., Darrow, C.W. and Blaurock, M. 1939. Blood pressure and palmar sweat (galvanic) repsonses of psychotic patients before and after Insulin and Metrazol therapy: a physiologic study of 'resistant' and cooperative attitudes. *Psychosomatic Medicine*, *1*(1), 118–137.

Starks, H.A. 1938. Subjective experiences in patients incident to Insulin and Metrazol therapy. *Psychiatric Quarterly*, *12*(4), 699–709.

Widenmeyer, H., Dr. 1937. Die Insulin- und Cardiazolschockbehandlung der Schizophrenen. *Geisteskrankenpflege. Monatsschrift für Geisteskranken- und Krankenpflege*, *41*(12), 161–165.

Wyllie, A.M. 1940. Convulsion therapy of the psychoses. *The British Journal of Psychiatry*, *86*, 248–259.

Ziskind, E. 1941. Memory defects during Metrazol therapy. *Archives of Neurology and Psychiatry*, *45*(2), 223–234.

Chapter 16
American Medical Psychiatry: A Contemporary Case of Lysenkoism

David H. Jacobs

In a 2005 publication, Robert Spitzer, the psychiatrist who spearheaded the APA's official paradigm shift to unsullied medicine, admitted that the false positive problem in psychiatry has proven to be insoluble. A symptoms-only approach to the problem of psychiatric diagnosis, although consistent with medical reasoning, ignores *background* and is thus blind to adversity and to the false positive problem. I argue that recognizing the reality of adversity, which can only be ascertained via dialogue and which ineradicably includes first-person subjective components, cannot be assimilated to either medicine or science. Indeed the psychiatrist-patient encounter, in contrast to the physician-patient encounter, is nothing *but* social interaction, dialogue, and interpretation. The difference is so obvious and dramatic that it is hard to see how the claim that the psychiatrist-patient encounter is a *medical* encounter can be presented seriously. Recognizing the reality of adversity shifts the subject matter from medicine and science to something else entirely. I argue that the APA's paradigm shift at the end of the 1970s should be understood sociologically, i.e., in terms of the profession's adaptation to external threats and demands that were too powerful to ignore. I end by arguing that it is barely possible that the *DSM-5* Task Force's insistence on applying medical reasoning to all aspects of life may have created an enduring backlash among the non-medical mental health professions.

Introduction

In a 2005 publication (Zimmerman and Spitzer 2005) on the topic of psychiatric diagnosis, Robert Spitzer, the guiding spirit of the *DSM-III* revolution, admitted that the false positive problem in psychiatry has proven to be insoluble. He also noted that the problem and its insolubility is not a topic that commands much interest or discussion in psychiatry. He reasoned as follows: (a) it is unrealistic to overlook the possibility that the patient's "clinically significant" distress or social disability may be the result of adversity the patient has faced or is facing, and (b) there is no objective, scientific method for determining if the patient's reaction to adversity is or is not warranted, justified, proportionate, and so on. In short, a mental disorder diagnosis must be an arbitrary conclusion, meaning a conclusion that is not reached on the basis of objective scientific evidence. The fact that a patient may be judged to meet the criteria for this or that mental disorder diagnosis is irrelevant because the issue of whether the adversity the patient has faced justifies the symptoms or entitles the patient to the symptoms is not addressed merely by noting that the patient's symptoms fulfill the listed criteria for this or that mental disorder. Notwithstanding his admission that deciding whether or not a person has a mental disorder is arbitrary, Spitzer expressed no doubt that some people do suffer from a mental disorder. Evidently he is not impressed by the argument that a concept that does not lend itself to distinguishing between true and false positives on the basis of objective evidence cannot claim to be designating something that has an independent existence of its own. Presumably he thinks there is something to discover as opposed to something to judge or have an opinion about (contrast discovering the cause of type 1 diabetes to deciding that a painting is a masterpiece or that Joyce's *Ulysses* is or is not pornographic). He said he hopes that future discoveries in evolutionary psychology will shift what are now arbitrary decisions to evidence-based scientific decisions. (I consider this grasping at straws; see Jacobs 2010.) But note that he does not elide the issue of adversity in a person's life and its connection to "symptoms." By admitting that adversity cannot realistically be overlooked he has, *de facto*, as I will discuss, turned away from the position he was so instrumental ushering in, namely the position that the subject matter of psychiatry are medical conditions that announce their presence exclusively as far as anyone can tell by producing troubling social behavior (such as complaining of feeling depressed).

Adversity is a word (concept) that does not fit easily or at all into a medical or scientific framework of thought. Spitzer surely realizes this. It only makes sense to say that a *person* has faced or is facing adversity, so it would seem that all of the conceptual and linguistic apparatus of medicine and science becomes immediately irrelevant when what is at issue or under discussion is at the person-level and not the body/organism level. The adversity a person has faced or is facing cannot be adequately/realistically described from an external, third-person perspective. Adversity cannot be described impersonally and objectively. Description depends upon first-person disclosure. Third-person access to first-person-experienced adversity depends upon dialogue; third-person observation by itself cannot be adequate. Adversity connotes a first-person, subjective component that cannot be overlooked. Since third-person access to first-person-experienced adversity depends on disclosure and dialogue, depiction of adversity can always be amended during the course of real-time dialogue or at any point after at the discretion of the informant. Since disclosure depends on social interaction and dialogue, the informant may say different things to different interlocutors. Since speech must be interpreted, the original interlocutor's understanding of what was said may diverge from the understanding of others who read the transcript or watch the videotape. Since the informant's description of adversity will frequently include reference to or connote or imply what could be called "symptoms," it is unnecessary and indeed misconceived to think of symptoms as an effect that is independent of the cause of the symptoms. For example, describing death of a loved one as a horrifying loss that left the informant alone and bereft in the world can hardly be considered a cause that is independent of its effects. In short it is misconceived to think that cause-effect reasoning is applicable here, and if this is the case then the subject matter falls outside of scientific explanation, i.e., no impersonal causal process is involved, so no impersonal causal process can be discovered.

Small wonder that medical psychiatry shies away from endeavoring to surface, through dialogue, the patient's exposure to adversity (and related considerations: situation, predicament, history, background, backstory, etc.). As soon as adversity and related considerations are allowed on stage the jig is basically up in so far as the claim that the subject matter at hand is medicine or that scientific research and explanation are pertinent. Once adversity and related considerations begin to be discussed there is no hiding that what is primarily occurring is social interaction, disclosure, dialogue, interpretation, interviewing, and so on. It will be apparent that no disclosure can be considered definitive in the sense that there is nothing left to say that might be pertinent, that the specific clinician as interlocutor and interpreter of what the patient says plays an active and irreproducible role in what emerges in the interview, that whether the patient is entitled to his "symptoms" given the background he reveals is an unabashedly ad hoc moral interpretation on the part of the clinician or anyone else who has access to the transcript, that the clinician's written summary of a series of interviews or sessions has basically the same relation to what the client literally said as a book review has to the book reviewed, and so on. In short, as soon as adversity and related considerations are allowed on stage it is more than apparent that the encounter between psychiatrist and patient is anything but a medical encounter. Unlike the physician-patient encounter, in the psychiatrist-patient encounter there is nowhere to go except more talking.

The psychiatrist can prescribe drugs, but that does not, except in a circular *ex juvantibus* sense, bear on what was the matter in the first place (see, for example, Moncrieff 2008). Healy (2012) emphasizes that the sponsoring pharmaceutical companies themselves both strongly influence if not *de facto* create the definition of psychiatric disorders and develop assessment of treatment measures that are designed to favor the effects of the drug they wish to promote. In numerous publications (e.g. 2000), Healy has pointed out that unambiguously positive indications of treatment outcome, like returns to work or discharge from hospital, have been rejected by the entire psychiatry-Pharma-NIMH-FDA complex in favor of rating scales. The use of rating scales permits claims of treatment "success" in randomized, placebo-controlled drug studies on the basis of what may be clinically insignificant statistical differences between active drug and placebo group. Large, multi-site drug studies which enlist hundreds or thousands of subjects allow very small rating-scale differences between active medication group and placebo group to reach statistical significance. The outcome measure of note is almost always the supposedly blinded assessment of the researcher who administered the drug and asked about side effects throughout the course of the typically very short drug treatment study. Quality of life measures are frequently administered but rarely reported. Adverse drug effects are under-scrutinized and under-reported. Since the pharmaceutical industry itself is primarily in charge of the design, execution, interpretation, and promotion of drug studies, hanky panky has basically run riot (e.g., see Cohen and Jacobs 2010, Jacobs and Cohen 2010).

The only way to sidestep the glaringly moral-interpretive issue concerning to what extent the patient's background justifies or entitles her to her distress or quirks or social difficulties is to make up supposedly discrete mental disorders conceived as idiopathic medical conditions defined exclusively on the basis of "symptoms" and to essentially turn a blind eye to adversity and related considerations. Although no actual medical discoveries bearing on psychiatric diagnosis occurred between *DSM-III-R* and the publication of *DSM-IV*, the APA officially banished psychogenesis from existence in *DSM-IV* (see the definition of primary mental disorder in *DSM-IV:* 165). A careful reading of the *DSM* offers only the barest suggestion that psychiatric patients have faced conditions of living that are worth remarking upon. This is, of course, entirely in keeping with the position that psychiatric disorders are in fact impersonal medical conditions, presumably endogenous neurological flaws. If adversity is acknowledged, as in PTSD and Adjustment Disorder, it is none the less taken for granted that the suffering individual is literally sick or disordered, since according to medical reasoning it would be absurd to argue that the suffering person's experience of adversity entitles him to his distress or social difficulties. It may be perfectly ordinary to say that a bereaved person is entitled to grief, but this is not medical reasoning. From the perspective of medical reasoning, "entitled to" is a foreign and absurd idea; the body is never entitled to fail to function as desired and expected. It does not matter what situation an individual might be in – the pancreas, for example, is never "entitled to" produce less insulin than is needed to maintain good health. Diabetes cannot be excused by circumstances; it is always considered disease. If medical reasoning is applied to people, not just to organisms, then there can be no excuse for distress or social difficulty regardless of circumstances. This is why PTSD and Adjustment Disorder are considered mental disorders, and this is why the *DSM-5* Task Force is inclined to reduce the bereavement exception from two months to two weeks (it was a year in *DSM-III)* – distress or disability that does not quickly remit is disease or disorder regardless of circumstances. This is medical reasoning.

It can be highly serviceable to think about the operation of the body/organism without considering *social* circumstances, but it is never serviceable (valid, realistic, useful) to think about a person and social behavior minus social circumstances. The two subject areas – the organism and the person – are in different realms. Different forms of reasoning are required and apt in one realm but not the other. The recent debacle on the part of the *DSM-5* Task Force concerning eliminating the bereavement exception that excited so much lay and professional outrage demonstrates that it is intuitively obvious to practically everyone not on the *DSM-5* Task Force that, at least when it comes to bereavement, the reasoning that applies to the body/organism does not apply to the *person*. Social behavior, of course, may be distorted or disabled by disease (e.g., precipitous drop in blood sugar level may bring about strange and unwarranted behavior), but it certainly will not do to consider deviations from normatively expected and desired behavior in general as brought about by idiopathic medical disease and, by so doing, terminate the usual interest when speaking about a person on background, circumstances, and so on. It is legitimate to suspend person considerations when physical evidence reveals that a causal disease or disorder explanation is called for, but in the absence of such evidence, suspending interest in person considerations does the person a great injustice and should be considered a form of violence.

DSM-5 will once again be obliged to diagnose all disorders unique to psychiatry exclusively in terms of first-person complaints and third-person observations and interpretations of behavior (it would be more precise to say that observations conveyed in words *are* interpretations.) Obviously this is not what the authors of *DSM-III* (published in 1980) expected by 2013. Psychiatry has "rejoined medicine" only in name and in *form*, not in substance. The complete failure of psychiatry to become medical in fact since the great leap forward has only inspired intellectual leaders in psychiatry to remark that the problems facing medical psychiatry have turned out to be harder than they looked from the perspective of the late 1970s when the great leap forward was being planned (e.g., Insel 2009). To grasp why the APA is committed to psychiatry is medicine despite an unbroken record of failure since *DSM-III* was published, it is enlightening to review the situation of psychiatry as a profession in the 1970s. What will come into view is that the reasons that led the leadership of the APA to abandon the Myerian framework of thought at the end of the 1970s continue to prevail today and will continue to prevail for the foreseeable future.

The Psychiatry Profession Meets the Corporate World and the Government

The most straightforward and convincing answer is to follow the money. I will draw first on what I think is the most respected and most frequently cited analysis concerning why the APA gave up Myerian psychiatry and officially adopted neo-Kraepelinism in 1980, namely Mitchell Wilson's 1993 piece in the *American Journal of Psychiatry.* In preparing this piece Wilson had numerous discussions with Robert Spitzer and access to documents in Spitzer's possession, and also access to APA archival documents. Wilson's published analysis emphasized psychiatry's *professional* problems in the 1970s and its realpolitik solution to its professional problems. According to Wilson's analysis the APA essentially adapted to demands on the part of external players too powerful to ignore. The adaptation—neo-Kraepelinism—solved psychiatry's urgent *professional* problems, but at the cost of adopting a framework of thought that is manifestly ill-suited to the subject matter. By *professional* problems Wilson is speaking unambiguously about access to money and external threats to access to money. This is clearly an unflattering view of the APA's decision to develop a revolutionary break with the past, so one has to wonder about it being published in the APA's own house organ. I cannot answer this question, although I can make the observation that Wilson's analysis had no effect on the content of *DSM-IV*, published in 1994, or on any other practical matter as far as I know. Of course this would be consistent with his thesis – what matters most to a profession are professional considerations (individuals may take a stand on principle or conscience, but a professional organization exists to foster the interests of the profession).

The two major external threats to the profession in the 1970s that Wilson identifies are (1) the federal government did not like psychosocial research into the causes of human distress and social difficulties and, in consequence, federal research money to psychiatry had been declining 5percent per year from 1965 to 1972. Unfortunately, Wilson provides practically no analysis of the federal government's antipathy towards psychosocial research. The reason cannot simply be that the Myerian framework did not easily lend itself to epidemiology, as he suggests. If one is writing critically and analytically about the policies of the federal government the topic of politics obviously cannot be avoided, but Wilson says nothing about politics (imagine avoiding political commentary when it comes to discussing federal policies during the 1960s, a period of unprecedented political and social upheaval; however, see Jacobs 1995). Perhaps Wilson thought the reasons for the federal government's antipathy towards psychosocial research were too obvious to discuss; (2) third-party payers, specifically the private insurance industry and the federal government in its capacity as third-party payer, made it clear to the APA that it would no longer tolerate (i.e., continue to pay for) the unstandardized and unreliable nature of psychiatric diagnosis. From the perspective of third-party payers reimbursing psychiatrists for treatment, this issue put them (third-party payers) in the position of paying for something amorphous, an intolerable position, especially as demand for psychotherapy kept growing. There must be accountability, meaning standardization. In addition, diagnosis must distinguish between real medical conditions and problems in living, which should not be covered under medical insurance. The Myerian emphasis on the psychosocial causes of distress and disability, its acceptance of a fuzzy and basically non-existent boundary between personal distress and mental illness, and its narrative (i.e., non-categorical, non-entity) approach to diagnosis were extremely problematic to the federal government as provider of research money into the causes of personal distress and social difficulties, and to the private insurance industry and the federal government as third-party payers for psychiatric treatment. It is intrinsic to Wilson's analysis that the parties demanding reform were not amenable to persuasion and were too big and important to ignore. The profession of psychiatry was in the position of having to reform or suffer severe consequences. The solution was abandoning the Myerian framework and adopting a conventional medical disease framework. In Wilson's view (and mine) the cost was high – the profession essentially abandoned a realistic framework of thought for its subject matter – but the *professional* reward was survival and growth.

There were other important contributions to psychiatry's shift to a conventional medical framework of thought that Wilson does not discuss, namely the growing competition for the psychotherapy dollar from non-medical professions and the FDA's demand for distinct clinical entities in order to approve new drugs (Mayes and Horwitz 2005). With regard to the latter, it could be argued on historical grounds that the FDA's requirements from psychiatry in terms of identifying distinct clinical entities were lax enough to continue with the Myerian framework of thought. But the Myerian framework was incompatible with aggressively promoting psychiatric problems as genuinely medical and therefore requiring drug treatment to address the actual cause of the problem. This position not only rendered psychiatrists immune to competition from the non-medical psychotherapy professions but opened the floodgates to the largess of the pharmaceutical industry. Over time the influence of the pharmaceutical industry on how psychiatric drug treatment research is conducted and on basic concepts of what is really the matter with people who seek psychiatric care has grown so large that it could be argued that the profession has *de facto* become an arm of the pharmaceutical industry (Cohen and Jacobs 2010, Jacobs and Cohen 2010).

If Wilson's analysis is taken seriously then it is appropriate to think of American medical psychiatry primarily as a sociological phenomenon rather than primarily as a *bona fide* scientific research endeavor and an applied science medical practice. Certainly there are research and practicing psychiatrists who fully believe that psychiatric problems are genuine medical diseases (based on biological faults, dysfunction, etc.), but that is beside the point. The point is that the existence of such beliefs among a minority of psychiatrists in the 1970s was not the main reason that the APA refashioned itself as a conventional medical specialty (i.e., diseases and medicines). A year after Wilson's paper was published, comments and rejoinders were published in the Letters to the Editor section (March 1994), including a rejoinder from Robert Spitzer (Spitzer and Williams 1994). What is noteworthy is that none of the published commentaries and rejoinders even acknowledged Wilson's major thesis, which was that the APA was basically pressured into dropping the Myerian framework by external players in the mental health industry, players whose interests were political and financial, not scientific or clinical. The closest Spitzer (Spitzer and Williams 1994) came to actually addressing Wilson's thesis was to admit that the majority of diagnostic categories in *DSM-III* lacked sufficient reliability data; the bulk of diagnostic categories included in *DSM-III* were present because clinicians needed them (to get reimbursed, although Spitzer is content not to complete the sentence). Having published Wilson's basically sociological analysis, the Editors declined to further honor it by demanding that published comments actually address and presumably attempt to refute his main thesis. What I want to emphasize is that the professional literature has largely followed suit – in the main there is no mention of the financial and political forces that in effect demanded a conventional medical paradigm in psychiatry. It is only a slight exaggeration to say that American medical psychiatry is a case of Lysenkoism, with the qualification that political and financial forces as opposed to exclusively political forces were operant. The overarching point I want to make is that attention to political and financial influences at work in shaping contemporary American medical psychiatry should have the effect of de-mesmerizing reactions to the unceasing stream of propaganda projected from the psychiatry-Pharma-NIMH complex.

Conclusion

In medicine, first-person complaints and/or third-person observation of the body or behaviour can serve as a *clue* to further investigation and diagnosis based on physical evidence (McHugh and Slavney 1988). In psychiatry, in the realm of primary mental disorders, first-person complaints and third-person observations (of social behaviour, which are actually interpretations) only lead to further talk in so far as diagnosis (what is the matter?) is concerned. It is misleading, not to say a farce, to call what occurs between psychiatrist and patient a medical encounter once actual medical disease has been ruled out on the basis of physical examination and negative physical evidence. The psychiatrist as a physician can prescribe drugs, but even if the drugs bring about a certain amount of relief from some features of the patient's complaints without too great a cost in physical and psychosocial adverse effects, this does not show that a genuine medical condition was the problem in the first place (Moncrieff 2009). It would be a somewhat different matter if psychiatric drugs were actually curative, but this is not the case (a frank admission of this can be found in a 2009 paper by the current head of NIMH, Thomas Insel); indeed it is not even the case that psychiatric drugs routinely outperform placebo in industry-controlled drug treatment studies, despite industry control of all aspects of the study, including interpretation of outcome data. This is not even to mention adverse drug effects. I cannot emphasize too strongly that adverse drug effects are not the focus of psychiatric drug treatment studies and are given short shrift (see Jacobs and Cohen 1999). In the absence of positive physical evidence that the patient's problem is really a medical condition, calling and treating the patient's difficulties a medical condition invalidates the person *as such* and should be considered a form of violence. This form of violence has become accepted as normal in American society. The consequences of invalidating the person qua person are limitless.

Think of depicting a bereaved patient's problem without reference to the patient's loss and without including any information concerning the nature, quality, and importance of the relationship between the patient and the deceased as far as the patient is concerned and what it means to the bereaved patient that the deceased is gone. This is not even a parody of the official line the APA has taken to grasping the patient's problem (i.e., a symptoms-only formulation of the patient's problem). It is true that Axis IV exists, but its use is officially optional (*DSM-IV-TR:* 27–37), the patient's history beyond one year ago is regarded as usually irrelevant, and finally and most importantly, the overall point of the manual is to advance the idea that mental disorders are impersonal medical conditions, albeit idiopathic medical conditions (see the definition of primary mental disorders). Although Axis IV continues to be included in the manual, psychogenesis was officially banned beginning with *DSM-IV*, which sends a clear message concerning the importance of psychosocial history-taking, as does the fact that Axis IV is optional. The person is considered the host of an idiopathic medical condition that announces its presence exclusively via behavioral symptoms (that is, complaints of psychological distress and/or troubling or disappointing social behavior). Considerations that would ordinarily pertain to understanding a person's thinking, feeling, and behavior are considered irrelevant because psychiatry is medicine and identifies and treats medical conditions. Meanwhile all disorders unique to psychiatry are identified without benefit of biological information or evidence of any kind. Nothing of a non-linguistic, non- interpretive nature has any bearing whatsoever on psychiatric diagnosis. Yet patients are informed they are suffering from a genuine medical illness and prescribed drugs in the spirit of being directly treated via drugs for what is really the matter with them as opposed to some narrative that is much closer to the truth. When adversity is acknowledged, as in PTSD and Adjustment Disorder, the distressed person is considered literally mentally disordered *because* she is distressed. It makes sense in medicine to see persistent bodily distress or functional disability as disorder, but discussion of the individual as a person must recognize that a person is responsive to important developments in his life as he sees it. Evaluations such as whether or not a tragedy has occurred and what feelings and behaviors tragedy does and does not entitle a person to are ad hoc moral-interpretive evaluations, not medical science. Medical reasoning cannot sensibly be applied to discussion of a person per se. The realm of person discussion cannot be replaced with medical reasoning. Pretending it can on the basis of a combination of professional self-interest, profit seeking, and political expediency can be called Lysenkoism.

Is there any hope for reform? As I write this chapter there is widespread lay and professional dismay and alarm concerning various *DSM*-5 Task Force recommendations. Numerous professional mental health organizations are threatening to boycott *DSM*-5 (this is actually practicable because by treaty the International Classification of Diseases trumps the *DSM*, although I don't think most mental health professionals realize this). The Chair of the *DSM-IV* Task Force, Allen Frances, has publically opined (as part of his larger mea culpa, as I see it), that the APA can no longer be trusted to be the official owner of psychiatric diagnosis in America. He has not come right out and said that the APA has been purchased by the pharmaceutical industry (although numerous others have), but he keeps making the point that *DSM-5* Task Force recommendations will create a new bonanza for the pharmaceutical industry while putting many people in danger. Reform is not in the interests of the major players in the mental health industry. This means that reform can only be brought about by persistent pressure, threat, and disruption from below, i.e., from the vast majority of mental health professionals who are not psychiatrists and who presumably do not have a vested interest in medical dominance of the mental health industry. Is there any possibility that the present widespread disaffection with how the APA is handling its *de facto* mandate to create an official diagnostic manual for everyone else will persist and develop once *DSM-5* is published in 2013? The historical record shows that the non-medical mental health professions have been content to permit an organization whose interests are undisguisedly self-promoting to call the shots for the entire industry. This is probably based on the fact that everyone wants to bill medical insurance and the insurance industry is not likely to turn to non-physicians to create an official system of *medical* diagnosis. Is there a way out of this? A way out will only materialize if there is sufficient pressure from below. The outlook is dim but large changes do occur when widespread disaffection passes a certain threshold.

References

Cohen, D. and Jacobs, D.H. 2010. Randomized controlled trials of antidepressants: Clinically and scientifically irrelevant. *The Journal of Mind and Behavior, 31*, 1–22.

Healy, D. 2000. The assessment of outcome in depression. *Reviews in Contemporary Pharmacotherapy, 11*, 295–301.

Healy, D. 2012. *Pharmageddon.* Berkeley: University of California Press.

Insel, T.R. 2009. Disruptive insights in psychiatry. *Journal of Clinical Investigation, 119*, 700–705.

Jacobs, D.H. 1995. Psychiatric drugging. *The Journal of Mind and Behavior, 16*, 421–470.

Jacobs, D.H. 2010. Is there really mental disorder? *The Humanistic Psychologist, 38*, 355–374.

Jacobs, D.H. and Cohen, D. 1999. What is really known about psychological alterations produced by psychiatric drugs? *International Journal of Risk and Safety in Medicine, 12*, 37–47.

Jacobs, D. H. and Cohen, D. 2010. The make-believe world of antidepressant randomized controlled trials. *The Journal of Mind and Behavior, 31*, 23–36.

McHugh, P.R. and Slavney, P. 1998. *The Perspectives of Psychiatry.* Baltimore: Johns Hopkins University Press.

Mayes, R. and Horwitz, A.V. 2005. DSM-III and the revolution in the classification of mental illness. *Journal of the History of the Behavioral Sciences, 41*, 249–267.

Moncrieff, J. 2008. *The Myth of the Chemical Cure.* London: Palgrave.

Spitzer, R.L. and Williams, J.B.W. (1994). Letter to the editor. *American Journal of Psychiatry, 151*, 459–460.

Wilson, M. 1993. DSM-III and the transformation of American psychiatry: A history. *American Journal of Psychiatry, 150*(3), 399–410.

Zimmerman, M. and Spitzer, R. 2005. Psychiatric classification. In B.J. Sadock and V.A. Sadock (Eds). *Comprehensive Textbook of Psychiatry*. Philadelphia, PA: Lippincott, Williams, & Wilkins, 1003–1033.

Chapter 17

The Evolution of Sex Offender Treatment: From Confinement to Consent

Natasha M. Knack and J. Paul Fedoroff

Introduction

The severe and lasting harm that results from the commission of sexual offenses makes the control and management of sexual offenders (SOs) a societal priority. Despite evidence that current treatments are effective, debate continues about whether the benefits of treatment surpass those of incarceration and/or incapacitation. In this chapter we argue that any controversy about treatment effectiveness is neither a reasonable justification for abandoning efforts to treat, nor an indication that SOs are untreatable. This is especially true when one considers that many of these controversies are based on studies using single cases, outdated treatments, or interventions that do not match the specific needs of individual SOs. Controversy about treatment effectiveness may be unrelated to the specific treatment interventions being studied, and instead may be due to inconsistent or inappropriate research methodologies. An important concern is whether incarceration assists or impedes the treatment of SOs. Although some research has found that correctional treatments can lead to a reduction in recidivism, there are multiple ethical and practical issues regarding treatment provided to SOs while in custody. Finally, we suggest that current management strategies used with SOs released into the community, including sex offender registries, parole/probation conditions, and residency restrictions, invoke ethically questionable practices that may cause some of these interventions to be more problematic than protective.

This chapter includes a brief summary of the various treatments currently used with SOs and a review of how these have evolved. It will then discuss some of the most prevalent myths about SOs, and how these myths, along with ineffective treatment interventions and inappropriate research methodologies, have played a role in diminishing the apparent efficacy of SO treatments. The chapter also includes a critical analysis of the ethical and practical issues involved in providing treatment for SOs in correctional versus community settings, as well as concerns about coercive and mandated treatment interventions. Finally, the community management strategies currently used with SOs will be reviewed and potential problems with these strategies will be explored. The overall aim of this chapter is to critically analyze SO treatment interventions and their effectiveness in order to determine why the literature on this topic is so inconsistent, as well as draw attention to issues that treatment providers and correctional staff working with SOs should address.

Evolution of Treatment Interventions

Due to changing perspectives on the causes of problematic sexual interests and behaviors, as well as the availability of new therapies for these problems, the treatment of SOs has evolved substantially. The four most well-known perspectives on the causes of problematic sexual interests include the disease, behavioral, dimensional, and life-story perspectives (see Fedoroff 2009 for a review). The behavioral and dimensional perspectives are especially important in the evolution of SO treatment because they provided explanations for sexual disorders that are not based solely on the presence of a disease, and therefore opened the door for non-medical treatment interventions for this population. In the 1930s, treatments for SOs were often based on psychoanalytic theory, which was the predominant theory of the era (Brooks-Gordon, Bilby, and Wells 2006). In the 1950s, when behavioral therapies were gaining prominence, SO treatments began to incorporate new approaches such as operant conditioning and other learning-based approaches (Dollard and Miller 1950). While behavioral therapies were likely more effective than psychoanalytic treatments, by definition they focused primarily on behaviors and therefore overlooked important factors such as SOs' phenomenological experiences and self-perceived explanations for their problems. It was not until the mid-1970s that treatment programs for SOs started to acknowledge these other fundamental issues, and began to integrate pre-existing approaches with established treatments for concurrent problems such as substance abuse, sexual dysfunction, social skills deficits, anger, and a variety of other mental health issues (Marshall et al. 1991).

Cognitive therapy, which was introduced in the 1970s, added a new aspect to SO treatment by attending to the thoughts that preceded problematic behaviors, rather than just the behaviors themselves (Mandeville-Norden and Beech 2004). Since the establishment of CBT programs, this approach has become the most commonly used treatment for SOs (Conroy 2006) and has been shown to be one of the most empirically supported therapies for reducing recidivism in SOs (Prescott and Levenson 2010). In the quest to find the most effective treatments for SOs, CBT has sometimes been combined with hormonal therapies such as anti-androgen medications and gonadotropin releasing hormone (GnRH) analogues. The use of hormonal therapies is often referred to as "chemical castration," as these medications lead to a decrease in testosterone and are associated with a reduction of sexual fantasies and urges. The effects of chemical castration are reversible once the hormonal therapies are discontinued. In contrast, surgical castration involves surgically removing a man's testes, and was first used to diminish sexual urges in SOs in the 1800s by Dr. Harry Sharp (Scott and Holmberg 2003). Unlike chemical castration, surgical castration is irreversible. Despite the availability of hormonal therapies, as of 2006, surgical castration was still offered in four American states (California, Florida, Louisiana, and Texas) (Norman-Eady 2006).

While the first reported use of hormonal therapy to treat sexual behaviors was in 1944 (Scott and Holmberg 2003), it was not until the 1960s that psychiatrists began more frequently prescribing medications such as medroxyprogesterone acetate (MPA) and cyproterone acetate (CPA) to their patients (CPA is not available in the United States but is used in Canada and Europe) (Codispoti 2008). Since the 1960s, new hormonal treatments have been found to be effective with SO populations, leading to the increased use of these treatments. In fact, some US states have even enacted legislation that allows the courts to include chemical castration, as well as voluntary surgical castration, into the judicial sentences of certain SOs (Scott and Holmberg 2003, Norman-Eady 2006). This ethically questionable practice is prohibited in Canada, where the courts are not permitted to sentence offenders to any specific forms of treatment, since they do not have medical licenses and cannot prescribe medications. Other studies have found that Selective Serotonin Reuptake Inhibitors (SSRIs, usually combined with psychotherapy) can be an effective treatment for SOs, and are thought to work by treating co-morbid problems such as depression, anxiety, and obsessive compulsive disorder (Conroy 2006). One of the newest approaches to the treatment of SOs is the Good Lives Model (GLM), first described in a publication by Tony Ward in 2002. The GLM is based on the concepts of primary goods (basic human needs) and secondary goods (means to secure primary goods) (Willis and Grace 2008). SOs are thought to have the same primary goods as the rest of humanity, but for one reason or another, these individuals use inappropriate and often unacceptable (morally and/or legally) methods to obtain these goals (Wormith et al. 2007). Treatments using the GLM aim to change problematic methods by ensuring that SOs are provided with the necessary information, resources, and social skills, to satisfy their primary needs through pro-social secondary goods. An important theme of GLM therapies is an emphasis on fostering positive features as opposed to simply attempting to suppress negative ones. For a comprehensive review of SO treatments, see Murphy, Bradford and Fedoroff (in press).

Myths about Sex Offenders

The myths and assumptions about people who commit sexual offenses are not only prevalent and extremely condemning of anyone labeled as an SO, it is possible they may have influenced the approaches to treating this population (see Fedoroff 1997 for a review of SO myths). One of the most problematic generalizations about SOs is that they are all the same, with similar motivations for sexually offending. It is therefore assumed that all SOs will respond the same way, to the same treatment(s). Assumptions like these have contributed to the adoption of a "one size fits all" treatment approach for this population. However, SOs are actually very heterogeneous, with a wide range of mental health issues, sexual interests, motivations, and lifestyle issues. Therefore, treatment interventions should be specialized for SO populations in general, as well as designed to focus on the individual offender's specific needs (Baerga-Buffler and Johnson 2006). The false assumption that all SOs are incorrigible, 'dangerous monsters' who are unable and/or unwilling to control their sexual desires may explain why incarceration has often been favored over treatment (Roseman et al. 2008). The decision to incarcerate may also be related to the unverified belief that all SOs will reoffend. In reality, even without treatment, the majority of SOs are not known to reoffend, especially first-time offenders (Cowburn 2005). Based on the mistaken belief that all SOs will reoffend, it is not surprising there is also an assumption that treatment for SOs is ineffective, and that this population will only accept treatment if it is forced upon them. While the results of treatment effectiveness are mixed, there is substantial evidence that treatment programs specifically designed for SOs can lead to lower recidivism rates (Lösel and Schmucker 2005). Furthermore, despite the belief that SOs require external motivation to enter treatment, it has been found that many SOs voluntarily seek treatment, and SOs' self-reports indicate they find treatment helpful (Prescott and Levenson 2010).

Germany's Prevention Project Dunkelfeld (PPD) is an example of SOs and people with problematic sexual interests seeking treatment, in spite of the lack of any legal coercion to do so. PPD is a Berlin-based program that uses mass advertising to encourage people with problematic sexual interests to seek treatment before they have offended, or been charged, or convicted. Initial reports from the PPD initiative have shown that an average of 15–20 people per month travelled to Berlin for the program, resulting in a total of more than 800 people seeking treatment independent of any legal coercion (Beier et al. 2009). The Sexual Behaviors Clinic (SBC) at The Royal in Ottawa, Canada, also treats individuals who have never offended, or who have never been charged or convicted of a sexual offense. The number of people who have self-referred to the SBC, in order to get help for their problematic sexual interests before offending, continues to rise. It seems that the real problem may not be that SOs don't want help, but that they are not sure how or where to get it, or that they fear the legal consequences of admitting their deviant sexual interests. A survey of people who self-identified as being attracted to minors found that 40% (n=159) of participants stated that they wanted treatment for this issue, but did not seek it out due to fears that they would be misunderstood (85%), treated with disrespect (54%), or that the treatment provider would be judgmental (63%), unethical (46%), or not respect confidentiality (51%) (Testa and West 2010). Together, these findings suggest that the reason many SOs and people with problematic sexual interests do not seek treatment may be due to the fact that they fear the implications of disclosing their sexual interests or behaviors. Primary prevention of sexual offenses and development of non-criminal sexual interests and behaviors are the ultimate treatment goals for this population. Further efforts to correctly amend SO treatment programs in order to achieve and verify these aims seem more prudent than simply locking up SOs until they are re-released into the community, along with the false message that they are untreatable and certain to reoffend.

The Debate over Treatment Effectiveness

In spite of the continued downward trend in the prevalence of sex offences and SO recidivism (Brennan 2012, Department of Justice 2012), some studies on treatment effectiveness show mixed results (Lösel and Schmucker 2005). There are many possible explanations for these findings that have little to do with the treatment approach itself. The varieties of treatments for SOs are considerable in number, and even within a specific type of intervention, there is a broad range of available therapeutic tools and techniques (Bilby, Brooks-Gordon and Wells 2006). Multiple studies have suggested that only treatment programs designed to specifically target the specific needs of individual SOs will significantly affect recidivism (Lösel and Schmucker 2005).

Treatment programs that use similar interventions for all different subtypes of SOs (i.e. rapists, child molesters, etc.) rather than acknowledge and address the distinct needs and motivations of these diverse groups, may have also influenced the debate over the effectiveness of SO treatment. Despite the well-accepted finding that treatment programs for SOs must be specially designed in order to be effective, multiple studies have shown that SO treatment programs are actively targeting factors that have been found to be *unrelated* to recidivism. For example, empathy for victims and denial of the offense are two dynamic factors that are often addressed in SO treatment programs, despite findings from multiple studies indicating that these issues do not predict recidivism (Conroy 2006). A meta-analysis of SO recidivism rates found that many of the elements that treatment programs often focus on actually have little, if any, correlation with sexual recidivism (Hanson and Morton-Bourgon 2005). The treatment provider also plays an important role in whether the treatment intervention will be effective, with studies showing that 25% of the variance in CBT treatment effectiveness can be attributed to the strength of the therapeutic relationship between the patient and the treatment provider (Collins and Nee 2010). This is consistent with research by Grady and Brodersen (2008), which reviewed five qualitative studies examining the personal perspectives of SOs in treatment and found that in all five studies, participants considered the therapeutic alliance to be one of the most important aspects of the program.

In addition to the influence of individual treatment programs and therapists, the debate around treatment effectiveness for SOs is also thought to be influenced by factors that are unrelated to the actual treatment interventions. These factors involve disparities in the research studies themselves, most commonly resulting from inconsistencies in research methodologies. Recidivism is frequently used to evaluate the success of a treatment program, and may be based on sexual, violent, or general (any) recidivism. Using recidivism as a measure of treatment effectiveness can be problematic, as "recidivism is a unified concept without a unified definition" (Wormith et al. 2007: 880). For research purposes, the term "recidivism" can encompass a broad range of definitions, including arrests with or without subsequent convictions, re-incarcerations, convictions for new offenses, or violations of probation or parole conditions. The definition of recidivism that researchers select for their particular studies can lead to a substantial variation in the study results, due to the considerable differences that exist between the rates of re-arrest versus re-convictions for SOs (Schneider et al. 2006). Using rates of re-arrest without conviction or certain parole/probation violations (such as failure to abstain from alcohol) to assess SO treatment programs is misleading, and may result in furthering the assumption that SOs cannot be effectively treated. Similarly, recidivism studies that combine both sexual and non-sexual re-offenses may overestimate recidivism rates for this population, again supporting the assumptions that treatment is not effective and that SOs have high rates of recidivism. Moreover, recidivism data typically does not take into account the severity of the re-offense, making it difficult to determine if SO treatment reduces the severity of the offenses, even if it does not completely prevent them.

Studies that examine SOs as one large homogeneous group, rather than distinct subtypes comprised of diverse individuals, may be unreliable as they result in generalized recidivism rates for anyone labeled as a SO, despite their specific offense or diagnosis. These studies simultaneously preclude true ascertainment of overall treatment effects, as well as make it difficult to identify which subtypes are truly at a high risk for recidivism (Schneider et al. 2006). Another issue related to research on SO treatments involves the period when the studies were conducted, and the length of time that SOs were followed up in the community. One of the explanations for the continuing controversy about treatment effectiveness likely results from when the research was conducted, and the treatment interventions that were in use during the timeframe covered by the particular study. Considering that more modern treatment approaches, such as CBT, are commonly found to be more effective for treating SOs than older approaches (some of which are now obsolete), it is not surprising that studies conducted at different times differ in terms of apparent efficacy (Wormith et al. 2007). Therefore, it is possible that the debate over whether or not treatment is effective for SOs is actually a reflection of two underlying issues: *what* treatments are effective and specifically *who* are they effective for?

Prison-Based Treatment versus Community-Based Treatment

Most convicted SOs are incarcerated for at least part of their sentence, with SOs representing almost one quarter of the entire population of state prisoners in the United States (McGrath et al. 2003). In Canada, the number of federally incarcerated SOs increased approximately 50% between 1990 and 1995 (John Howard Society 1997). While studies on the effectiveness of prison-based treatments for SOs have been conflicting, some older studies have reported positive findings (see Polizzi, MacKenzie, and Hickman 1999 for a review). However, a more recent review by Brooks-Gordon et al. (2006) evaluated nine randomized control trials to determine the effectiveness of psychological interventions for SOs, and concluded that although there are indications that prison-based approaches may be promising for treating SOs, there was insufficient evidence to establish this finding with certainty.

One problem arising in the treatment of incarcerated SOs is that "truly voluntary participation does not exist in the criminal justice system because there is always some degree of external pressure" (Parhar et al. 2008: 1111). For example, SOs may feel coerced into treatment if their participation could lead to a reduction in the length or severity of their sentence, or result in increased privileges while incarcerated. This may have serious implications for treating SOs, especially considering that a meta-analysis of studies examining general offenders found that both coerced and mandated treatments in custodial settings had no effect on recidivism (Parhar et al. 2008). In addition to the inherently coercive nature of custodial settings, prison-based treatment programs also operate within environments that strip individuals of their rights and freedoms, and are replete with conflicting messages, as well as tensions between punishment and treatment goals. James Waldram (2008) provides an apt description of the underlying conflicts faced by SOs receiving prison-based treatment: "They remain 'inmates' even while undergoing treatment as 'patients' and their everyday interactions with inmates from other units during common recreational periods exists as a constant reminder that they are the lowest of the low" (pp. 423–424).

Incarcerated SOs must interact with correctional staff members, who may exhibit inconsistent beliefs about SOs, resulting in SOs being treated differently by various prison employees. A recent survey of Correctional Service Canada (CSC) employees (from prison guards to policy makers) contained a question regarding "treating offenders with respect as human beings," which actually had to be dropped from the survey's end results due to substantial discrepancy among the 2200 participant responses (Campbell 2013). The final results of this survey indicate that CSC employees may have significantly different beliefs with regard to respecting offenders and, "without proper training, employees rely on what is deeply ingrained in their beliefs to mould how they treat offenders" (Campbell 2013: 1). Incarcerated SOs must undergo treatment in an atmosphere that clearly values security over rehabilitation (Collins and Nee 2010). For example, it can be extremely difficult for therapists to treat incarcerated SOs, since their movement within the facility may be controlled by prison guards, and they may be subject to strictly planned time schedules or lock-down conditions. The physical layout and décor of correctional settings are rarely based on what would be appropriate for efficacious interventions, and these environments often fail to provide safe and therapeutic environments (Schneider et al. 2006). SOs may also be hesitant to reveal their offense(s) due to fear that they will be overheard or exposed, since becoming known as an SO (especially a child molester) can lead to being downgraded even lower in the prison hierarchy, and may also result in threats or physical injuries. Finally, there is something problematic and hypocritical about treatment programs that emphasize the necessity of consent within an inherently coercive and non-consensual environment. Based on this information, it is not surprising that correctional environments are not typically found to be mentally healthy environments (Schneider et al. 2006).

A qualitative study by Hudson (2005), which used interviews with incarcerated SOs to obtain participants' perspectives on treatment, found that due to feeling pressured to conform to treatment program models, as well as feeling unable to voice opposing opinions, some participants simply learned the responses that treatment providers wanted to hear rather than making any intrinsic changes. These results are consistent with findings from Waldram's (2007) qualitative study on SOs in a prison-based treatment facility. Drapeau et al. (2005) also conducted interviews with incarcerated SOs and found that participants reported that they were likely to disengage with therapy if they perceived themselves to be unsafe or unsupported in the treatment process. A review of five qualitative studies examining offenders' subjective perspectives, including the studies by Hudson (2005) and Drapeau et al. (2005), concluded that the program content used in treatment interventions for SOs may actually be less important than the climate in which it is provided (Grady and Brodersen 2008). This review also found that the role of peers is meaningful for the treatment of SOs. This is consistent with research by Hanson and Harris (2000), which found that SOs who reoffended had significantly fewer positive peer relationships in their life, and more negative peer relationships than did non-recidivists (Willis and Grace 2008). Based on these findings, and on the fact that studies have consistently shown that antisocial peer relationships are associated with general recidivism, the fact that incarcerated SOs have only other convicted offenders as their peers could result in an increase in their overall criminality, as well as increase their risk of sexual recidivism (Willis and Grace 2008).

It may also be an issue that prison-based treatment programs rarely give much thought to what happens to SOs once they are released from custody. Considering that substance abuse, as well as physical and mental health problems, have consistently been found to be overrepresented in prison populations, it is rational to assume that offenders who are released into the community without being connected to appropriate resources for these issues are more likely to reoffend. It also seems reasonable that for SOs to become pro-social, functioning members of society, they need access to suitable accommodation and gainful employment. In fact, employment has not only been found to be an important aspect of community integration (Alexander 2010), a meta-analysis by Hanson and Morton-Bourgon (2005) identified employment instability as a significant risk factor for sexual recidivism.

Unfortunately, many SOs have extreme difficulty finding accommodation and employment after they are released due to their criminal records, stigmatization if their offenses are known, and various forms of correctional SO management (e.g. conditions, SO registries). Clearly, it is extremely difficult for SOs to reintegrate into society after they are released, and it is possible that including reintegration plans in prison-based treatment programs may help in reducing recidivism rates for this population. In order to determine the effect of reintegration planning on sexual recidivism, Willis and Grace (2008) conducted a retrospective study comparing the file information of 39 child molesters who had reoffended after participating in a specialized prison-based treatment program in New Zealand, with a group of 42 non-recidivists matched on static risk level and release date. They found that the mean scores for reintegration planning were significantly higher for the non-recidivists with regards to the specific issues of accommodation, employment, and secondary goods (as identified by the Good Lives Model); however, these results were no longer significant when controlling for the influence of IQ and overall deviance. Nonetheless, these results suggest that reintegration planning may play a role in preventing sexual re-offenses and indicates an important area for future research.

While incarceration for these offences is an effective punitive measure, research and clinical initiatives have shown that it is often not a sufficiently effective method to prevent initial or recurrent child sexual abuse (Farkas and Stichman 2002). Furthermore, incarceration is often a rather short-term solution. In his study of federally incarcerated sexual offenders, Waldram (2007) found that the average sentence length for sexual assault (on women or children) was between three to six years. Consequently, it is important that community-based treatment programs are available for SOs released from incarceration, as well as for offenders who are given community sentences and individuals with problematic sexual interests who have never offended or never been convicted (Wormith et al. 2007). Even more important is that these treatment programs are effective in reducing recidivism for those SOs who are residing in the community. A meta-analysis of treatment effectiveness for SOs by Lösel and Schmucker (2005) found outpatient programs had larger treatment effects than programs administered in correctional settings, and determined that the outcome of a program is at least partly dependent on the context in which treatment is delivered. These findings are consistent with a review of psychological interventions for SOs by Brooks-Gordon et al. (2006), which concluded that community-based treatment programs are effective in reducing recidivism for this population.

Compared to prison-based approaches, fewer ethical and procedural issues appear to surround community-based treatment programs for SOs. However, a community-based approach to treating this population does have its own difficulties. For example, it is possible that SOs in the community may still be coerced or mandated to attend treatment, whether through the courts as part of sentencing, as a condition of probation/parole, or due to other external pressures such as that from family and friends. Glaser (2003) asserts that, "most sex offender treatment programs are administered as specific components of punishment ordered by a court, parole board, or similar body" (p. 144). While we do not necessarily agree that these agencies are intending to further punish those who have sexually offended, we do believe it is possible that SOs who are mandated to attend community-based treatments may perceive this as a continuation of their punishment. Consequently, it is important that therapists providing treatment in the community not only strive to gain the trust of their clients in order to develop a therapeutic relationship, they should also help SOs to understand the true role of treatment in their recovery and how it is different from punishment. One review of general offender populations found that, unlike prison-based programs, community-based treatments were effective in reducing recidivism despite the presence of coercion (Parhar et al. 2008). The same review also discusses the idea that offenders are likely to perceive custodial settings as more coercive than community settings, despite the actual degree of coercion. This indicates that attending a community-based treatment program may be associated with greater levels of perceived personal choice and freedom compared to attending prison-based treatment programs, even if the community-based treatment is also mandated. Therapists in these settings have an advantage if they can link personal choice to personal responsibility.

Some community-based programs are entirely voluntary, such as Circles of Support and Accountability (CoSA). CoSA is intended for SOs released from federal penitentiaries, and operates by assigning three to five trained volunteers to a released SO (referred to as a 'Core Member'), and having these volunteers regularly meet with their Core Member in various places in the community, such as a coffee shop (John Howard Society 1997). Volunteers are given the necessary skills to assist their Core Member with community reintegration (e.g. finding employment/ accommodation), solving everyday problems, as well as challenging the Core Member's offense-related beliefs and actions, while still providing emotional support and acknowledging successes (CoSA Website). Problems with the CoSA model can theoretically arise when the volunteers attempt to move from the role of providing community support and begin acting as the Core Member's therapist or probation officer, despite their lack of training in these areas. Problems can also arise if CoSA volunteers become employed with Correctional Services Canada (CSC) or other agencies that would put them into a dual role. The concept of dual roles essentially refers to one person having obligations toward two different individuals or agencies, which may have contradictory intentions or goals. Dual roles are likely quite common in community-based treatments, and may lead to unethical interventions for SOs. For example, consider a SO who, as part of his probation, must see a psychologist employed by Correctional Services Canada. Psychologists in this position are in a dual role, since on the one hand they are treatment providers with standard obligations to their patients, but at the same time they are employees of CSC, with obligations to protect the community at all costs. Other problems with community-based treatment include treatment compliance and access to services. Outpatient SOs with serious mental illnesses or developmental delays may have difficulty remembering to keep their appointments or may not be able to access the mental health and social services that they need due to their living situations.

Issues Involving Sex-Offender Management

Due to the severe and potential lifelong harm that can result from sexual offenses, it is understandable that SOs released into the community must adhere to conditions and regulations, which are intended to help protect the community (and the offender) by helping to prevent reoffending. Strategies used to manage SOs in the community include parole/probation conditions, sex-offender registries, and residency restrictions. Taken at face value, these strategies appear to be useful for community protection; however, closer examination indicates that they may also inadvertently hinder the successful reintegration of SOs. Considering that SOs are already one of the most marginalized groups in society, who are likely to have difficulties with reintegration simply due to severe stigmatization, inappropriate management strategies could actually become a risk factor for recidivism. As Ward (2007) points out, "current policies and legislation continue to further ostracize and demonize sex offenders" (as cited in Grady and Brodersen 2008: 342).

Parole and probation conditions are rules that are placed on offenders once they are released into the community as part of a conditional sentence. We believe that some conditions can actually be useful, as they may help SOs avoid places and situations that could result in recidivism, or that others may perceive as leading to reoffending. The ideal set of conditions would be those which, after being removed, do not result in significant changes to an individual's daily routine. However, certain conditions can be extremely difficult for SOs to live with, considering that some conditions can impact the ability to secure gainful employment (e.g. no Internet access) or acquire suitable accommodation (e.g. cannot live near schools, parks, daycares, etc.). In Texas, SOs released into outpatient community treatment programs are regularly given 97 conditions, making it the state with the largest number of standard conditions for SOs (Conroy 2006). Although 97 seems like an especially high number, SOs are often given a large number of conditions as part of their probation or parole, and having these many conditions may be confusing for some SOs (especially those who are illiterate), and could result in an accidental breach. One of the reasons for the high number of conditions placed on SOs may be that courts have a predetermined list of conditions that are applied to anyone labeled an SO, regardless of the specific details of their offense. This would explain why some conditions seem irrelevant, such as weapons bans for SOs who have never owned/used a weapon, while others seem quite illogical, such as hands-on offenders with Internet bans and child pornography offenders who are allowed to freely access the Internet. Considering that being banned from using the Internet seems to be one of the most common and most challenging conditions, it is interesting to note that the Internet was recently declared an essential service in Germany (Hudson 2013). Finally, parole and probation conditions are often extremely vague, and thus may result in significantly different interpretations depending on who is doing the interpreting (e.g. police vs. parole/probations officers).

In Canada, sex offender registries (SORs) require convicted SOs to register their address annually, as well as when they move, and also to alert the authorities if they will be out of town for a certain period of time. It is interesting to note that registries do not exist for any other types of crime, despite the extreme violence associated with other offenses such as murder and assault. This may be due, in part, to the myths examined at the beginning of this chapter, such as the assumption that all SOs will reoffend. Individuals on the SOR receive annual visits from police officers in order to ensure that they are living at their specified address. In order to avoid identifying, and consequently stigmatizing SOs, police officers who conduct these home visits are advised to do so in plain clothes and with an unmarked car. However, despite this advice, SOs continue to report that police officers come to their homes or places of employment in uniform, sometimes leading to these individuals being questioned by their housemates, neighbors, or employers. SORs are very different in Canada compared to the U.S. In the U.S., Megan's Law was enacted in 1996, making it possible for anyone in the community to obtain personal information on registered SOs, often through public access websites, or notifications through local media outlets (Office of the Attorney General 2004). Despite the belief that public SORs protect the community, research has found that public registries and notification laws have had little to no impact on SOs overall recidivism rates, which continue to be higher in the U.S. compared to Canada, where SORs are private and can only be accessed by specific criminal justice officials (Murphy, Fedoroff, and Martineau 2009a). Public SORs also seem to enhance a self-fulfilling prophesy based on the belief that SOs will be non-compliant with registration laws, which often results in these individuals going 'underground' and thus losing contact with the criminal justice system. In 2000, an estimated 40% of SOs in Iowa were supposed to be on the SOR but were not, and in 2003, California reported that it had 'lost track' of 44% of SOs who were supposed to be on it (Murphy et al. 2009b). In comparison, SORs in Canada have a compliance rate of approximately 95% (Murphy et al. 2009b). A final issue with SORs is that some SOs are required to register for life, which supports the assumption that SOs never change, even if they receive treatment.

Residency restrictions (RRs) may be the most problematic of all the management strategies, as many SOs have a hard time finding suitable and affordable accommodation that meet these restrictions. As of 2010, RRs had been enacted in 30 states (Prescott and Levenson 2010) and in Canada they are encompassed in a prohibition order (i.e. a 161 Order) that is given to most SOs, preventing them from attending places where there is a reasonable assumption that children will be present. The severity of RRs in the U.S. has resulted in many SOs becoming homeless, or forced to live in inhumane conditions. For example, many SOs in Miami, Florida, have no choice but to live under bridges, as the majority of other housing options are within areas restricted to them (Prescott and Levenson 2010). Similarly, in Southampton, New York., 40 SOs are currently being housed in two trailers, each with a fridge, stove, and bunk beds, but with only one shower for all 40 men to share (the trailer did not even have a shower until 2010) (Schwirtz 2013). These living conditions do not seem to be conducive to successful reintegration, nor to mental and emotional wellbeing. Furthermore, RRs can actually prevent SOs from moving in with supportive family members (Willis and Grace 2008), or may force the families of SOs to uproot and relocate if they want to stay together. RRs may also require SOs to live in remote areas, making it difficult, if not impossible, to access the social services and treatment resources that they require. Finally, it is well-established in the literature that sexual offenses are most often committed by someone known to the victim and RRs do nothing to protect incest victims or prevent offences against someone already known to the offender. Although some measure of controlling where SOs live may be warranted, even Laura Ahearn, the executive director of Parents for Megan's Law and Crime Victims Center, stated, "When you propose a law restricting sex offenders to 1000 feet from any bus stop, that's just not going to work. You have to be reasonable" (Schwirtz 2013: 1).

Conclusion

Myths about SOs, including the belief that they are homogeneous and will all reoffend, may have played a role in the development of treatment interventions that are ineffective for this population. These ineffective treatments, along with inconsistent and sometimes flawed study methodologies, have likely contributed to the idea that SOs cannot change, consequently leading to false expectations. An especially controversial aspect of this issue concerns the effectiveness of prison-based and/or coercive treatment interventions for SOs. However, even if these interventions are successful in reducing recidivism in SOs, many ethical and practical issues make coercive and correctional-based treatments problematic. This is also true for SO management strategies. While some of the current strategies may help to protect the community, as well as the SO, they can also result in SOs being stigmatized, ostracized, and forced to contend with significant barriers to successful reintegration.

Since all sex crimes involve breach of consent, it seems reasonable that effective treatments will be based on consent. The issue of consent is a problem for treatment interventions offered to SOs who are in custody, and even to those on probation and parole. It is especially problematic for therapists who have a dual role, requesting the SO to be honest about problems, for example, while also reporting possible breaches. One solution to this problem has been adopted by the SBC. SBC therapists report only legally mandated issues (e.g. potential harm to an identifiable child) but not other issues that can be dealt with in therapy (e.g. an urge to resume using illegal drugs). By modeling scrupulous respect for consent, therapists can demonstrate to SOs why it is important, and how valuing consent can actually improve their everyday lives and relationships.

Despite the plethora of research on SOs, many areas still warrant further investigation, such as the impact of environment on treatment effectiveness, and whether some management strategies actually increase risk of recidivism by preventing successful reintegration. With regard to treatment, interventions for this population need to move toward primary prevention, which would eliminate the problems associated with correctional-based treatment programs. In order for SO treatments to evolve successfully, researchers and treatment providers in this field must strive to correct the mistaken beliefs about SOs, as it seems unlikely that future interventions will be more effective if they continue to be based on myths and incorrect assumptions.

References

Alexander, R. 2010. Collaborative supervision strategies for sex offender community management. *Federal Probation, 74*, 16–19.

Baerga-Buffler, M. and Johnson, J.L. 2006. Sex offender management in the federal probation and pretrial services system. *Department of Justice Press Release.*

Beier, K.M., Neutze, J., Mundt, I.A., Ahlers, C.J., Goecker, D., Konrad, A., and Schaefer, G.A. 2009. Encouraging self-identified pedophiles and hebephiles to seek professional help: First results of the Prevention Project Dunkelfeld (PPD). *Child Abuse & Neglect, 33*, 545–549.

Bilby, C., Brooks-Gordon, B., and Wells, H. 2006. A systematic review of psychological interventions for sexual offenders II: Quasi-experimental and qualitative data. *The Journal of Forensic Psychiatry & Psychology, 17*, 467–484.

Brennan, S. 2012. *Police-reported crime statistics in Canada, 2011.* [Online]. Available at: http://www.statcan.gc.ca/pub/85–002-x/2012001/article/11692-eng.htm [accessed: July 26, 2012].

Brooks-Gordon, B., Bilby, C., and Wells, H. 2006. A systematic review of psychological interventions for sexual offenders: Randomised control trials. *The Journal of Forensic Psychiatry and Psychology, 17*, 442–466.

Campbell, W. 2013. Canada's prison guards lack 'common understanding' on basic human respect for inmates. *The Huffington Post—Canada.* [Online]. Available at: http://www.huffingtonpost.ca/2013/03/31/canada-prison-guards_n_2988443.html [accessed: April 1, 2013].

Codispoti, V.L. 2008. Pharmacology of sexually compulsive behavior. *Psychiatric Clinics of North America, 31*, 671–679.

Collins, S. and Nee, C. 2010. Factors influencing the process of change in sex offender interventions: Therapists' experiences and perceptions. *Journal of Sexual Aggression, 16*, 311–331.

Conroy, M.A. 2006. Risk management of sex offenders: A model for community intervention. *The Journal of Psychiatry & Law, 34*, 5–23.

Cowburn, M. 2005. Hegemony and discourse: Reconstructing the male sex offender and sexual coercion by men. *Sexualities, Evolution, and Gender, 7*, 215–231.

Dollard, J., and Miller, N.E. 1950. *Personality and Psychotherapy: An Analysis in Terms of Learning, Thinking, and Culture.* New York, NY: McGraw Hill.

Department of Justice—Federal Bureau of Investigation. 2012. *Uniform crime report: Crime in the United States, 2011.* Clarksburg, WV. [Online]. Available at: http://www.fbi.gov/about-us/cjis/ucr/crime-in-the-u.s/2011/crime-in-the-u.s.-2011 [Accessed: April 11, 2013].

Fedoroff, JP. 2009. The Paraphilias. In M. Gelder, N. Andereasen, J. Lopez-Iber and J. Beddes (Eds). *The New Oxford Textbook of Psychiatry* (2nd ed.). New York: Oxford University Press, 832–842.

Fedoroff, J.P. and Moran, B. 1997. Myths and misconceptions about sex offenders. *The Canadian Journal of Human Sexuality*, *6*, 263–276.

Glaser, B. 2003. Therapeutic jurisprudence: An ethical paradigm for therapists in sex offender treatment programs. *Western Criminology Review*, *4*, 143–154.

Grady, M.D. and Brodersen, M. 2008. In their voices: Perspectives of incarcerated sex offenders on their treatment experiences. *Sexual Addiction & Compulsivity*, *15*, 320–345.

Hudson, A. 2013. German court rules internet "essential." *Reuters*. [Online]. Available at: http://www.reuters.com/article/2013/01/24/us-germany-internet-idUSBRE90N15H20130124 [Accessed: January 24, 2013].

John Howard Society of Alberta. 1997. Community based sex offender treatment programs.

Lösel, F. and Schmucker, M. 2005. The effectiveness of treatment for sexual offenders: A comprehensive meta-analysis. *Journal of Experimental Criminology*, *1*, 117–146.

Marshall, W.L., Jones, R., Ward, A., Johnston, P., and Barbaree, H. 1991. Treatment outcome with sex offenders. *Clinical Psychology Review*, *11*, 465–485.

McGrath, R.J., Cumming, G., Liningston, J. and Hoke, S. 2003. Outcome of a treatment program for adult sex offenders: From prison to community. *Journal of Interpersonal Violence*, *18*, 3–18.

Murphy, L., Bradford, J.M. and Fedoroff, J.P. (In press). Treatment of paraphilias and paraphilic disorders. In G. Gabbard, A. Clayton and R. Balon (Eds). *Gabbard's Treatment of Psychiatric Disorders* (5th ed.). Arlington, VA: American Psychiatric Publishing.

Murphy, L., Fedoroff, J.P., and Martineau, M. 2009a. Canada's sex offender registries: Background implementation and social policy considerations. *Canadian Journal of Human Sexuality*, *18*, 61–71.

Murphy, L., Brodsky, D., Brakel, J., Petrunik, M., Fedoroff, J.P., and Grudzinskas, A. 2009b. In F. Saleh, A. Grudzinskas Jr., J. Bradford and D. Brodsky (Eds). *Sex Offenders: Identification, Risk Assessment, Treatment and Legal Issues*. New York: Oxford University Press, 412–424.

Norman-Eady, S. 2006. *Castration of Sex Offenders*. (Research Report No. 2006-R-0183). Hartford, CT: Office of Legislative Research. [Online]. Available at: http://www.cga.ct.gov/2006/rpt/2006-R-0183.htm [Accessed: April 10, 2013].

Office of the Attorney General, Department of Public Law and Safety. 2004. *Megan's Law*. [Online]. Available at: http://www.about-megans-law.com/index.html [Accessed: March 20, 2013].

Parhar, K.K., Wormith, J.S., Derkzen, D.M., and Beauregard, A.M. 2008. Offender coercion in treatment: A meta-analysis of effectiveness. *Criminal Justice and Behavior*, *35*, 1109–1135.

Polizzi, D.M., MacKenzie, D.L., and Hickman, L.J. 1999. What works in adult sex offender treatment? A review of prison- and non-prison-based treatment programs. *International Journal of Offender Therapy and Comparative Criminology*, *43*, 357–374.

Prescott, D.S. and Levenson, J.S. 2010. Sex offender treatment is not punishment. *Journal of Sexual Aggression*, *16*, 275–285.

Roseman, C.P., Yeager, C., Korcuska, J.S., and Cromly, A. 2008. Sexual behavior intervention program: An innovative level of care in male sex offender treatment. *Journal of Mental Health Counseling*, *30*, 297–310.

Schneider, J. Tay Bosley, J., Ferguson, G., and Main, M. 2006. The challenges of sexual offense treatment programs in correctional facilities. *The Journal of Psychiatry & Law*, *34*, 169–196.

Schwirtz, M. 2013. In 2 trailers, the neighbors nobody wants. *The New York Times*. [Online]. Available at: http://www.nytimes.com/2013/02/05/nyregion/suffolk-county-still-struggling-to-house-sex-offenders.html?pagewanted=all&_r=0 [Accessed: February 4, 2013].

Scott, C.L. and Holmberg, T. 2003. Castration of sex offenders: Prisoners' rights versus public safety. *Journal of the American Academy of Psychiatry and the Law*, *31*, 502–509.

Testa, M. and West, S.G. 2010. Civil commitment in the United States. *Psychiatry* (Edgemont), *7*, 30–40.

Waldram, J.B. 2007. Everybody has a story: Listening to imprisoned sexual offenders. *Qualitative Health Research*, *17*, 963–970.

Waldram, J.B. 2008. The narrative challenge to cognitive behavioural treatment of sexual offenders. *Culture, Medicine, and Psychiatry*, *32*, 421–439.

Willis, G.M. and Grace, R.C. 2008. The quality of community reintegration planning for child molesters: Effects on sexual recidivism. *Sexual Abuse: A Journal of Research and Treatment*, *20*, 218–240.

Wormith, J.S., Althouse, R., Simpson, M., Reitzel, L.R., Fagan, T.J., and Morgan, R.D. 2007. The rehabilitation and reintegration of offenders: The current landscape and some future directions for correctional psychology. *Criminal Justice and Behavior*, *34*, 879–892.

Index